IMMUNODEFICIENCY

IMMUNODEFICIENCY
Its Nature and Etiological Significance in Human Diseases

Proceedings of the International Symposium on Immunodeficiency held September 13–15, 1976, Tokyo

Edited by
Noboru Kobayashi

UNIVERSITY PARK PRESS
Baltimore

JAPAN MEDICAL RESEARCH FOUNDATION
PUBLICATION NO. 5

UNIVERSITY PARK PRESS
Baltimore

Library of Congress Catalog Card Number   78-56872
ISBN   0-8391-1291-2

Originally published by
UNIVERSITY OF TOKYO PRESS

Foreword

The development of modern medicine has contributed to clarifying the etiology and treatment of various diseases as well as to improving public health and welfare. However, there are many diseases of unknown etiology, for which there is no known treatment, which still leave large numbers of patients in a chronic incurable state. In order to promote research on the etiology and treatment of such diseases, non-governmental funding, as well as governmental support, is very important. The Japan Medical Research Foundation has been in existence since October 1973 in order to meet such needs with aid from non-governmental financial sources.

The subject of this symposium is immunodeficiency, its nature and etiological significance in human diseases. Immunodeficiency is related to various intractable chronic diseases, such as SLE rheumatoid arthritis, myasthenia gravis, multiple sclerosis, Behçet disease, leukemia, malignant tumors and others.

The Japan Medical Research Foundation is very pleased to sponsor this symposium, and I am hopeful that the publication of its proceedings will make its work available to a wide scientific readership.

February 10, 1978

Masayoshi Yamamoto
President
Japan Medical Research
Foundation

Preface

It was a great pleasure and honour for all of us, the "immunophylic" pediatricians and physicians, and related investigators in Japan, to hold this symposium with distinguished investigators in this field from the U.S.A. and Europe. This symposium has certainly had a strong impact on us and has stimulated activity in this field in Japan.

Unfortunately a typhoon hit Japan at the beginning of the symposium and the transportation was collapsed, which meant that some of the foreign guests and a number of the Japanese participants were delayed. Nevertheless our discussions here were instructive and fruitful and the friendships between Japanese and foreign investigators will remain warm.

The purpose of this symposium was to clarify the nature of primary immunodeficiency syndrome and the etiological links between this syndrome and various chronic intractable diseases such as autoimmune-collagen diseases, malignancy and others. With that as our purpose, this symposium is not the end, but rather just the end of the beginning of investigation into this area. Combined with recent advances in immunology in general, the lessons from this symposium are of great value for future contributions to those presently unclarified problems of modern medicine.

With the cooperation of all the participants, the proceedings of symposium are now being compiled into a book. As the chairman of the organizing committee of this symposium, I know that this is a great pleasure for us. The information gathered here is of great value to Japanese investigators and we hope of equal value to investigators abroad.

Finally I would like to express my gratitude to Prof. J. Yata, the Toho university and assistant Prof. H. Hayakawa, Branch Hospital, University of Tokyo, for their editorial assistance on this Volume.

Noboru Kobayashi, M.D.

Preface

Contents

I. PATHOLOGY AND PATHOGENESIS OF IMMUNODEFICIENCY

II. ETIOLOGICAL SIGNIFICANCE OF IMMUNODEFICIENCY AND ITS IMPLICATIONS FOR PATHOGENESIS OF HUMAN DISEASE

III. COMPARATIVE AND ANALYTICAL EPIDEMIOLOGY OF IMMUNO-
    DEFICIENCY

IV. NATURE AND EFFECTIVENESS OF THE TREATMENTS FOR
    IMMUNODEFICIENCY

Opening Remarks

The Japan Medical Research Foundation is about to open its Fourth International Symposium, "Immunodeficiency, Its Nature and Etiological Significance in Human Diseases." The Foundation was established in 1973 for the promotion of medical research in Japan, particularly for research on the so-called "nanbyo"—that is, the chronic, intractable and most threatening diseases of man, such as collagen dieseases, autoimmune or allergic diseases, malignancies and so forth.

We are very fortunate to have 10 distinguished foreign investigators as guests. In addition to the Japan Medical Research Foundation, the U.S. National Science Foundation, the International Congress of Hematology and the Japan Allergy Foundation have generously provided financial support to cover a part of the expenses. Thus our symposium is bigger and more exciting than the Foundation originally planned. However, it is unfortunate that Dr. Rosen of Boston was unable to be here. We have more than 100 participants from Japan and the majority of them are members of the project team on "immunodeficiency syndrome," supported by a grant from the Ministry of Health and Welfare. In addition, we have leading investigators from fields related to this condition as well as to "nanbyo."

We know that the majority of cases of primary immunodeficiency are genetically determined, but the relation between the inheritable pattern of the disease and immune-regulatory genes is not clear. We know that virus infection causes immunodeficiency or immunological abnormality and also autoimmunity and even malignancy in experimental systems as well as in humans, although this is only in a limited number of conditions. We know that autoimmune disease and lymphoid malignancy are developed from a primary immunodeficiency at a higher frequency than from the general population. For this reason, primary immunodeficiency is unique among the various types of "nanbyo," since it is one of the "experiments of nature." It is no surprise that studies on "experiments of nature" bring us valuable informations, and this is also true for primary immunodeficiency.

The Foundation has selected "immunodeficiency" as the theme of the 4th International Symposium. As all of you here know, primary immunodeficiency, which is the major topic of this symposium, is a rare disease, but scientific information obtained from studies on this particular disease is now being used to improve understanding of the so-called "nanbyo," and also to provide a scientific basis for analysis, diagnosis and interpretation of the interrelationships among the so-called "nanbyo." By the definition formulated by the Ministry of Health and Welfare and the project teams, "nanbyo" includes SLE, rheumatoid arthritis, myasthenia gravis, multiple sclerosis and Behcet's disease, and in general also includes allergic diseases and malignancies such as leukemia, lymphoma and of course primary immunodeficiency. The etiology and pathogenesis of these conditions have still not been clarified, but primary immunodeficiency is etiologically unique in its position among them.

The purpose of this symposium is to bring together foreign and Japanese researchers on immunodeficiency to exchange scientific knowledge and ideas on this condition, particularly knowledge on primary immunodeficiency, especially on its nature and etiological significance in human disease. Since some sporadic studies of immunodeficiency started in the early 1960's in Japan and the project team was organized only two years ago, we on the Japanese side will derive great benefit from this symposium. We, the organizing committee, sincerely hope that we will have fruitful presentations and discussions at this symposium. I thank you.

Noboru Kobayashi, M. D.

Chairman of the Organizing Committee
of the Japan Medical Research Foundation
Symposium on "Immunodeficiency, Its
Nature and Etiological Significance in Human Disease"

Representative of the All Japan
Immunodeficiency Registration Center

Professor and Director
Department of Pediatrics
University of Tokyo

I. PATHOLOGY AND PATHOGENESIS OF IMMUNODEFICIENCY

Clinicopathologic Correlations in Immunologic Deficiency Diseases of Children, with Emphasis on Thymic Histologic Patterns

Benjamin H. LANDING, Ida L. YUTUC, and Virginia L. SWANSON

Although the relation of the thymus to maturation and function of lymphoid tissues, and thymic abnormality found in certain "immunodeficiency" syndromes, are well known, general pathologic classification and clinicopathologic correlation in this area of disease have been hampered by lack of certainty of the histologic criteria of thymic dysplasia, of the effect of "stress" on thymic development, and of the regularity of association of different abnormal thymic histologic patterns with specific diseases. For disorders including T or B lymphocyte dysfunction, the possible production of the same functional state by deficient helper, or by excessive suppressor, effects of T lymphocytes on B cell function, and vice versa, further complicates clinicopathologic analysis, as does the possibility of transplacental or other white cell implantation, with or without graft-versus-host reaction.

In an effort to elucidate some of these matters, and to analyze differences in thymic involutionary patterns in disorders of either short or protracted duration, with or without chronic infection, malnutrition, or steroid hormone treatment, we have analyzed material available in the Department of Pathology, Childrens Hospital of Los Angeles, from those categories of patients listed in Table 1. For each of the patients, hematoxylin-eosin stained sections of thymus, spleen and lymph nodes were reviewed, and the number and pattern of distribution of apparent T and B lymphocytes were recorded, as well as the presence of germinal (secondary) lymphoid centers, the number of plasmacytes, eosinophils and macrophages, and the presence of certain other histologic features discussed below. The findings in each group were reviewed for regular or repetitive features, and these were compared for the various groups of patients.

Severe combined immunodeficiency disease (SCID). This category may

Departments of Pathology and Pediatrics, Childrens Hospital of Los Angeles and University of Southern California School of Medicine, Los Angeles, California, U.S.A.

TABLE 1.   Categories of immunodeficiency and other syndromes reviewed

	Accepted	Questionable
Combined immunodeficiency	2	4
Pure T cell deficiency	8	4
Pure B cell deficiency	10	—
Ataxia telangiectasia	6	—
Zinsser-Cole-Engman syndrome	1	—
Septic granulomatosis	8	1
Histiocytosis/lymphohistiocytosis	12	—
Graft-versus-host disease	1	—
Systemic hyalinosis	3	2

Other syndromes reviewed

Hodgkin's disease	9
Biliary atresia	22
Juvenile rheumatoid arthritis	3
Systemic lupus erythematosis	16
Mixed connective tissue disease	1
Chronic hemodialysis/renal transplant/ chronic renal disease	11
DiGeorge syndrome	2
Thalassemia major	9
Thalassemia trait	1
Infantile Gaucher's disease	1
Infantile Niemann-Pick disease	3
Juvenile Niemann-Pick disease	1

include three patterns of thymic abnormality. The pattern called in this study "pinealoid" (Fig. 1), the classical pattern of thymic dysplasia, resembles that seen in the nude mouse. As Figs. 1–3 show, patients with this thymic pattern showed a larger number of lymphocytes in spleen and lymph nodes especially in loci typical for T lymphocytes ("collars" around small splenic arteries; parafollicular cortical zone of lymph nodes) (Fig. 3) than did the patient with SCID which was due to adenosine deaminase (ADA) deficiency or a similar patient (#2 of Table 2) whose ADA level was not determined. They also showed poorly developed primitive B cell centers in lymph nodes (Fig. 3) and serum immunoglobulins (A, G and M) in the low normal to normal range. This pattern of thymic dysplasia has been considered by other workers to occur in some patients with SCID who may thus correspond to the group of patients with SCID who have less severe lymphocyte deficiency and who respond better to immunologic reconstitution. If they have SCID, patients 1–3 of Table 2

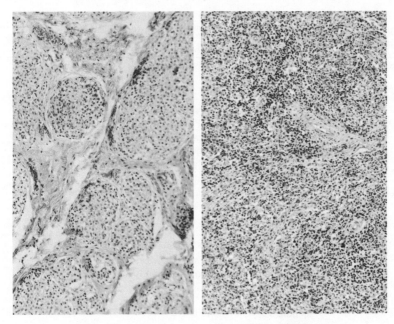

Fig. 1   Fig. 2

FIG. 1. "Pinealoid" pattern of thymic dysplasia. This may occur in both severe combined immunodeficiency disease and in pure T cell deficiency (Nezelof syndrome) (pt. 1, group 1, Table 2). (H & E, × 50)

FIG. 2. Spleen of same patient as in Fig. 1, showing diffusely distributed lymphocyte population, without germinal (B-cell) centers, and with very poor "collar" (T-cell) grouping. (H & E, × 80)

probably should be considered to have the X-linked recessive form. Although both T and B lymphocyte populations in spleen and lymph nodes of patients with the "pinealoid" pattern of thymus were abnormal it may be more appropriate to consider this disorder as primary T-deficiency without immunoglobulin deficiency (Nezelof syndrome), the pathologic features perhaps reflecting severe lack of "helper" effect of T on B cells. It is of interest that Huber[1] has recently reported that normal fetal thymus implanted into patients with "pinealoid" thymic dysplasia acquires the "pinealoid" thymic lesion. This finding indicates that this lesion is not the result of a primary genetically determined defect in the program for thymic maturation but is the result of an "environmental" effect on the thymus possibly from deficient or abnormal "feed-back" from the peripheral lymphoid tissues.

TABLE 2.   Severe combined immunodeficiency disease (SCID)
Thymic dysplasia, "pinealoid" pattern [? X-linked recessive SCID, ? T-deficiency with
immunoglobulins (Nezelof syndrome)]

Age	Sex	Thymic pattern	Infection	Gamma globulin levels
1 4 m	M	pinealoid	CMV, Candida Pseudomonas	A,G,M normal for age
2. 11 m	M	pinealoid	(Pneumocystis, parainfluenza; malignant lymphoma)	A,G,M low normal
3. 1 8/12	M	pinealoid	Candida	A,G,M normal
		Thymic epithelial "stem only" pattern		
4. 4 m	F	stem only, pale matrix	E. coli Pseudomonas	skeletal dysplasia adenosine deaminase deficiency (has affected sib)
5. 11 m	F	stem only, pale matrix	Pseudomonas	
		Small lobule/small dark cell pattern (? actually T-deficiency)		
6. 1 y	M	small lobules, small dark spindle cell matrix, HC-O	CMV	

The thymic pattern in ADA-negative SCID (Pts. 4 and 5 of Table 2) (Fig. 4)
is quite different, with better formation of the thymic epithelial stem, although
with little or no formation of true Hassall's corpuscles. As is implied above,
the spleen and lymph nodes of such patients show more severe lymphocyte
deficiency than do those of patients with "pinealoid" thymus (Fig.5). Whether
the small dark spindle-cell appearance of the thymus in patient #6 of Table 2
is truly associable with SCID, or whether this patient is mis-assigned because
of inadequate clinical data, cannot be stated; although this pattern has been
described in autosomal recessive SCID it is apparently more typical of
T-lymphocyte deficiency (Fig. 6).

T-lymphocyte deficiency.   With the possible exception of the patients with
"pinealoid" thymus, as discussed above, those patients assigned to this
category are summarized in Table 3. As can be seen, the most typical thymic
patterns with this functional state are a pattern of small thymic lobules composed
of small dark spindle-shaped cells with very few or no Hassall's corpuscles and
a pattern which is essentially the same but with a cleft or small cyst formation
in what appears to be a poorly differentiated thymic epithelial stem (Figs. 7 and

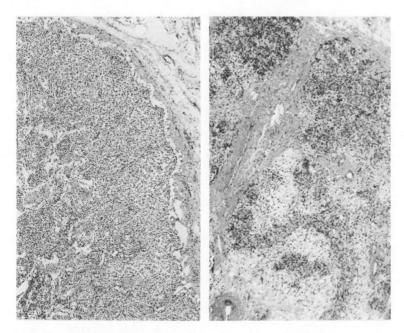

Fig. 3   Fig. 4

FIG. 3. Lymph node of same patient as in Figs. 1 and 2, showing low numbers of both B and T lymphocytes, but with irregular outer border of cortex ("B-bumps") indicative of very primitive B-cell grouping. (H & E, × 32)

FIG. 4. Thymus of patient with SCID due to adenosine deaminase deficiency (pt. 4, group 2, Table 2) showing thymic epithelial stem surrounded by pale myxoid matrix, without definite formation of Hassall's corpuscles. (H & E, × 50)

8). Whether these patterns should be separated cannot be decided on the basis of present information since none of the patients of this series was studied for the presence of nucleoside (inosine) phosphorylase deficiency which causes a T-lymphocyte deficiency disease.[2] However the relative uniformity of these pathologic patterns of the thymus in patients accepted in this review as having pure T-cell deficiency may suggest that there is a specific disease which is the most common cause of this condition. A relatively better survival of patients with pure T-lymphocyte deficiency (average age at death, 57 months) than that of those with SCID (average age at death 6, 8 or 10.3 months) is apparent in Table 3.

20

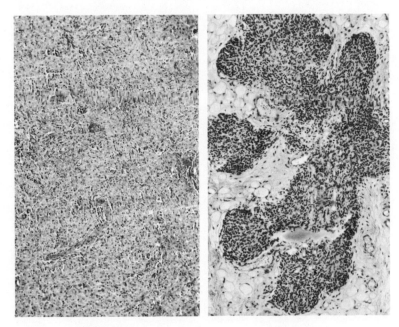

Fig. 5   Fig. 6

FIG. 5. Spleen of same patient as in Fig. 4, showing "empty" pulp, with neither T nor B cell aggregations. (H & E, × 50)

FIG. 6. Small dark spindle-celled pattern of thymus of pt. 6, group 3, Table 2. Whether this pattern actually occurs in SCID, or should be considered to indicate only T-lymphocyte deficiency, is uncertain. (H & E, × 50)

DiGeorge syndrome. One of two patients with DiGeorge syndrome in this study showed a hypoplastic thymus (so-called partial DiGeorge syndrome) with basically normal microscopic pattern (Fig. 9). The peripheral lymphoid tissues however showed distinct T-lymphocyte deficiency (Fig. 10). Whether this observation indicates that the amount of thymus present in this patient was not enough to permit peripheral T-cell proliferation, or whether it indicates that such thymuses do not produce thymic hormone(s), is not known.

B-lymphocyte deficiency. Included in Table 4 are patients with both agammaglobulinemia in the sense of having low values for immunoglobulins A, G and M, and those with dysgammaglobulinemia, in the sense of having low values for one or two of gammas A, G or M, and normal or elevated values for the others, on the assumption that dysgammaglobulinemia indicates partial

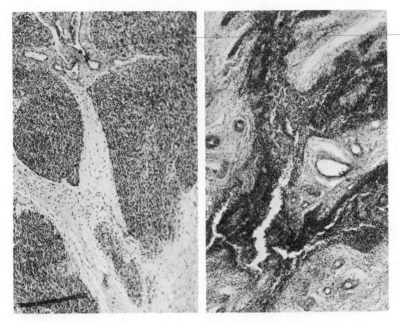

Fig. 7   Fig. 8

FIG. 7. Small dark spindle-celled pattern of thymus in T cell deficiency (pt. 1, Table 3). (H & E, × 32)

FIG. 8. Small dark-celled thymus with clefting of central zones ("stem cystosis") in T-cell deficiency (pt. 6, Table 3). (H & E, × 32)

(clonal or lacunar) B cell deficiency. Five males presumably had Bruton X-linked agammaglobulinemia, the most common disorder in this category. Thymuses of such patients show normal involutionary changes, with Hassall's corpuscles within normal range for age (Fig. 11), and lymph nodes showing absence of B-centers (Fig. 12). Whether the "central Hassall's corpuscle" pattern of the thymus, more typical of dysgammaglobulinemia, is truly a diagnostic feature will require further study (Fig. 13). Since three of the four patients with dysgammaglobulinemia were female, the X-linked dysgammaglobulinemia described by Stiehm and Fudenberg may not have been represented in this series.

Ataxia-telangiectasia. Table 5 summarizes the patients with this well-known autosomal recessive form of T-lymphocyte deficiency. The relative lack of major symptoms of this disorder in infancy and early childhood are well known, and the much longer survival of patients with ataxia-telangiectasia,

TABLE 3. T cell immunodeficiency patients (see also Patients 4–6, Table 2)
Accepted diagnosis

	Age	Sex	Thymic pattern	Infection	Other
1.	5 m	M	small dark cell, HC-O	Candida	
2.	1 1/12	F	small dark cell/stem cystosis, HC±		
3.	1 5/12	M	small dark cell, HC-O	Myxovirus Mitis Diphtheria	
4.	1 8/12	M	HC±	Candida	
5.	2 8/12	F	HC-O		hydrocephalus
6.	2 10/12	F	small dark cell/stem cystosis, HC-O	Herpes, broncho- pneumonia	
7.	12 4/12	M	small dark cell/stem cystosis, HC±		
8.	15 y	F	small dark cell/stem cystosis, HC-O	? Actinomycosis	

Questionable diagnosis

	Age	Sex	Thymic pattern	Infection	Other
1.	1 5/12	M	HC±		hydrocephalus, ? fetal alcohol syndrome
2.	3 y	M	stem cystosis, HC±	Candida, E. coli	aplagtic anemia
3.	6 6/12	M	HC±		
4.	8 6/12	M	stem cystosis, HC-O		"histiocytic lymphoma"

(HC-O = No Hassall's corpuscles;
HC ± = Hassall's corpuscles very rare)

compared to those with T-lymphocyte deficiency listed in Table 3, is apparent.
The severe deficiency of thymic tissue typical of such older patients with A-T
is illustrated in Fig. 14, but, clearly, definitive study of the thymic anatomy of
such patients in infancy is needed before the genesis of their thymic lesion can
be understood. Pathologic sequences in their lymph nodes are also not clear
(Fig. 15).

Zinsser-Cole-Engman syndrome (X-linked congenital dyskeratosis with pancytopenia).   The one patient with this distinctive disease included in this study
is also summarized in Table 5. Although T-lymphocyte deficiency may be a
basic feature of the disorder, and deficient immunologic surveillance may
contribute to the liability of these patients to malignant tumors, a decision on
the pathogenesis of their thymic lesion awaits further study (Fig. 16).   As with

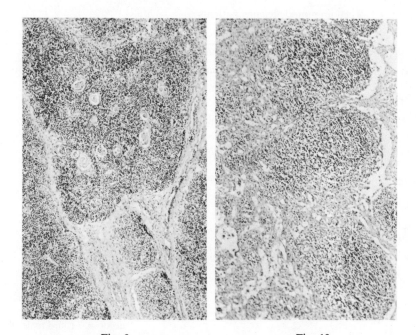

Fig. 9   Fig. 10

FIG. 9. Thymus of patient with "partial DiGeorge Syndrome", showing pattern of moderate chronic involution, with reduction in corticomedullary demarcation, but with normal number of Hassall's corpuscles. (H & E, × 50)

FIG. 10. Lymph node of same patient as in Fig. 9, showing prominent peripheral B-cell centers, but marked deficiency of parafollicular T-lymphocyte population. (H & E, × 50)

ataxia-telangiectasia, the Zinsser-Cole-Engman syndrome typically permits longer survival than does typical T-lymphocyte deficiency. Hypoplastic anemia was also observed in this review in a patient with Bruton agammaglobulinemia; whether the anemia of the Zinsser-Cole-Engman syndrome can be attributed to abnormal B cell function due to deficiency of helper T-lymphocytes would appear to merit study.

Hodgkin's disease. Hodgkin's disease is generally considered to include T-lymphocyte deficiency, and the pathologic similarity of the thymus of many patients with Hodgkin's disease to that of patients with ataxia telangiectasia is illustrated in Fig. 17. The large amount of central thymic epithelium present in

TABLE 4.   B cell immunodeficiency patients
Accepted diagnosis

	Age	Sex	Thymic pattern	Infection	Etc.
1.	3 w	F	involution 3+, HC+	Candida	dysgammaglobulinemia (low G, high A, M)
2.	1 m	M	Involution 2+, HC 2+		neutropenia
3.	6 w	F	involution 3+, HC 2+	Klebsiella	dysgammaglobulinemia (low A, M, high G)
4.	4 m	M	involution 3+, HC+	CMV	dysgammaglobulinemia (low G, high A, M)
5.	7 m	F	involution 3+, HC+	Pneumocystis	dysgammaglobulinemia (low A, G, normal M)
6.	9 m	F	involution 3+, HC 2+		no Ig determination
7.	9 m	M	involution 3+, HC 2+	CMV, Pneumocystis	sib of # 10
8.	9 m	M	involution 3+, HC 2+	Staphylococcus	
9.	11 y	M	involution 3+, HC+		hypocomplementemic chronic lobular glomerulonephritis
10.	13 y	M	involution 2+, HC 2+		hypoplastic anemia sib of # 7 (third male sib also affected)

TABLE 5.   Ataxia-telangiectasia patients

	Age	Sex	Thymic pattern	Other
1.	13 y	F	marked general "hypoplasia", HC-O	malignant lymphoma
2.	16 1/12	M	HC ±	
3.	16 10/12	M	HC-O	malignant lymphoma
4.	17 y	F	HC-O	
5.	19 8/12	M	HC-O	
6.	31 y	M	HC-O	malignant lymphoma, basal cell carcinomas

Zinsser-Cole-Engman syndrome

	Age	Sex		Other
1.	11 1/2	M	marked general "hypoplasia", HC-O	chronic hypoplastic anemia hemosiderosis

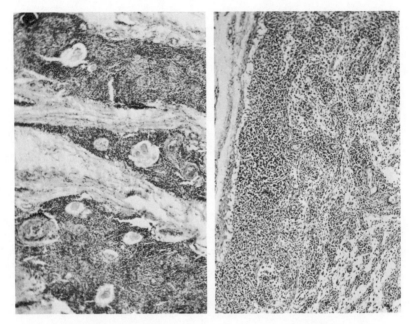

Fig. 11　　　　　　　　　　　　Fig. 12

FIG. 11. Thymus of 13-year-old boy with Bruton agammaglobulinemia (pt. 10, Table 4), showing appearance of chronic involution, with abundant Hassall's corpuscles. (H & E, × 50)

FIG. 12. Lymph node of 9-month-old boy with Bruton agammaglobulinemia, a sib of the patient illustrated in Fig. 11. Note the smooth
cortical surface of the node (absence of "B-bumps"), with diffuse
pattern of cortical T-cells. (H & E, × 50)

the one infant in this series (the patient died of bacterial sepsis after having had
splenectomy) may indicate that the deficiency of Hassall's corpuscles seen in
five of the patients in Table 6 is the result of "acquired" loss of thymic epithelium, and study of the thymic anatomy of patients with Hodgkin's disease at
as early an age as possible would be of great interest. That the lymph nodes of
treated patients with Hodgkin's disease appear to show a greater relative
deficiency of T-lymphocytes than does the spleen is also of interest, but study
of these relations before treatment is needed. As is implied above, the findings
in Hodgkin's disease may shed light on the pathogenetic sequences in ataxia-
telangiectasia and the Zinsser-Cole-Engman syndrome, but the data of this
study do not permit definite conclusions.

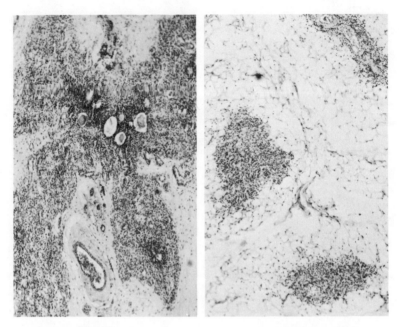

Fig. 13   Fig. 14

FIG. 13.   Thymus of 4-month-old male with dysgammaglobulinemia (pt. 4 of Table 4), showing "central Hassall's corpuscle"
pattern. (H & E, × 50)
FIG. 14.   Thymus of 17-year-old girl with ataxia-telangiectasia (pt.
4 of Table 5), showing very small thymic lobules, fatty replacement
of bulk of thymus, and absence of Hassall's corpuscles. (H & E, × 50)

The findings in the patients discussed in the three preceding sections have
raised the question of the occurrence of "acquired", but possibly programmed,
loss of central thymic epithelium, with clinical and laboratory evidence of T-
lymphocyte deficiency in certain diseases. Whether thymic epithelial loss is
always associated with demonstrable T-cell deficiency is not known, and it is
not generally assumed to date that this association is mandatory, although
thymic deficiency secondary to the severe malnutrition-infection syndromes
seen in infants in less developed countries is accepted by some workers.[6]
Whether malnutrition, infection (in general, or by specific agents, *e.g.* measles
virus), or young age is most important in producing this outcome cannot be
stated from available data. However, the material of this study suggests that
biliary atresia and Letterer-Siwe disease may be of interest in possibly provid-

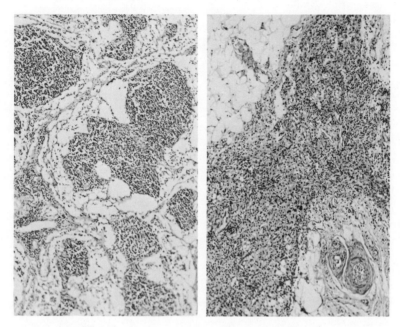

Fig. 15   Fig. 16

FIG. 15. Lymph node of same patient as in Fig. 14, showing nodules of B-lymphocytes, without secondary centers, diffusely distributed through the node. These nodules are less superficial than are normal cortical B-centers, and the surface of the node is smooth. (H & E, × 50)

FIG. 16. Thymus of patient with congenital dyskeratosis with pancytopenia (Zinsser-Cole-Engman syndrome), showing lack of corticomedullary demarcation and of Hassall's corpuscles. (H & E, × 50)

ing more reliably programmed models of "attrition" of the thymus-T lymphocyte system.

Biliary atresia.   The patients with extrahepatic biliary atresia reviewed in this study are summarized in Table 7, and the apparently progressive loss of thymic epithelium which occurs with this disease (Fig. 18) is diagrammed in Fig. 19. Studies of T-lymphocyte number and function over the course of this disorder are needed. The data of this study suggest that the loss of thymic epithelium progresses over about 18 months.

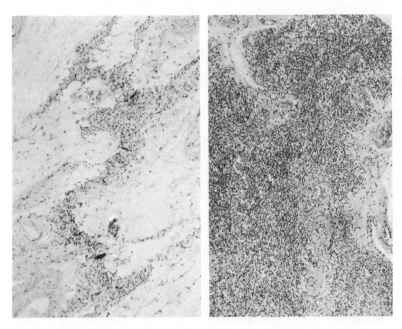

Fig. 17   Fig. 18

FIG. 17.   Thymus of patient with Hodgkin's disease (pt. 4, Table 6), showing very small lobules lacking Hassall's corpuscles. (H & E, × 50)

FIG. 18.   Thymus of patient with biliary atresia, showing marked deficiency of Hassall's corpuscles. (H & E, × 50)

TABLE 6.   Hodgkin's disease patients

	Age	Sex	Thymus	Spleen	Nodes
1.	2 y	M	HC3+, stem hyperplasia	—	? B > T
2.	5 6/12	M	stem only, HC-O	T > B	B > T
3.	9 3/12	F	AT-like, HC-O	T > B	both deficient; infection
4.	12 9/12	M	AT-like, HC-O	both deficient	both deficient; scar
5.	12 10/12	M	stem cystosis, HC2+	T only	? T only
6.	13 3/12	F	stem cystosis, HC+	both deficient	both deficient; scar
7.	15 y	M	HC+	(B > T)	B > T
8.	15 11/12	M	stem cystosis, HC ±	both deficient	B > T, infection
9.	18 6/12	M	stem only, HC-O	T only	extensive scar

(   ) Splenectomy performed earlier

T > B: T lymphocyte population better preserved than B-population

B > T: B lymphocyte population better preserved than T-population

TABLE 7. Biliary atresia patients

Age	Sex	Hassall's corpuscles
1 w	F	2+
1.5 m	F	2+
2 m	M	2+
2 m	F	2+
3.5 m	M	2+
3.5 m	F	2+
6 m	F	+
6 m	F	+
6.5 m	F	±
7 m	F	2+
8 m	F	+
9 m	F	2+
9 m	F	±
10 m	M	+
11 m	F	±
1 y	F	+
1 11/12	F	±
3 2/12	M	±
3 4/12	M	−
3 6/12	F	±
3 6/12	F	−
4 y	F	±

Letterer-Siwe disease. The eight patients with Letterer-Siwe disease (disseminated histiocytosis X) reviewed in this study are summarized in Table 8. That at least some patients diagnosed as having Letterer-Siwe disease have primary SCID, with transplacental implantation of maternal immunocytes and secondary graft-versus-host disease, has been shown.[7] To what extent this phenomenon is a more general explanation of Letterer-Siwe disease is not known. It is of considerable interest therefore that all eight patients with this disorder in the material of this study show thymic epithelial deficiency; apparently the absence of Hassall's corpuscles was total in six (Fig. 20). If acquired, this thymic epithelial deficiency is apparently the most rapidly progressive of any form included in this review. Studies of immunocyte number and function in patients with Letterer-Siwe disease published to date have given conflicting results, and much further study of this issue is needed. The data of Table 8 suggest that patients with Letterer-Siwe disease do not regularly show deficiency of both T and B lymphocytes, but study of their lymphoid tissues before treatment is necessary. The male preponderance shown in Table 8 could be compatible with the Eichwald phenomenon (greater rejection of

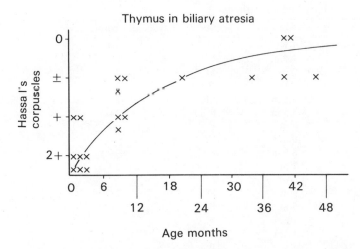

FIG. 19.   Relation of number of Hassall's corpuscles in thymus to age at death for patients with biliary atresia, showing progressive decrease in number of Hassall's corpuscles with age. (Code for Hassall's corpuscles is : 0 = none; ± = very few; + = few; 2+ = moderate number.)

male tissue by female immunocytes than vice versa), but the rarity of familial Letterer-Siwe disease, and the apparent lack of occurrence of SCID or T-cell deficiency in the siblings of patients with Letterer-Siwe disease, cast doubt on a general relation of primary immunodeficiency to this disorder.

Graft-versus-host (GVH) disease.   Only one patient with GVH disease, a two-month old male with typical clinical and pathologic "runt disease" following exchange transfusion, was available for this review. His central thymic epithelium appeared adequate (Fig. 21). Study of more such patients will be necessary before decision as to whether this finding suggests that GVH disease is not a frequent explanation of Letterer-Siwe disease can be reached.

Lymphohistiocytosis.   Although at least four different forms of lymphohistiocytosis have been described, it is of interest that the patients with lymphohistiocytosis reviewed in this study (Table 8) all showed deficient thymic epithelium and Hassall's corpuscles (Fig. 22). (The condition called in some reports "familial Letterer-Siwe disease" is included in this category, as "erythrophagocytic lymphohistiocytosis".) The relation, if any, between this group of dis-

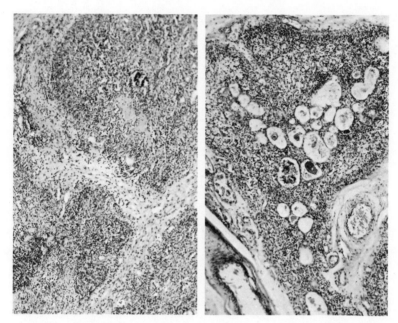

Fig. 20   Fig. 21

FIG. 20. Thymus of 4-month-old patient with Letterer-Siwe disease (pt. 4, Table 8), showing severe deficiency of Hassall's corpuscles. Hyalinosis of lobular stroma is not shown well at this low magnification. (H & E, × 50)

FIG. 21. Thymus of patient with graft-versus-host disease (Table 8), showing involuted appearance with prominent cystic central Hassall's corpuscles (cf. Fig. 13). (H & E, × 50)

orders and the entity discussed above as Letterer-Siwe's disease, and the mechanism of thymic epithelial deficiency in both, cannot yet be stated.

Septic granulomatosis.   Not an immunodeficiency disease in the strict sense, this disorder of polymorphonuclear and macrophage phagocytic function is included in this review as a disorder causing severe chronic or recurrent infection in infancy and early childhood. As Table 9 shows, septic granulomatosis does not regularly cause the degree of thymic epithelial deficiency seen in Letterer-Siwe disease, late biliary atresia, or other entities discussed above. The patient with questionable septic granulomatosis is the only one observed to date in this hospital with *M. tuberculosis* infection; the presence of thymic

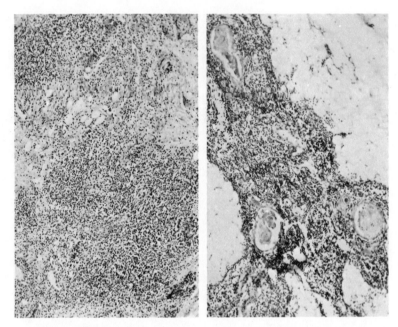

Fig. 22   Fig. 23

FIG. 22.   Thymus of patient with lymphohistiocytosis (pt. 3, group 3, Table 8) showing reduction in thymocytes and lack of Hassall's corpuscles. (H & E, × 50)

FIG. 23.   Thymus of patient with systemic lupus erythematosus, showing large cystic Hassall's corpuscles (pt. 2, Table 10). (H & E, × 50)

hyalinosis raises the question that the patient had the disorder, systemic hyalinosis, discussed below. The eight typical patients appear to have had the x-linked recessive form of chronic granulomatous disease.

Systemic lupus erythematosus.   This disorder, despite producing severe chronic illness and liability to infection, and leading to protracted steroid treatment, does not reliably produce severe, nor apparently progressive, thymic epithelial loss (Table 10). The Hassall's corpuscles seen in the thymus in patients with SLE are typically larger and more cystic than those in juvenile rheumatoid arthritis or mixed connective tissue disease (Fig. 23).

Juvenile rheumatoid arthritis, Mixed connective tissue disease, Chronic renal insufficiency with chronic hemodialysis, renal transplantation, or both.   Like

TABLE 8.   Letterer-Siwe disease

Age	Sex	Thymus	Spleen	Nodes
1. 3 m	M	HC-O	T > B	both deficient
2. 4 m	M	HC±, hyalinosis	T > B	B > T
3. 8 m	F	HC-O	both deficient	both deficient
4. 1 2/12	M	HC-O	B = T	B > T
5. 1 7/12	M	HC-O	T > B	T > B
6. 1 8/12	M	HC-O	T > B	—
7. 2 y	F	HC ±	—	—
8. 2 8/12	M	HC-O	T > B	T > B

Runt (graft-versus-host) disease

1. 2 m	M	HC 2+	post-exchange	transfusion

Lymphohistiocytosis

1. 3 m	M	HC-O	T > B	T > B
2. 7 6/12	F	HC±	—	both depleted
3. 9 3/12	M	HC-O	B > T	? T proliferation
4. 15 5/12	F	HC±	T deficiency	T deficiency, lymphoma

TABLE 9.   Septic granulomatosis patients
Accepted diagnosis

	Age	Sex	Thymic pattern	Infection
1.	3 y	M	PLH3+, HC±	Pseudomonas
2.	4 y	M	PLH+, HC+	Nocardia
3.	5 y	M	PLH2+, HC2+	Nocardia
4.	5 4/12	M	PLH4+, HC±	?
5.	6 y	M	PLH2+, HC+	Salmonellosis
6.	6 6/12	M	PLH2+, HC-O	? Staphylococcus
7.	7 8/12	M	PLH3+, HC±	Candida
8.	8 y	M	PLH2+, HC+	Paracolon

Questionable diagnosis

1.	1 y	M	hyalinosis + PLH±, HC-O	Tuberculosis

PLH = Pigmented lipid histiocytes

SLE, these conditions of protracted illness, with increased frequency of infections, and with extensive steroid treatment, do not lead to regular disappearance of the thymic epithelium. Thymic lymphocyte depletion was much less marked in the patient with mixed connective tissue disease, a disorder only recently separated from systemic lupus, than was the case in any of the patients with SLE (Fig. 24). As was mentioned above, the Hassall's corpuscles in juvenile rheumatoid arthritis were typically not so large nor so cystic as those in SLE (Fig. 25).

TABLE 10. Systemic lupus erythematosus patients

	Age	Sex	Thymus	Spleen	Nodes
1.	6 6/12	F	HC+, large	B def.	T > B
2.	12 y	F	HC+, moderate	B def.	—
3.	12 y	M	HC+, large	B def.	T > B
4.	12 6/12	M	HC2+, large	T > B	T > B
5.	14 y	F	HC+, small	T > B	B def.
6.	14 y	M	HC+, variable	T > B	T > B
7.	14 6/12	F	HC±, moderate	T > B	T > B
8.	15 y	F	HC2+, large	—	T > B
9.	15 y	F	HC+, large	B def.	diffuse pattern
10.	15 y	F	HC+, large	B > T	B > T
11.	15 6/12	F	HC-O	B def.	B def; plasmacytosis
12.	16 4/12	F	HC+, moderate	B def.	diffuse pattern
13.	16 8/12	F	HC+, small	T > B	diffuse pattern
14.	17 y	F	HC+, large	T > B	B > T
15.	18 y	F	HC+, variable	both def.	T > B
16.	18 y	M	HC2+, large	B def.	T > B

TABLE 11. Juvenile rheumatoid arthritis patients

	Age	Sex	Thymus	Spleen	Nodes	Diagnosis
1.	4	F	HC±	T > B	B > T	
2.	6 9/12	M	HC2+	T > B	B > T	
3.	15 2/12	M	HC+	—	B > T	

Mixed connective tissue disease

	Age	Sex	Thymus	Spleen	Nodes	
1.	16 y	F	HC+	B deficiency	both +	

Chronic renal insufficiency (with chronic hemodialysis and/or renal transplantation)

	Age	Sex	Thymus	Spleen	Nodes	Diagnosis
1.	4 8/12	M	HC+	B > T	B > T	obstructive uropathy
2.	9 9/12	F	HC-O	T > B	T > B	chronic Bright's disease
3.	12	M	HC±	T = B	T = B	obstructive uropathy
4.	12	M	HC±	—	—	infantile polycystic disease
5.	12 7/12	M	HC+	T > B	B > T	chronic glomerulonephritis
6.	14	F	HC2+	T > B	T > B	chronic glomerulonephritis
7.	15 y	F	HC-O	T = B	T = B	rapidly progressive glomerulonephritis
8.	15 3/12	F	HC2+	T > B	T = B	chronic Bright's disease
9.	15 3/12	M	HC2+	T > B	B > T	chronic Bright's disease
10.	18 2/12	M	HC+	T > B	B > T	chronic Bright's disease
11.	21	F	HC±	T > B	T = B	membranoproliferative glomerulonephritis

TABLE 12.   Systemic hyalinosis patients

	Age	Sex	Thymic pattern	Other involvement
1.	1 3/12	F	hyalinosis, HC-O	skin, GI, nodes, adrenal, parathyroid, muscle (sib of #3)
2.	1 6/12	F	hyalinosis, HC±	skin, GI, lung, pancreas, adrenal, muscle
3.	1 8/12	F	hyalinosis, HC+	skin, GI, nodes, bladder, adrenal, ovary, heart, muscle

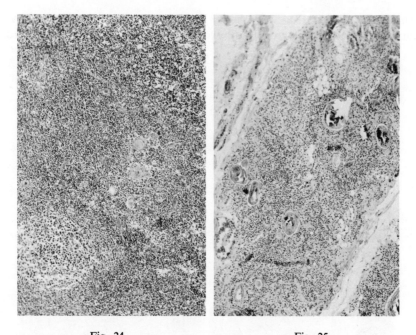

Fig. 24   Fig. 25

FIG. 24.   Thymus of patient with mixed connective tissue disease, showing abundant lymphocytes, with suggestion of early germinal center (B-cell center) formation, and abundant small Hassall's corpuscles. (H & E, × 50)

FIG. 25.   Thymus in juvenile rheumatoid arthritis (pt. 2, Table 11), showing small Hassall's corpuscles, many mineralized. (H & E, × 50)

Systemic hyalinosis.   Three patients, all female infants, with this rare
disorder, of which liability to infection is a feature, are summarized in Table
12.[8] Whether the susceptibility to infection reflects thymic deficiency, lymph
node involvement, malnutrition due to severe hyalinosis of small intestinal
mucosa, or other possible mechanisms, cannot be stated. The presence of the
disease in two siblings suggests that this is a valid entity. Additional patients
who may have had systemic hyalinosis are also listed under Letterer-Siwe
disease (patient #2, Table 8) and septic granulomatosis (Table 9). Pathogenetic mechanisms in this disorder are still very poorly understood (Figs. 26 and
27).

Thalassemia (Table 13).   Although liability to infection is not a major
feature of thalassemia, factors leading to infection in patients with this disorder

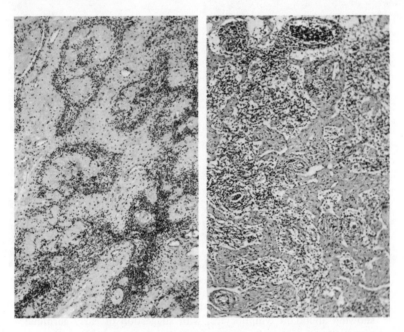

Fig. 26   Fig. 27

FIG. 26.   Thymus of patient with systemic hyalinosis, showing extensive deposition of hyaline material and absence of Hassall's corpuscles (pt. 1 of Table 12). (H & E, × 50)
FIG. 27.   Lymph node of same patient as in Fig. 25, showing
hyalinosis, with relative sparing of subcapsular B-centers. (H & E,
× 50)

TABLE 13.   Thalassemic patients
Thalassemic patients

	Age	Sex	Thymus	Spleen	Nodes
1.	9 y	M	HC2+	(B > T)	B > T
2.	10 10/12	M	HC+	T > B	B > T
3.	11 11/12	M	—	(B > T)	B > T; calcinosis
4.	13 y	F	HC2+	(?B > T)	B > T
5.	15 y	F	—	—	B > T; T zone hemosiderosis
6.	15 y	M	HC-O	(B = T)	B > T; T zone hemosiderosis
7.	18 11/12	F	HC±	(B > T)	?B > T; calcinosis
					siderosis 4+
8.	19 10/12	M	HC+	(B only)	B > T
9.	23 y	F	HC+, with B centers	(B > T)	B > T; T zone hemosiderosis

Thalassemia trait

1.	8 6/12	M	HC2+, large	—	B > T

(   ) Splenectomy performed at earlier age
— Tissue not available for study

include high tissue and serum iron levels, reticuloendothelial blockade by hemosiderin, and splenectomy. Relatively selective involvement of the parafollicular T-lymphocyte regions of lymph nodes by hemosiderosis is illustrated in Fig. 28. Relatively poor T-zone development may be a basic feature of the disease, however, since it was seen in nodes in five patients in the absence of severe nodal siderosis, and in the spleens of six of eight at splenectomy a number of years before death. Strangely, it was also found in one patient with thalassemia trait who died of other causes. No data on lymphocyte function in these patients are available.

Lysosomal Storage Diseases (Gaucher and Niemann-Pick diseases) (Table 14). Reticuloendothelial blockade as a cause of liability to infection has been mentioned above for thalassemia major. Macrophage dysfunction has also been considered a contributing factor to infection in patients with reticuloendothelial storage diseases like Gaucher and Niemann-Pick diseases, although splenectomy appears also to be a factor in many patients with classical or "adult" Gaucher's disease. No patients with this latter disease were included in the material of this review, but one patient with infantile Gaucher's disease showed absence of thymic Hassall's corpuscles (Fig. 29). Two of the patients with classical "infantile" Niemann-Pick disease showed lipid histiocytosis of B-centers and of T-zones in spleen and lymph nodes (Fig. 30). Whether the third patient listed under infantile Niemann-Pick disease actually had one of

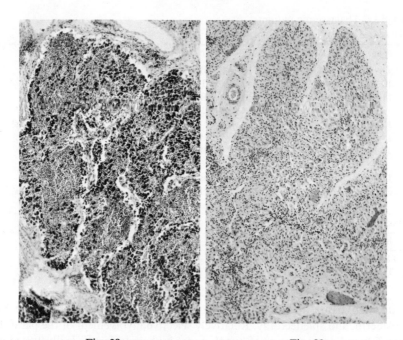

Fig. 28   Fig. 29

FIG. 28.   Lymph node in advanced thalassemia major (pt. 6, Table 13) showing extensive hemosiderosis, which tends to spare the B-cell centers. (H & E, × 50)

FIG. 29.   Thymus of patient with infantile Gaucher disease (Table 14), showing heavy infiltration by Gaucher cells, and lack of Hassall's corpuscles. (H & E, × 50)

the two juvenile Niemann-Pick diseases cannot be stated, but the greater involvement of T-lymphocyte zones than of B-centers in spleen and nodes resembles the pattern seen in the patient with juvenile disease (Fig. 31). Detailed study of peripheral blood lymphocyte numbers, types and functions in these and other lysosomal storage diseases would be of interest, and the results possibly of diagnostic value.

Association of thymic epithelial deficiency with malignant tumors.   Among the patients listed in Tables 1–14, malignant tumors were observed in the following:

SCID, pt. #5   -   malignant lymphoma
? T deficiency, pt. #4   -   "histiocytic lymphoma"
ataxia-telangiectasia, pts. #1, 3, 6   malignant lymphoma

TABLE 14. Lymphoid tissues in storage diseases

Disease	Age	Sex	Thymus	Spleen	Nodes
Infantile Gaucher	9.5 m	F	HC-O, marked histiocytosis	Histiocytosis T & B deficiency	—
Infantile Niemann-Pick	10.5 m	M	T cells few HC± moderate histiocytosis	—	T cells present B center histiocytosis
	2.5 y	F	T cells + HC ± moderate histiocytosis	T cells few B center histiocytosis	T cells present B center histiocytosis
	2.5 y	F	T cells + HC+ marked histiocytosis	B cells ± T zone histiocytosis	B cells ± T zone histiocytosis
Juvenile Niemann-Pick	10 7/12	F	HC± marked histiocytosis	T zone histiocytosis B cells +	T zone histiocytosis B cells +

pt. #6 - basal cell carcinomas
lymphohistiocytosis pt. #4 - malignant lymphoma
Other patients with malignant tumors who were observed to show absence of Hassall's corpuscles were found in the files of the Department of Pathology, Childrens Hospital of Los Angeles, during the same period from which the material for this review was drawn, and are shown in Table 15 (the four patients with Hodgkin's disease and absence of Hassall's corpuscles are also included in Table 6). The eight patients with leukemia represent only a small fraction of the patients with leukemia autopsied over this period, possibly a significant association, but not an indication that primary immunodeficiency is an important cause of leukemia in children in general. The association of absence of Hassall's corpuscles with malignant lymphoma is higher (6 of 30 = 20% in the CHLA autopsy series), and deserving of further study.

TABLE 15. Tumors with absent Hassall's corpuscles

	Number in base population
Leukemia, lymphocytic	5)
myeloid	1) 400
monomyeloid	2)
Lymphoma	6 – 30
Hodgkin's disease	4 – 9
Wilms' tumor	1 – 30

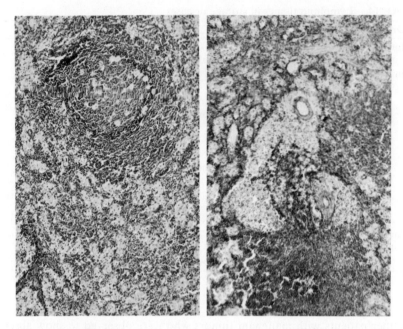

Fig. 30   Fig. 31

FIG. 30.   Spleen of patient with infantile Niemann-Pick disease (pt. 2, Table 14), showing extensive lipid histiocytosis of red pulp, with involvement also of germinal centers. (H & E, × 50)

FIG. 31.   Spleen of patient with juvenile Niemann-Pick disease (Table 14), showing heavy foam cell infiltration around smaller vessels (areas of T-cell collars); foam cells are not seen in the germinal centers. (H & E, × 50)

CONCLUDING REMARKS

Table 16 illustrates that at least nine different thymic patterns can be identified in the material reviewed in this paper. The "pinealoid" pattern of thymic dysplasia may occur in both adenosine deaminase positive severe combined immunodeficiency disease and in pure T cell deficiency, whereas the "thymic epithelial stem only" pattern is typical of adenosine deaminase-deficient severe combined immunodeficiency disease. The regular association of the "small dark cell" thymus, with or without stem cystosis, with T cell deficiency suggests that a single disorder, possibly (although *not* proven on any of the patients in this series) nucleoside (inosine) phosphorylase deficiency, is the most common cause of this functional state. The regular occurrence of

TABLE 16. Thymic patterns in diseases reviewed in this study

Thymic Pattern	SCID	T-deficiency	B-deficiency	Ataxia telangiectasia	Z-C-E syndrome	Hodgkin's disease	Letterer-Siwe disease	Lymphohistiocytosis	Septic granulomatosis	SLE	JRA	Chronic renal disease	Systemic hyalinosis	Thalassemia	Biliary atresia
"Pinealoid"	?3	?3													
Epithelial core-pale matrix	2														
Small lobules-small dark cell	1	6													
Small lobules, small dark cell, stem cystosis		6													
Variably involuted, with HC-0				5	1	4	6	2	2	1	1	2	1	1	2
HC±				1		1	2	2	3	1	1	3	1	1	7
HC+			4			2			3	11	1	3	1	2	5
HC2+			6			1			1	3	1	3	1	2	8
HC3+						1									
HC deficient (0 or ±)	6(?3)	12(?15)	–	6	1	5	8	4	5	2	1	5	2	2	9
HC adequate (+ or more)	–	–	10	–	–	4	–	–	4	14	2	6	1	4	13

30   B. H. Landing *et al.*

deficiency of thymic epithelium and Hassall's corpuscles in ataxia-telangiectasia, Letterer-Siwe disease and lymphohistiocytosis, its frequent occurrence
(± 50%) in Hodgkin's disease, septic granulomatosis, chronic renal insufficiency (especially with hemodialysis and renal transplantation) and biliary
atresia, and its general non-occurrence in B cell deficiency, systemic lupus
erythematosis and thalassemia are summarized in the lower portion of Table 16.
The data presented suggest strongly that loss of thymic epithelium progresses
over about 18 months in biliary atresia, and less strongly that it also progresses with age in Hodgkin's disease, although whether or not this T cell attrition begins before or after the onset of the disease itself cannot be stated.
The lack of evidence of progression of thymic epithelial deficiency with age or
duration of disease in septic granulomatosis, chronic renal insufficiency,
systemic lupus erythematosis, juvenile rheumatoid arthritis and thalassemia
raise questions as to the pathogenetic mechanisms believed to be responsible
for the "acquired immunodeficiency" considered by some workers to be a
sequel to severe malnutrition/infection, especially in infancy (Fig. 32). Biliary

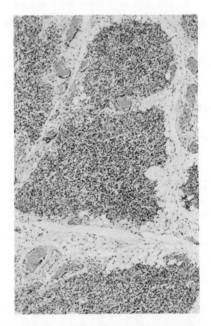

Fig. 32.   Thymus of 4-month-old Vietnamese orphan with Pneumocystis pneumonia, possibly an example of loss of Hassall's corpuscles
due to severe malnutrition and infection in infancy. (H & E, × 50)

atresia, Hodgkin's disease, Letterer-Siwe disease and the lymphohistiocytosis syndromes may, however, be examples of "thymic epithelial attrition" sufficiently reliably programmed to be of value in the elucidation of the pathogenetic mechanisms at issue in this area of disease. The findings in the thymus in systemic lupus erythematosis, juvenile rheumatoid arthritis and mixed connective tissue disease do not particularly suggest that primary immunodeficiency of the thymic "control system" is a basic feature of any or all of these disorders, but do indicate that they differ in the behavior of the thymus, despite similarities in course of illness and in treatment with steroids, and thereby imply the existence of basic differences in pathogenetic mechanisms among these "collagen diseases". That systemic hyalinosis is a distinct entity, and that T or B lymphocyte number or function may be abnormal in thalassemia, Gaucher's disease and Niemann-Pick disease, are suggested.

Specific suggestions on areas of deficient information warranting further study:
1. Regularity of association of nucleoside phosphorylase deficiency with pure T-cell deficiency;
2. production of thymic hormone(s) in partial DiGeorge syndrome;
3. regularity of association of the "central Hassall's corpuscle" thymic pattern with dysgammaglobulinemia;
4. thymic anatomy in ataxia-telangiectasia in infancy;
5. thymic anatomy in Zinsser-Cole-Engman syndrome in infancy;
6. thymic anatomy in Hodgkin's disease in infancy, before onset of disease, and before treatment;
7. T-lymphocyte number and function in biliary atresia;
8. further study of lymphocyte function in Letterer-Siwe disease;
9. thymic anatomy and lymphocyte function in early lymphohistiocytosis;
10. pathogenetic mechanisms in systemic hyalinosis;
11. T-lymphocyte number and function in thalassemia and thalassemia trait;
12. lymphocyte number and function in Gaucher, Niemann-Pick and other reticuloendothelial lysosomal storage diseases.

REFERENCES

1. Huber, J. and Gelfand, E. W.: Failure of differentiation of implanted thymic tissue in a patient with severe combined immunodeficiency disease. Abstr. 11th International Congress, Intern. Acad. Pathol., Washington, D.C., October, 1976.
2. Giblett, E. R., Ammann, A. J., Wara, D. W., Sandeman, R., and Diamond, L. K.:

32   B. H. Landing *et al.*

Nucleoside-phosphorylase deficiency in a child with severely defective T-cell
immunity and normal B-cell immunity. *Lancet* (May 3): 1010, 1975.
3. Stiehm, E. R., and Fudenberg, H. H.: Clinical and immunologic features of dysgammaglobulinemia type 1. *Am. J. Med.* **40**: 805, 1966.
4. Ortega, J. A., Swanson, V. L., Landing, B. H., and Hammond, G. D.: Congenital
dyskeratosis. Zinsser-Cole-Engman syndrome with thymic dysplasia and
aeplastic anemia. *Am. J. Dis. Child.* **124**, 701, 1972.
5. Eltringham, J. R. and Kaplan, H. S.: Immunodeficiency in Hodgkin's disease.
in: Immunodeficiency in Man and Animals, National Foundation. Birth
Defects: Original Article Series Vol. 11, No. 1, 1975, p. 278.
6. Dutz, W., Rossipal, E., Ghavami, K., and Vessal, K.: Persistent acquired cell-
mediated immunodeficiency following infantile diarrhea during the first 6
months of life. Abstr. Pediat. Path. Club, New Orleans, Louisiana, March
1975.
7. Cederbaum, S. D., Niwayama, G., Stiehm, E. R., Neerhout, R. C., Ammann,
A. J., and Berman, W. J.: Combined immunodeficiency presented as the
Letterer-Siwe syndrome. *J. Pediat.* **85**: 466, 1974.
8. Alfi, O. S., Heuser, E. T., Landing, B. H., Robinson, R. E., Nadler, S., and Don-
nell, G. N.: A syndrome of systemic hyalinosis, short-limb dwarfism
and possible thymic dysplasia. *In*: New Chromosomal and Malformation
Syndromes. National Foundation. Birth Defects: Original Article Series,
Vol. 11, No. 5, 1975, p. 57.

DISCUSSION

Dr. GOOD: As we permit everybody else to get wound up, I would like to say that
the real difficulty in dealing with post mortem material largely has been the
extraordinary influence of secondary involution, of losses of germinal centers,
extraordinary depletion of the thymus, even epithelial depletion, and although
I have been on record advising against any further extensive efforts to obtain
lymphoid tissues during life and following stimulation, I am not sure that we do
not need to try to compare in these various entities the lymphoid tissue during
life with that at post mortem.
Dr. LANDING: As we will come to later on, the problem of the loss of thymic
epithelium and so on is a major one. I know there are people who believe in it
strongly. As we will show, there are many syndromes with severe illness leading to
death and major treatment by immunodepressive agents, which do not produce
that outcome in the lymphoid tissue. It is not quite as simple as that chronic
illness can do it.
Dr. HITZIG: I should like to make a comment in the same direction. We have
described a family in 1971 where three boys were affected. They survived
three months, four months, and, I think, fifteen months, and we had some
evidence that the thymus became more involuted the longer they survived.
Now later on when ADA deficiency (i.e., adenosine deaminase deficiency) became known, we tested the family and both parents were carriers of the genes,

so it is very probable that these boys were ADA-deficient; we then made the theory that the thymus was involuted because of intoxication, or, that is, by a deficiency of the enzyme. It seems to me that we have in this case both a quiet atrophy or involution of the thymus and hereditary disease. ADA deficiency is not a stem cell disease. Apparently the stem cells are normal; the thymus is, at birth, probably normal, but it is involuted because of the deficiency of the enzyme. This is a challenge and it is a hypothesis, but I think it might be one of the major objects of our discussion.

Dr. YAMAMURA: I think this may be a strange question from a biochemist, but in order to bring out the questions from the Japanese, I should like to ask one question. Are there any special features to identify, or to differentiate, a primary immunodeficiency and one secondary to infection?

Dr. GOOD: I think in those situations where we can actually identify an enzyme abnormality, or a genetic pattern, I think we have a handle. I think also, early in the course of the disease, the study of the lymphoid tissue by biospy, and clearly, the study of the lymphoid cells in the circulating blood in after-coming members of a family, provide diagnosis without any evidence of infection. So that these are not all consequences of infection. In Bruton's original case, it is very suggestive that an infection may have played a role in the pathogenesis, rather than in just revealing the disease. Dr. Aiuti has a question.

Dr. AIUTI: What I want to point out is that there is a variation in the lymphoid picture in pure T-cell deficiency. In these patients' spleen, there is always the presence of more lymphoid cells, and in the bone marrow, plasma cells are always present.

Dr. GOOD: I should like to ask Dr. Aiuti, did you have or did you see in the pure T-cell deficiency germinal centers in any of the nodes, true germinal centers?

Dr. AIUTI: After antigenic stimulation with vaccine, we saw germinal centers in the nodes.

Dr. GOOD: The reason for emphasizing this is that one of the striking things in the nude mouse, or in the neonatal thymectomized mice that are athymic, when you really do not have any T-cells, you do not get germinal centers. I mean, we have really seen that, and this is, I think, very consistent.

There are several points in this that we have been trying to address from the other perspective of looking at functions of the immunocytes in patients with these various diseases. For example, in Hodgkin's disease studying patients between nine and twenty-five years after complete recovery from Hodgkin's disease, we are still able to demonstrate abnormalities of the function of the lymphoid system. Now we do not know whether that means that there is a latent Hodgkin's virus or what is producing that abnormality, or even if it is a consequence in some way of the therapy, but there it is, nine to twenty-five years after Hodgkin's disease, you can regularly demonstrate an abnormality of function.

In the patients with the chronic granulomatous disease, from an immunological point of view, when you get members of the family very early in their life and

recognise the patient before he has any chronic granulomatous disease, or any
septic granulomatosis they seem to be quite normal immunologically. But once
they have begun to have problems with infection, you can regularly demonstrate
appurtabation. I am always embarrassed by the lipid histiocytosis, which you
have emphasized and were the first really to clearly point out. There it was, and I
had pointed it out to our pathologists, and they had said, 'Oh, that is always
seen when you have chronic inflammation', but it is not. Not in this disease. But
the lymphoid system, the distribution of cells, I do not think are too surprising
with a chronic inflammation. What you find is tremendous plasmacytosis in the
marrow and in the red part of the spleen. Although there is a 3-cell deficiency,
you find this very great terminal differentiation of the B-lymphocytes, which I
think goes along very well with their hypogammaglobulinemia. I think we need
some more studies on that. But I am impressed by the fact that you are able,
now, with this systematic and careful look at the lymphoid system, to show us
that there is something more here than just a disease chronicity and the consequences of stress. I think we need to look at these issues now in the experimental
perspective and see whether we do have the capacity to induce secondarily the
sorts of changes you talk about. There is no question in my mind that in rabbits
and in mice, where I have worked with this, that I can produce a virtual absence
of Hassall's corpuscles by long exposure to hydrocortisone in very large doses,
and I can certainly do it with starvation. But what the real mechanisms are, and
why you have such differences in patients on immunosuppressive therapy,
when in certain other diseases one does not find this, I think really now is going
to take us back to the laboratory for analysis.

Dr. HITZIG: I have a very naïve question. I am not a pathologist, but we are now
looking at the Hassall's corpuscles twenty-five years or so later. What are they
really, what do they mean? What can you learn from the Hassall's corpuscles,
if you are paying so much attention to them?

Dr. GOOD: The Hassall's corpuscles have been around for a long, long time, for
more than eighty years, very regularly described. They have been around pyro-
genetically for at least four hundred million years, because every single animal
that has a thymus, with all of the pyrogenetic deviations, has Hassall's corpuscles.
And yet, the amount of information about Hassall's corpuscles is infinitesimally
small. I mean, many people have described these things, but we really do not
know very much about them.

The thymus seems to contain, when you look for it, nuclear and cellular debris,
and some, or all, of it has some kind of disposal mechanism, but there is no real
evidence for this. There was a thesis from Utrecht, in which they seemed to be
able to relate the numbers of Hassall's corpuscles in an experimental situation to
a stimulus for self-mediated immunity, and that looked very impressive, but I
have not seen confirmation of that, or any real developments. I do not think at
all that this is just some sort of a quantified consequence of the epithelial structure. I really think they must have a function. They are preserved through many,

many pyrogenetic lines and we really need to have as hard a look at Hassall's corpuscles as possible, as Dr. Landing's presentation here provokes me to think. And I think that experimental approaches are going to be the way, just as with the thymus where really we had completely erroneous ideas until we began studying it, and I think we have got to begin moving the Hassall's corpuscles in the directions that your pathological analysis suggests may be possible.

Two Types of Defects in the Suppression of Antibody Response

Tomio TADA, Masaru TANIGUCHI, and Toshitada TAKEMORI

ABSTRACT

In this paper, we have described two types of defects in the expression of suppressor and acceptor molecules on T cells among various mouse strains. One example is A/J which does not produce the KLH-specific suppressor factor despite being able to accept the factor produced by histocompatible strains. The other type of suppressor defect was found in B10 congenic lines and D2.GD mice which can produce but cannot accept the factor. Both strains are known to be high responders to KLH. If A/J (nonproducer) were crossed with B10.A (nonacceptor) having the same H-2 haplotype, their F_1 hybrids could both produce and accept the factor, indicating that both expressions are dominant traits. These results suggest that certain defects in the immunoregulatory system could be explained by defective expression of either the suppressor or acceptor gene. Either defect may lead to an abnormal responsiveness to a given antigen, and thus may be included in immunodeficiency states. Some implications of these defects on the induction of autoimmune phenomena are discussed.

INTRODUCTION

Suppression of immune responses by T cells and their products is under the control of genes which are located in the *I* region of *H-2* complex. Our previous studies indicated that an *in vitro* secondary IgG antibody response against dinitrophenylated keyhole limpet hemocyanin (DNP-KLH) was greatly suppressed by an extract of thymocytes or spleen cells from syngeneic mice that had been immunized with a relatively high dose of KLH.[1-3] The active factor was recently identified as a product of a gene present in a newly defined *I* subregion (*I-J*), which is intercalated between *I-B* and *I-C* subregions.[4] This factor could suppress the responses of mice which share identical *I-J*

Laboratories for Immunology, School of Medicine, Chiba University, Chiba, Japan subregion with the donor of the suppressive T cell factor but not those of *I-J* incompatible strains, indicating that the acceptor site for the suppressive T cell factor is also encoded by a gene in the *I-J* subregion.[4] The results suggest that the suppressor phenomena are determined by the phenotypic expressions of paired genes perhaps closely linked with each other and located in the same *I-J* subregion.

Since it is now widely recognized that the suppression of antibody response by T cells is a physiologic mechanism involved in the regulation of the immune response, it may not be irrelevant to discuss the defects in the suppressor mechanism as examples of immunological dysfunction. In fact, it has been suggested that defective regulatory function leads to certain immunological abnormalities, such as autoimmune diseases and hypergammaglobulinemia (reviewed in 5). In addition, cases of immunodeficiency disease (common variable agammaglobulinemia) have been shown to result from an overfunction of suppressor T cell.[6] Therefore, we would like to demonstrate two types of defects in the physiologic suppressor mechanism in certain strains of mice, and further discuss possible implications in human immunologic abnormalities.

Histocompatibility requirement for effective suppression by T cell factor

In a previous publication, we have shown that the suppressive T cell factor obtained from one strain of mice could effectively suppress the responses of mice sharing the same histocompatibility antigen.[3] This genetic requirement was found to be directed to *I-J* subregion compatibility,[4] and thus combinations in which *I-J* subregion is identical between given strains could induce effective suppression regardless of differences in other subregions in *H-2* complex.[4] The simplest explanation for this histocompatibility requirement is that the acceptor site on the target cells for the suppressive T cell factor has a structure complementary to the suppressor molecule, with which effective and efficient suppression is made possible. It is predicted that both the suppressor and acceptor molecules on T cells are coded for by paired genes both present in the same *I* subregion, one of which is selectively expressed on the suppressor or acceptor T cell.

In various strain combinations including several recombinant mice, it has been proved that *I-J* compatibility is, in fact, both necessary and sufficient for effective suppression. The general rule for this will be found in Table 1 which indicates that syngeneic and semisyngeneic (parents and F_1) combinations are always effective in inducing suppression. It is also apparent that the acceptor sites for the factors derived from parent strains are codominantly expressed on T cells of the F_1 mice, and that F_1 mice produce separate molecules which suppress either parental strain response.

TABLE 1. Suppression of *in vitro* antibody response by the T cell factor from histocompatible strains

Donor strain	Recipient strain	Identities*	% suppression of indirect PFC
BALB/c	BALB/c	K,I,S,D	86
	A/J	S,D	0
	(BALB/c × A/J)F₁	$\underline{K,I,S,D}$	75
	(BALB/c × CBA)F₁	$\underline{K,I,S,D}$	92
	CBA	none	0
CBA	CBA	K,I,S,D	93
	C3H	K,I,S,D	81
	(BALB/c × A/J)F₁	$\underline{K,I}$	94
	A/J	K,I	74
	BALB/c	none	0
(BALB/c × CBA)F₁	(BALB/c × CBA)F₁	K,I,S,D	91
	BALB/c	$\underline{K,I,S,D}$	88
	CBA	$\underline{K,I,S,D}$	75
	A/J	$\underline{K,I}$	76
	SJL	none	0

*Semisyngeneic regions are underlined.

Defective expression of the suppressive T cell factor or acceptor site in certain strains

During the course of this study, we found that there are two types of defects in the expression of suppressor phenomena. One example is the A/J strain which does not produce the KLH-specific suppressor factor despite being able to accept the factor produced by histocompatible strains. As shown in Table 2, the T cell extract from KLH-primed A/J mice could not suppress the responses of both syngeneic A/J and *I* region compatible C3H mice. We have repeated

TABLE 2. Failure to produce suppressive T cell factor in A/J and (BALB/c × A/J)F₁ strain

Donor strain	Recipient strain	Identities*	% suppression of indirect PFC
A/J	A/J	K^k,I^k,S^d,D^d	0
	C3H	K^k,I^k	0
	BALB/c	S^d,D^d	0
(BALB/c × A/J)F₁	A/J	$\underline{K^k,I^k}$	0
	C3H	$\underline{K^k,I^k}$	0
	BALB/c	$\underline{K^d,I^d,S^d,D^d}$	70
	(BALB/c × A/J)F₁	$K^{d/k},I^{d/k},S^d,D^d$	70

*Semisyngeneic regions are underlined.

several experiments using different immunization regimens with a constant failure to produce the KLH-specific suppressor factor in A/J strain.

Even more peculiar is the genetic trait for the inability to produce the suppressive T cell factor in A/J mice. When (BALB/c × A/J)F₁ was used as the donor of the T cell factor, the factor from this F_1 could suppress responses of both (BALB/c × A/J)F₁ and BALB/c, but not the response of the other parental partner A/J. The F_1 factor also failed to suppress the responses of *H-2^k* mice (CBA and C3H). Therefore, the production of the suppressive T cell factor *per se* is genetically dominant, but the produced factor is strictly strain specific, and thus the inability to produce the *H-2^k* reactive factor of A/J mice is also inherited by the F_1 mice.

The other type of suppressor defect was found in B10 congenic lines and D2.GD mice. Quite the contrary of A/J, these strains can produce the factor but are unable to accept the suppressor factor produced by syngeneic or *I-J* compatible strains. Table 3 shows such an example observed in B10.S mice. There are striking differences in the sensitivity to the suppression by *H-2^s* factor in SJL and B10.S spleen cells. The response of SJL spleen cells was markedly suppressed by the T-extract derived from either SJL or B10.S, indicating that both strains could produce the suppressive T cell factor which can act on SJL responding cells. However, the response of B10.S spleen cells was not suppressed by the T-extract from either B10.S or SJL which had been shown to suppress the response of SJL under the identical conditions. Furthermore, B10.S factor consistently enhanced the response of B10.S spleen cells, while it suppressed the response of SJL spleen cells. We have later found that all the congenic strains of B10 background can produce the suppressor factor which is reactive with histocompatible spleen cells, but the acceptor for the syngeneic or histocompatible suppressor factor is lacking in all cases examined. This inability to accept the suppressor factor is most likely due to a defect in the expression of acceptor for the KLH-specific T cell factor. Since all the B10 congenic lines could not accept the suppressive T cell factor, it is suggested that

TABLE 3.   Failure to accept the suppressive effect of the H-2^s factor in B10.S mice

Donor strain	Recipient strain	Identities	% suppression of indirect PFC
SJL	SJL	K,I,S,D	72
	B10.S	K,I,S,D	0
	CBA	none	0
B10.S	SJL	K,I,S,D	63
	B10.S	K,I,S,D	0*
	CBA	none	0

*Definite enhancement.

the expression of *I* region genes is influenced by other genes not linked to the *H-2* complex.

It is interesting to note that C57BL/6J can accept the *H-2^b* factor, while C57BL/10 (B10) lacks the acceptor site. The genetic differences between these two strains are known to be very small.

The genetic trait of the suppressor-acceptor expressions

Since A/J and B10.A, both having the same *H-2* haplotype, lack one of the expressions of the suppressor or acceptor, we crossed these strains to obtain their F_1 hybrid. The ability of the (A/J × B10.A)F_1 to produce the suppressive T cell factor as well as to accept the factor was tested by combinations of F_1 and parents as donor and recipient. As shown in Table 4, the (A/J × B10.A)F_1 could produce the T cell factor which can suppress both A/J and F_1 responses. The same factor could not suppress the response of the other parental partner strain B10.A which lacks acceptor site. Similarly the response of (A/J × B10. A)F_1 is suppressible by the factors derived from F_1 and B10.A but not from A/J, since A/J could not produce the suppressive T cell factor. Thus both the suppressor and acceptor are dominantly expressed on the cells of F_1 whose parents lack either one of the expressions.

TABLE 4. Dominant expressions of both the suppressor and acceptor genes on the cells of (A/J × B10.A)F_1

Donor strain	Recipient strain	% suppression of indirect PFC
(A/J × B10.A)F_1	A/J	75
(A/J × B10.A)F_1	B10.A	0
(A/J × B10.A)F_1	(A/J × B10.A)F_1	72
A/J	(A/J × B10.A)F_1	0
B10.A	(A/J × B10.A)F_1	73

DISCUSSION

It has been reported in various experimental systems that immunocompetent cell interactions are achieved by direct contact between functionally different cell types or by soluble factors elaborated by T cells.[7] In either case, there exist certain genetic restrictions on the effective interactions. Such restrictions are considered to be mainly determined by the expressions of the effector molecules (T cell factor) and the acceptor site on responding cell types for different T cell factors. Taussig and Munro[8] suggested that T and B cells interact with each other through complementary structures present on these cell types which are determined by genes in the *I* region of an *H-2* complex. They have found that there exist two types of nonresponders, T cell nonresponders and B cell nonresponders, thus proposing a two-gene model in T-B cell interaction. The results presented in this paper also strongly suggest that suppressor phenomena are determined by products of two genes closely linked to each other and present in the same *I* subregion (*I-J*). This model was strongly supported by the occurrence of special strains which lack one of the suppressor and acceptor expressions. Either defect may lead to an extremely high responsiveness to a given antigen. This idea is probably consistent with the observation made by Cerottini and Unanue,[9] who showed that A/J strain is a high responder to KLH, while CBA and BALB/c were rather poor responders, and that the responsiveness to KLH is not under H-linked Ir gene control.

This may also imply that A/J mice lack the expression of one of the paired genes to produce the suppressor factor, while the expression of the other gene for the acceptor site is intact. Alternatively, the expression of the suppressor molecule is determined by other unknown regulator genes which are not linked to *H-2* complex. In fact, we are aware of the fact that A/J strain is in many respects peculiar in its response to various complex antigens. It has been known that A/J strain naturally produces antinuclear antibody according to aging. Also, A/J can produce various idiotype-bearing antibodies, *i.e.* A5A, alsonate and KLH. Such genetic abnormalities may at least partially be due to the lack of expression of the suppressor molecule.

However, it is not known at the present time whether this lack of expression of the suppressor molecule is due to a point mutation in *I-J* subregion in A/J or to be attributed by non-*H-2* genes. On the other hand, since all the B10 congenic lines do not express KLH-specific acceptor site, this defect may be due to the effect of background non-*H-2* genes. In certain experimental systems histoincompatible animals were shown to accept the factor produced by other low responder animals.[10] Therefore, such defects may primarily depend on the antigen used to stimulate these cell types. More recently we have shown that the cell type expressing acceptor site for the T cell factor is the T cell having Lyt 1,2,3 alloantigens, which after acceptance of the T cell factor differentiates into new suppressor T cells having Lyt 2,3 alloantigen.[11] Therefore, the suppression of the antibody response is achieved via the intermediary of a novel T cell type which expresses acceptor site for the T cell factor. The importance of this intermediary cell type is discussed elsewhere.[11]

Since both producer and acceptor T cells play important roles in the induction of physiologic suppression of antibody response, a defect in either cell type may lead to an abnormal responsiveness to certain antigens, an example of which may be the production of autoantibodies. It has been suggested that autoimmune phenomena in NZB and (NZB × NZW)F$_1$ mice are due to a defect of suppressor mechanism.[12] It is important to determine which of the producer and acceptor cell types is affected in aged NZ mouse strains. Our current interest is to determine what type of gene defect is present in nonproducer and nonacceptor strains, and what human counterparts can be detected in autoimmune diseases.

The results presented in this paper suggest that certain defects in the immunoregulatory system could be explained by defective expression of either suppressor or acceptor genes. It is now of crucial importance to clarify the nature of these suppressor and acceptor molecules expressed on different subsets of T cells and determined by the same subregion of *H-2* complex, and the consequence of the interaction of the two *I* region gene products in the regulation of the antibody response. Such a study will give a clue for more precise understanding of the whole picture of the immunoregulatory system and the resultant abnormalities in immunological diseases.

Acknowledgements

We wish to express our sincere thanks to Drs. B. Benacerraf, C.S. David and R.S. Schwartz for their generous supply of alloantisera and recombinant strains. We are grateful to our colleagues Drs. K. Hayakawa, T. Tokuhisa and K. Yamauchi in the Laboratories for Immunology, Chiba University, who participated in the studies described herein. We also wish to thank Mr. H. Takahashi and Ms. Y. Yamaguchi for their excellent technical and secretarial assistance.

This study was supported by grants from the Ministry of Education, Science and Culture, and the Ministry of Health, Japan.

REFERENCES

1. Taniguchi, M., Hayakawa, K., Tada T.: Properties of antigen-specific suppressive T-cell factor in the regulation of antibody response of the mouse. II. *In vitro* activity and evidence for the *I* region gene product. *J. Immunol.* **116**:542, 1976.
2. Taniguchi, M., Tada, T., and Tokuhisa, T: Properties of the antigen-specific suppressive T-cell factor in the regulation of antibody response of the mouse. III. Dual gene control of the T-cell-mediated suppression of the antibody response. *J. Exp. Med. 144*:20, 1976.
3. Tada, T. and Taniguchi, M.: Characterization of the antigen-specific suppressive T cell factor with special reference to the expression of *I* region genes. in: The Role of Products of the Histocompatibility Gene Complex in Immune Responses. Academic Press, New York, 1976.

4. Tada, T., Taniguchi, M., and David, C. S.: Properties of the antigen-specific suppressive T-cell factor in the regulation of antibody response of the mouse. IV. Special subregion assignment of the gene(s) that codes for the suppressive T-cell factor in the *H-2* histocompatibility complex. *J. Exp. Med.* **144**: 713, 1976.
5. Allison, A. C.: Interactions of T and B lymphocytes in self-tolerance and autoimmunity. in: Immunological Tolerance, Academic Press, New York, 1975.
6. Waldman, T. A., Broder, S., Blease, R. M., *et al*: Role of suppressor T cells in pathogenesis of common variable hypogammaglobulinemia. *Lancet* **2**:609, 1974.
7. Katz, D. H. and Benacerraf, B.: Regulatory influence of activated T cells on B cell responses to antigen. *Adv. Immunol.* **15**:1, 1973.
8. Munro, A. J. and Taussig, M. J.: Two genes in the major histocompatibility complex control immune response. *Nature* **256**:103, 1975.
9. Cerottini, J. C. and Unanue, E. R.: Genetic control of the immune response of mice to hemocyanin. I. The role of macrophages. *J. Immunol.* **106**:732, 1971.
10. Kapp, J. A., Pierce, C. W., and Benacerraf, B.: Suppressive activity of lymphoid cell extracts from non-responder mice injected with the terpolymer L-glutamic acid[60]-L-alanine[30]-L-tyrosin[10] (GAT). In: The Role of Products of the Histocompatibility Gene Complex in Immune Response. Academic Press, New York, 1976.
11. Tada, T., Taniguchi, M., and Tokuhisa, T.: Suppressive T cell factor and its acceptor expressed on different subsets of T cells: A possible amplification loop in the suppressor system. In: Proceedings of Third *Ir* Gene Workshop, in press.
12. Talal, N.: Disordered immunologic regulation and autoimmunity. *Transplant. Rev.* **31**:240, 1976.

DISCUSSION

Dr. GOOD: Whenever we have a phenomenon that is Lyt 123 positive, one worries about the possibility that it is the precursor cell that you are detecting rather than the definitive cell, because as Cantor and Boyse have shown, the Lyt 123 can become either Lyt 23 or Lyt 1 in a matter of hours. How long did your assay take, and how have you assured yourself against this possibility?

Dr. TADA: Lyt 123 positive cells, which are adherent to nylon wool, could absorb the suppressive T-cell factor, and when those cells were killed, we could not get any suppression. I think there are two possibilities: one is that Lyt 123 cells just transmit the activity of a factor to the final target cells, and the other is that they are the amplifying device of the Lyt 23 cells to become effective. In our hands, Lyt phenotype is very stable, and does not change so easily.

Helper or Suppressor Effect on Mitogen Induced B Cell Differentiation of T Cells from Immune Disorders*

Junichi YATA, Toshiro NAKAGAWA,
Toshikazu SHINBO, Machiko SUGAWARA,
Utako HIEI, and Tadashi MATSUMOTO

It has been firmly established in experimental animals that T cells are divided into subgroups according to their functions. Helper T cells assist B cells to differentiate into antibody producing cells. Suppressor T cells regulate B cell differentiation by acting directly on B cells or via helper T cells. Killer T cells reject grafted allogeneic cells, virus infected cells and tumor cells. These killer T cells are controlled by helper and suppressor T cells. T cells are also effectors of delayed hypersensitivity reactions.

Each of these functions should be distinguished to establish our understanding of abnormalities in the immune systems of patients with immune disorders. Waldmann et al.[1] and Siegal et al.[2] reported that lymphocytes from patients with variable immunodeficiency suppressed immunoglobulin production by B cells from healthy individuals and suggested the role of suppressor T cells in the etiology of hypogammaglobulinemia.

We report here the effect on mitogen induced B cell differentiation of T cells from various types of immune disorders.

MATERIALS AND METHODS

1. Separation of T cells and B cell enriched population
   T cells and other cells were separated by rosette sedimentation.[3] The peripheral blood lymphocytes collected by Ficoll-Hypaque density gradient were mixed with sheep erythrocytes at 1:100. The cells were suspended in fetal calf

Departments of Pediatrics and Immunology, Toho University, Tokyo, Japan
   *Supported by a research grant from the Japanese Ministry of Education and Ministry of Welfare.

serum, centrifuged at 400*g* for 5 minutes and incubated in ice water for 1 hour to form rosettes. They were gently resuspended and centrifuged at the same density gradient. The cells forming rosettes were sedimented to the bottom and the others remained at the interface. The cells collected from the bottom were added with 0.83 % NH_4Cl to lyse the sheep erythrocytes. The cells thus obtained were mostly T cells (less than 1 % of B cells and no monocytes). The cells remaining at the interface were usually composed of 30–50 % B cells, 30–60 % monocytes and a small number of T cells (B cell enriched population, BRC).

2. Combination of the cells to test their interaction

Combination of the cells to test their interaction in B cell differentiation was carried out as follows:

1) Bn (2 × 10^5 BRC from normal individuals)
2) Tn (8 × 10^5 T cells from normal individuals)
3) Tp (8 × 10^5 T cells from patients)
4) Bn + Tn
5) Bn + Tp

In the cases where T cells were expected to suppress the appearance of immunoglobulin producing cells (Ig cells), normal BRC were mixed with normal T cells to elicit a certain number of Ig cells, and then the test T cells were further added to them.

6) Bn + Tn′ (2 × 10^5 T cells from normal individuals)
7) Bn + Tn′ + Tp

These cells were suspended in 1 ml of medium RPMI 1640 supplemented with 20 % fetal calf serum.

3. Induction of immunoglobulin producing cells

10 μg of poke weed mitogen was added to each combination of cells, and the cells were cultured at 37°C for 1 week in 5 % CO_2 incubator.

4. Estimation of immunoglobulin producing cells

The number of the cells was counted at the end of culture. The cells were then smeared on a UV glass slide, fixed with acetone and stained for cytoplasmic immunoglobulin by immunofluorescence. The percentage of the cells with cytoplasmic fluorescence (Ig cells) was scored under a fluorescence microscope and their absolute number was calculated according to the number of total cells. Thus Ig cells generated from the same number of BRC alone or BRC supplemented with different T cells can be compared.

5. Evaluation of helper function

The helper function of test T cells was expressed by the following formula:

$$\frac{Ig(Bn + Tp) - Ig(Bn)}{Ig(Bn + Tn) - Ig(Bn)} \times 100$$

Ig (Bn + Tn) indicates the number of Ig cells which appeared from (Bn + Tn) cell culture.

6. Evaluation of suppressor function

When the test T cells were expected to suppress the appearance of Ig cells, suppressor function of the cells was expressed by the following formula:

$$-\left(1 - \frac{Ig(Bn + Tn' + Tp)}{Ig(Bn + Tn')}\right) \times 100$$

RESULTS

1. Amplification of B cell differentiation by T cell

Only a very few Ig cells appeared from the culture of Bn alone. The appearance of Ig cells was, however, amplified very much in the presence of Tn (Fig. 1). It is, therefore, suggested that mitogen induced B cell differentiation is helped by T cells.

T cells alone elicited almost no Ig cells.

2. Comparison of the effect of allogeneic T cells and autologous T cells in the generation of immunoglobulin producing cells

The number of Ig cells which appeared from Bn added with allogeneic T cells (Tal) was compared with those from Bn supplemented with autologous T cells (Tau). No big difference was observed between the two. When the effect of Tal was expressed by percentages of the number of Ig cells from (Bn + Tal) to that of (Bn + Tau), their variation was $100\% \pm 22$ (SD) (Fig. 2).

This indicated that the mixed lymphocyte culture reaction (reactions between Bn and Tal) itself or the genetic barrier present between allogeneic T and B cells does not have much influence on the appearance of Ig cells helped by T cells in this system and that allogeneic combinations of T and B cells can be used to estimate the function of T cells.

3. Effect of T cells from immunodeficiency diseases

T cells from X-linked infantile agammaglobulinemia showed some helper

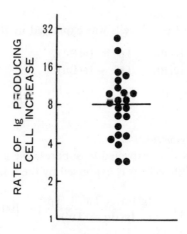

FIG. 1. Number of immunoglobulin producing cells (Ig cells) generated from B cells was increased by supplement of autologous T cells. Number in the graph indicates the ratio of increase in the number of Ig cells by addition of T cells.

effect but it was lower than that of healthy T cells. No Ig cells appeared from the T cell depleted population of the patients even in the presence of normal T cells (Fig. 3).

Most other congenital agammaglobulinemia of the sporadic type showed the same profile (Fig. 7). A small number of Ig cells appeared from BRC by adding normal T cells in 3 out of 7 such cases.

T cells from variable immunodeficiency suppressed the appearance of Ig cells from the culture of normal B and T cell mixture in 4 cases and showed a decreased but still some helper function in 2 cases.

Differentiation of patients' B cells was not recovered even by supplementing normal T cells in most cases (Fig. 4, Fig. 7).

In the case of severe combined immunodeficiency, its T cells showed neither helper nor suppressor effect (Fig. 7).

A small number of Ig cells appeared from BRC, but they were not increased by the addition of normal T cells.

T cells from 3 cases with Wiskott-Aldrich syndrome showed decreased helper function. A certain number of Ig cells appeared from their BRC (Fig. 5, Fig. 7)

4. T cells from hypergammaglobulinemia

Two cases which showed more than 7,000mg/dl of serum IgG levels and

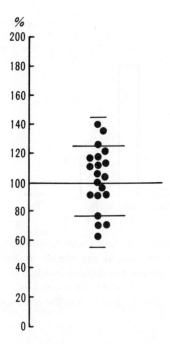

FIG. 2. Allogeneic T cells showed almost the same helper effect on B cells as autologous T cells in generation of immunoglobulin producing cells (Ig cells). Number in the graph indicates the percentage when the number of Ig cells which appeared from B cells helped by allogeneic T cells were compared with Ig cells from the same B cells helped by autologous T cells.

plasma cell hyperplasia in biopsied lymph node were studied. Although the etiology of hypergammaglobulinemia in these patients was obscure, increased immunoglobulin was polyclonal and the hyperplastic plasma cells did not seem to be morphologically of a malignant nature.

The helper function of the T cells from these patients was lower than normal, while their B cell differentiation occurred well with normal T cells (Fig. 6).

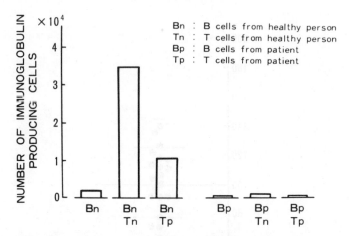

FIG. 3. Appearance of immunoglobulin-producing cells from various combinations of cells are shown in Fig.3 – Fig.6. T cells from a case of congenital agammaglobulinemia showed weaker helper effect as compared with T cells from normal individuals. B cells from the patient did not differentiate even in the presence of normal T cells.

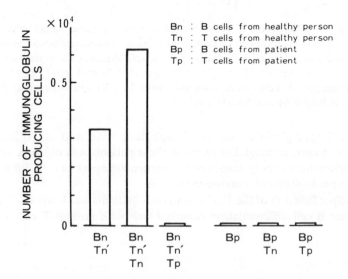

FIG. 4. T cells from a case of variable immunodeficiency suppressed the appearance of immunoglobulin producing cells from normal B cells helped by normal T cells. B cells of patient did not differentiate even with a supplement of normal T cells.

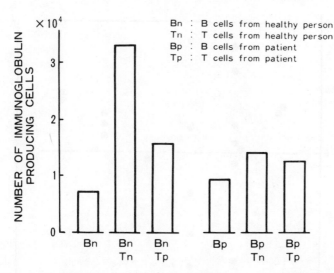

FIG. 5.   T cells from a case of Wiskott-Aldrich syndrome showed weaker helper effect.

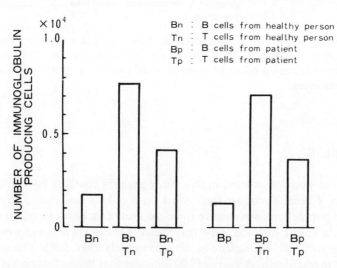

FIG. 6.   T cells from a case of hypergammaglobulinemia showed a rather weaker helper effect. B cells differentiated well with normal T cells.

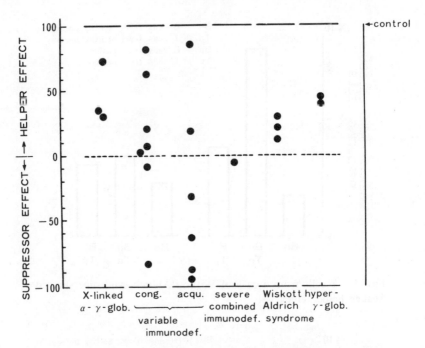

Fig. 7. Effect of T cells from immunological disorders on the generation of B cells. 100 $\pm$ 50 indicates normal helper effect. 0–50 indicates decreased helper function. 0~–100 indicates suppressor effect is dominant.

DISCUSSION

The T cell population used in this study perhaps contains both helper and suppressor T cells. Therefore their effect on B cells is the result of actions of these two populations which have quite opposite functions. In our scores expressing the helper function, zero may mean that helpers and suppressors are cancelling each other's functions or alternatively that both functions are abolished in test T cells. A score of 100 indicates that helper function is stronger than suppressor as in normal T cells.

In order to estimate the function of helpers or suppressors independently, we need a method for isolating each population in its pure form.

We do not so far have definitive cell markers to identify helpers and suppressors. Cooper *et al.* suggested that T cells with IgG Fc receptor correspond to suppressors and those with IgM receptor to helpers.[4]

These parameters may provide a method for purification of T cell subsets.

Allogeneic B cells are known to stimulate T cells, which may amplify the effect of T cells on B cell differentiation. Cytotoxic reaction of T cells against allogeneic B cells may have an influence on the generation of immunoglobulin producing cells. It has been proved in experimental animals that concordance of histocompatible alloantigens of T and B cells is a prerequisite for the cell interactions at least in some situations. Therefore, allogeneic T cells may not work as well as autologous or syngeneic T cells. These possibilities seemed not to have much influence on the appearance of immunoglobulin producing cells in our system since the effects of allogeneic T cells were not very different from those of autologous T cells. This would make it feasible to estimate the helper function of allogeneic test T cells by comparing the appearance of Ig cells from normal B cells helped by them with that of those helped by autologous normal T cells.

Decreased helper function observed in congenital agammaglobulinemia may be due to the feedback mechanisms to the helper T cell system from gammaglobulin passively administered as a supplemental therapy. Helper T cells may not develop well when the number of B cells, the target of their action, is decreased. It is also possible that some primary T cell abnormalities are present in some of the patients.

Suppressor T cells seemed to be increased in most variable immunodeficiency cases, as suggested by Waldmann and others.[1] B cells of most of these patients did not produce immunoglobulin in our study even when T cells of patients were replaced with normal T cells. This may mean that the B cells have lost their ability to differentiate into Ig cells or that the few very potent suppressor T cells remaining in the B cell enriched population still suppress the helper activity and then reduce B cell differentiation. If the latter is the case, complete eradication of abnormal T cells may provide for the recovery of B cell function.

T cells from a severe combined immunodeficiency case showed no effect on B cell differentiation. This perhaps indicates that even though some T cells remain in the patient, they do not express any function.

Decreased helper function observed in two hypergammaglobulinemia cases may reflect a feedback suppression of the helper T cells by increased gammaglobulin produced from plasma cells showing uncontrolled proliferation.

REFERENCES

1. Waldmann, T. A., Durm, M., Broder, S., et al: Role of suppressor T cells in pathogenesis of common variable hypogammaglobulinemia. Lancet 2:609–613, 1974.
2. Siegal, F, P,, Siegal, M., and Good, R. A.: Suppression of B-cell differentiation by leukocytes from hypogammaglobulinemic patients. J. Clin. Invest. 58: 109–122, 1976.
3. Yata, J., Desgranges, C., Tachibana, T., et al.: Separation of human lymphocytes forming spontaneous rosettes with sheep erythrocytes. Biomedicine 19: 475–478, 1973.
4. Cooper, M. D., Moretta, L., Webb, S. R., et al.: in this issue.

Defective Immunoregulatory T Cell
Function in Human Disease

T. A. WALDMANN, S. BRODER, and R. M. BLAESE

ABSTRACT

A series of suppressor cell systems has been described that appears to regulate virtually all immunological processes. Disorders of these immunoregulatory systems have been demonstrated in association with some of the primary immunodeficiency diseases. We have demonstrated these disorders using techniques that have been established to study the effect of regulatory cells on the pokeweed mitogen driven differentiation of peripheral blood B lymphocytes into plasma cells. As assessed by this technique patients with common variable immunodeficiency were heterogeneous in terms of their basic pathophysiological defect. The majority had an intrinsic defect in the cells of the B-cell-plasma cell series. In addition, 6 of 25 patients studied synthesized immunoglobulins *in vitro* when cultured in fetal calf serum but not in autologous plasma or mixtures of fetal calf serum and autologous plasma. These patients appear to have a circulating inhibitor of B cell differentiation and immunoglobulin synthesis. In a final subset of patients with this disorder there was an abnormal number or abnormal state of activation of circulating suppressor T cells which act to inhibit B-cell maturation and antibody synthesis. In many cases an intrinsic defect of B cells also exists and the suppressor T cells may be a secondary event. In some patients, however, the suppressor T cells may play a more primary role in the pathogenesis of the hypogammaglobulinemia.

When the *in vitro* biosynthesis technique was applied to the study of the peripheral blood lymphocytes of 14 patients with selective IgA deficiency, two patterns emerged. Eleven of 14 patients had an intrinsic defect in the maturation and IgA secretory capacity of B cells, whereas 3 of the 14 patients had an abnormality of IgA-specific suppressor cells that prevented B cells from maturing into IgA-synthesizing and -secreting cells.

Immune responses are similar to other complex biological processes in that

The Metabolism Branch, National Cancer Institute, National Institutes of Health, Bethesda, Maryland, U.S.A.

they are controlled by a series of negative as well as positive regulatory factors. A variety of suppressor cell systems have been implicated in virtually all of the immunologic regulatory mechanisms that are recognized.[1,2] Thus, suppressor cells have been shown to play an active role in the maintenance of immunological tolerance, in the phenomenon of antigenic competition, in the control of contact and delayed hypersensitivity reactions, in the genetic control of the immune response, in the phenomenon of chronic allotype suppression, and in the regulation of the antibody response to antigens.

More recently, it has been recognized that many immunological deficiency and autoimmune diseases are associated with disorders of the negative regulatory or suppressor cell systems.[2] An abnormal number or an abnormal state of activation of suppressor T cells has been demonstrated in some patients with agammaglobulinemia[3-6] or with selective immunoglobulin deficiency[8] as well as in animal models of agammaglobulinemia.[9] Non-T-cell suppressor cells have been implicated in the polyclonal immunodeficiency associated with multiple myeloma[4,9] and in the anergy associated with Hodgkin's disease[10] and with widespread fungal infections.[11] Suppressor cells have also been implicated in the immunological enhancement of tumor growth.[12] At the other end of the spectrum of immunological response, loss of suppressor cell activity has been implicated in the pathogenesis of autoimmune disorders.[13,14]

The object of the present study was to define disorders of suppressor mechanisms associated with the primary immunodeficiency diseases. These studies were performed utilizing techniques that we have established to study the terminal differentiation of B lymphocytes into plasma cells and to define the effect of regulatory cells on this process.[3,4]

Hypogammaglobulinemia in man

The primary immunological deficiency diseases in man associated with hypogammaglobulinemia have, in general, been thought of as primary disorders in the B cell-plasma cell series involved in antibody production. Patients with these diseases have defects at distinct positions in the sequence of development of bone marrow stem cells into immunoglobulin-producing and -secreting plasma cells. For example, patients with severe combined immunodeficiency disease appear to have a defect in the stem cell precursors of the immunocompetent cells, and the majority of patients with infantile X-linked agammaglobulinemia (Bruton type agammaglobulinemia) appear to have a defect in the differentiation of the stem cells into B lymphocytes. Most patients with common variable hypogammaglobulinemia have significant numbers of B lymphocytes, yet are unable to produce normal quantities of immunoglobulin *in vivo* and are thus viewed as having a defect in the terminal differentiation of

B lymphocytes into mature immunoglobulin synthesizing and secreting cells. To analyze this defect, we developed a technique to study the terminal differentiation of B lymphocytes *in vitro* using the polyclonal stimulant, pokeweed mitogen (PWM), to drive the B cells into terminal maturation.[3] In this technique, supernatant cells were obtained from 20–50 ml of heparinized blood sedimented at 37°C. In order to remove human serum immunoglobulins, the cells were washed four times through heat-inactivated fetal calf serum. Two million lymphocytes per ml were then incubated at 37°C in 5% CO_2 in loosely capped vials in the presence of pokeweed mitogen using RPMI 1640 medium supplemented with glutamine, penicillin, streptomycin, and 10% fetal calf serum. At the termination of the culture period, the tubes were centrifuged at 2500 rpm (1200 g) for 10 minutes. The amount of IgG, IgA, and IgM synthesized and secreted into the culture medium was then determined by double antibody radioimmunoassays. In a number of studies aliquots of cells obtained on the seventh day of culture were assayed for cytoplasmic immunoglobulin molecules by direct and indirect staining using fluorescein-labeled antibodies. Utilizing the *in vitro* biosynthesis technique, the peripheral blood lymphocytes of 22 normal individuals had geometric mean synthetic rates for IgG, IgA, and IgM of 1625 ng, 1270 ng, and 4910 ng/2×10^6 lymphocytes, respectively, over the 7-day culture period. In contrast, the peripheral blood lymphocytes of 19 of the 25 patients with common variable immunodeficiency synthesized and secreted less than 100ng of each class of immunoglobulin during the same period. The lymphocytes of 6 of the patients produced modest quantities of immunoglobulin. Immunoglobulin synthesis by the lymphocytes in short-term culture from some but not all agammaglobulinemic patients has also been observed by Wu et al.[15] and Geha et al.[16] It should be noted that the lymphocytes from one of the patients in our studies synthesized significant quantities of IgM cultured *in vivo* with pokeweed mitogen in fetal calf serum, but not when cultured in autologous plasma or in a mixture of fetal calf serum and autologous plasma. Normal cells failed to synthesize immunoglobulins when cultured in this patient's plasma. These observations suggest that this patient had a circulating inhibitor of B cell differentiation and immunoglobulin synthesis. A similar patient with hypogammaglobulinemia associated with a circulating inhibitor of B cell differentiation was reported by Geha and co-workers.[16] To determine whether the failure of immunoglobulin synthesis by the patients who did not synthesize gammaglobulin *in vitro* was due to an intrinsic defect in their B lymphocytes alone or whether it could be due to suppressor cells, we co-cultured the lymphocytes of the patients with lymphocytes from normal individuals. The synthesis of the immunoglobulins by the cells of the two subjects in co-culture was related to the sum of the expected contributions of the individual lymphocyte populations. The synthesis of immunoglobulins by normal cells was reduced by a factor of 75-100% when cultured with lymphocytes of 9 of the 13 hypogammaglobulinemic patients studied. All classes of immunoglobulins were affected. A comparable suppression of immunoglobulin synthesis by normal lymphocytes was observed when they were co-cultured with purified thymus derived lymphocytes (T cells) from the hypogammaglobulinemic patients. Thus, the synthesis of the three major immunoglobulin classes by normal lymphocytes was reduced by a factor of 85-100% when co-cultured with T cells from patients with this disorder. In control studies, lymphocytes of normals co-cultured with lymphocytes from unrelated normal individuals did not result in significant inhibition of immunoglobulin synthesis. Similarly, lymphocytes from patients with chronic lymphocytic leukemia, a B cell leukemia, or from patients with the Sezary syndrome, a T cell leukemia, did not inhibit immunoglobulin synthesis in co-culture with normal cells. Thus, the ability of moderate numbers of cells of one individual to inhibit immunoglobulin synthesis by cells from another is not a nonspecific phenomenon, but is a special feature of patients with hypogammaglobulinemia. Broom *et al.*[5] and Siegal, Siegal and Good[6] have subsequently made similar observations. In these studies, the mononuclear cells of the patients inhibited immunoglobulin synthesis by the cells of some but not all controls in co-culture. In addition, Siegal, Siegal and Good[6] showed that cells from one agammaglobulinemic patient suppressed the maturation of B cells from his normal identical twin, confirming that a mixed leukocyte reaction was not critically involved in the suppression observed in these co-culture studies.

An abnormality of suppressor T cells has also been demonstrated in association with other forms of humoral immunodeficiency associated with hypogammaglobulinemia. The lymphocytes from the three patients with thymoma and hypogammaglobulinemia studied by us[7] and from the patient studied by Siegal, Siegal and Good[6] did not synthesize immunoglobulin molecules of any class during the *in vitro* culture period with pokeweed mitogen. In addition, when lymphocytes of three of the four patients studied were co-cultured with normal lymphocytes and pokeweed mitogen, synthesis by the normal lymphocytes was markedly depressed. Similarly, incubation of the normal lymphocytes with purified T cells from the patients with a thymoma and hypogammaglobulinemia resulted in suppression of immunoglobulin synthesis by a factor of 73-100%. Thus, at least a significant subset of patients with thymoma and hypogammaglobulinemia have associated circulating suppressor T cells. In addition, immunoglobulin synthesis by normal lymphocytes was suppressed when they were co-cultured with lymphocytes of two out of four patients with X-linked agammaglobulinemia studied by us,[4] and two of three patients with this syndrome studied by Siegal, Siegal and Good.[6] Dosch and Gelfand[18] also demonstrated suppressor lymphocytes in patients with congenital agammaglobulinemia. It is possible that patients with X-linked agammaglobulinemia have an abnormality of supressors as the primary pathogenic mechanism causing the hypogammaglobulinemia, with the suppressors acting early in the differentiative process preventing maturation of stem cells into B cells. An alternative view is that patients with X-linked agammaglobulinemia have a primary defect in the maturation of stem cells into B cells and secondarily develop circulating suppressor T cells. Evidence for such secondary development of biologically significant T cell suppressors has been observed in the animal models of immunodeficiency such as that observed with one form of chronic allotype suppression[19] and that observed in the "infectious" agammaglobulinemia observed with bursectomized birds.[8] In a similar fashion, in some patients with hypogammaglobulinemia the development of circulating suppressor T cells could be a secondary event which would perpetuate diminished immunoglobulin synthesis. These suppressor T cells would be clinically significant, however, in that they would make the effective immunological reconstitution of these patients through transplantation of plasma cell precursors from HLA-MLC matched donors more difficult. Indeed the reported failure of transplanted marrow from a normal individual to reconstitute the humoral immune function of his agammaglobulinemic twin may have been due to the presence of such suppressor cells in the patient.[20]

A significant group of the patients with common variable hypogammaglobulinemia may have a primary B-cell defect with the secondary development of circulating suppressor T cells. However, in one subset of patients with common variable hypogammaglobulinemia we studied, the autologous suppressor T cell may play a more primary role in the pathogenesis of hypogammaglobulinemia. For these patients B cells and macrophages were largely, but not completely, freed of autologous T cells either by a sheep cell rosetting technique or by the use of affinity columns bearing antibodies to the Fab component of immunoglobulin molecules. Neither the unseparated lymphocytes nor the T lymphocytes of these patients were able to synthesize immunoglobulin molecules when cultured alone. In addition, they suppressed immunoglobulin synthesis of normal lymphocytes when co-cultured with them. In contrast, the B cells largely but not completely freed of T cells from the patients of this subgroup synthesized significant quantities of IgM when cultured with pokeweed mitogen *in vitro*. In addition, these B cells and macrophages from the patients did not suppress immunoglobulin synthesis of normal lymphocytes in co-culture. Finally, in a case studied extensively, when the T cell preparation of the patient was mixed with the patient's own purified B cells at a ratio comparable to that obtained *in vivo* (*i. e.* 20% B cells to 80% T cells), the IgM synthesis of the B cells was completely suppressed. These latter studies again appear to rule out any allogeneic effect as the cause of the demonstrated suppression. The inhibitory effect of suppressor T cells on B cell maturation and immunoglobulin synthesis by this patient could also be reversed by procedures that might ultimately be applied to therapy of hypogammaglobulinemia. In the patient studied, unseparated lymphocytes produced no immunoglobulins when cultured in the presence of pokeweed mitogen. However, when cells of the patient were cultured in the presence of 10^{-5} molar hydrocortisone succinate and pokeweed mitogen, they synthesized significant quantities of IgM. Following the lead obtained from these *in vitro* studies, a single patient was placed on a high dose of prednisone for a 7-day period. The lymphocytes removed from this patient on the seventh day of steroid administration synthesized normal quantities of IgM in culture without further *in vitro* fractionation or treatment. Furthermore, the patient's lymphocytes did not suppress immunoglobulin synthesis by normal cells when they were co-cultured with them. Thus, the lymphocytes of this patient who had not been able to synthesize immunoglobulins *in vitro* prior to prednisone treatment were able to synthesize IgM following therapy. In a patient studied by Soothill and co-workers[21] the serum levels of all classes of immunoglobulins were markedly reduced prior to therapy. Following the initiation of prednisone therapy the IgM level rose from approximately 10% of normal to 100% of the normal mean level, and there was a 4-fold rise in the IgG level from approximately 1 to 4 mg/ml. Following the cessation of therapy the IgM and IgG levels returned to their previous exceedingly reduced values. Taken as a whole, these studies suggest that this disorder, common variable hypogammaglobulinemia, is a very heterogenous group of immunodeficiency states with a variety of pathophysiological defects. In a subset of patients with this disease the abnormality of the immunoglobulin synthesis cannot be understood as an intrinsic defect in the B cell-plasma cell series alone, but is associated with a disorder of regulatory suppressor T cells which act to inhibit B cell maturation and antibody synthesis. In many cases a primary B cell defect also exists and the suppressor T cells merely act to perpetuate the disorder. In a small number of patients, however, the suppressor T cell may play a more primary role in the pathogenesis of the hypogammaglobulinemia.

Selective IgA deficiency

Selective deficiency of the immunoglobulin, IgA, is by far the most common of the primary immunodeficiency diseases occurring in 1:500–1:700 individuals

It is characterized by the essential absence of IgA from the serum and external secretions in individuals who have normal serum levels of the other major immunoglobulin classes and have normal cell-mediated immunity. When the technique for the study of *in vitro* immunoglobulin synthesis and secretion was applied to the study of peripheral blood lymphocytes of 14 patients with selective IgA deficiency, two patterns emerged.[7] Eleven of the 14 patients had an intrinsic defect in the terminal maturation of their B cells, whereas 3 of the 14 patients had an abnormality of IgA-specific suppressor cells that prevented the B cells from maturing into IgA-synthesizing and -secreting cells. The 11 patients of the first group studied synthesized and secreted normal quantities of IgG and IgM, but secreted virtually no IgA into the medium. The patients of this group did not have demonstrable abnormalities of helper or suppressor T cells. These studies suggest that the lymphocytes of this group of patients with selective IgA deficiency have a defect in the B cells that synthesize and secrete IgA. A second, smaller group of patients with selective IgA deficiency presented a different pattern. The cultured lymphocytes of these three patients, like those of the first group, synthesized and secreted normal quantities of IgM and IgG into the medium, but secreted less than 100 ng of IgA. They did not synthesize IgA in pokeweed mitogen-stimulated cultures as assessed by staining for cytoplasmic IgA using fluorescein-labeled anti-IgA antisera. To determine whether this failure of lymphocyte IgA synthesis by these patients was due solely to an intrinsic defect in the maturation of their B lymphocytes or whether it could be due to the presence of suppressor cells, the lymphocytes of the patients were co-cultured with lymphocytes from normal individuals. When the lymphocytes from these three patients were co-cultured with normal lymphocytes and pokeweed mitogen, the synthesis of IgA by the normal cells was suppressed by 80–100%. Synthesis of IgM and IgG was not suppressed in these co-cultures. Thus, it appears that this subgroup of patients with selective IgA deficiency developed IgA-specific suppressor cells either as a primary or secondary event and did not synthesize IgA molecules. These IgA-specific suppressor cells prevented B cells from maturing into IgA-synthesizing and -secreting plasma cells.

REFERENCES

1. Gerson, R. K.: T cell control of antibody production. *In*: Contemporary Topics in Immunobiology (M. D. Cooper and N. L. Warner, eds). Plenum Press, New York-London, 1974, p 1.
2. Waldmann, T. A. and Broder, S.: Suppressor cells in the regulation of the immune response. *In*: Progress in Clinical Immunology, Vol. 3 (R. Schwartz, ed), Grune and Stratton, New York, p. 155–199.

3. Waldmann, T. A., Broder, S., Blaese, R. M., Durm, M., Blackman, M., and Strober, W.: Role of suppressor T cells in pathogenesis of common variable hypogammaglobulinaemia. *Lancet* **2**:609, 1974.
4. Waldmann, T. A., Broder, S., Krakauer, R., MacDermott, R. P., Durm, M., Goldman, C., and Meade, B.: The role of suppressor cells in the pathogenesis of common variable hypogammaglobulinemia and the immunodeficiency associated with myeloma. *Fed. Proc.* **35**:2067, 1976.
5. Broom, B. C., De La Concha, E. G., Webster, A. D. B., and Janossy, G. L.: Intracellular immunoglobulin production *in vitro* by lymphocytes from patients with hypogammaglobulinaemia and their effect on normal lymphocytes. *Clin. Exp. Immunol.* **23**:73, 1976.
6. Siegal, F. P., Siegal, M., and Good, R. A.: Suppression of B-cell differentiation by leukocytes from hypogammaglobulinemic patients. *J. Clin. Invest.* **58**:109, 1976.
7. Waldmann, T. A., Broder, S., Krakauer, R., Durm, M., Meade, B., and Goldman, C.: Defects in IgA secretion and in IgA specific suppressor cells in patients with isolated IgA deficiency. *Clin. Res.* **24**:483A, 1976.
8. Blaese, R. M., Weiden, P. L., Koski, I., and Dooley, N.: Infectious agammaglobulinemia: Transmission of immunodeficiency with grafts of agammaglobulinemic cells. *J. Exp. Med.* **140**:1097, 1974.
9. Broder, S., Humphrey, R., Durm, M., Blackman, M., Meade, B., Goldman, C., Strober, W., and Waldmann, T. A.: Impaired synthesis of polyclonal (nonparaprotein) immunoglobulins by circulating lymphocytes from patients with multiple myeloma: Role of suppressor cells. *New Engl. J. Med.* **293**:887, 1975.
10. Twomey, J. J., Laughter, A. H., Farrow, S., and Douglass, C. C.: Hodgkin's disease: An immunodepleting and immunosuppressive disorder. *J. Clin. Invest.* **56**:467, 1975.
11. Stobo, J. D., Paul, S., Van Scoy, R. E., and Hermans, P.: Suppressor thymus-derived lymphocytes in fungal infection. *J. Clin. Invest.* **57**:319, 1976.
12. Fujimoto, S., Greene, M. I., and Sehon, A. H.: Regulation of the immune response to tumor antigens. I. Immunosuppressor cells in tumor-bearing hosts. *J. Immunol.* **116**: 791, 1976.
13. Gerber, N. L., Hardin, J. A., Chused, T. M., and Steinberg, A. D.: Loss with age in NZB/W mice of thymic suppressor cells in the graft-*vs*-host reaction. *J. Immunol.* **113**:1618, 1974.
14. Krakauer, R. S., Waldmann, T. A., and Strober, W.: Loss of suppressor T-cells in adult NZB/NZW mice. *J. Exp. Med.* **144**:662, 1976.
15. Wu, L. Y. F., Lawton, A. R., and Cooper, M. D.: Differentiation capacity of cultured B lymphocytes from immunodeficient patients. *J. Clin. Invest.* **5**: 3180, 1973.
16. Geha, R. S., Schneeberger, E., Merler, E., and Rosen, F. S.: Heterogeneity of "acquired" or common variable agammaglobulinemia. *New Engl. J. Med.* **291**:1, 1974.
17. Waldmann, T. A., Broder, S., Durm, M., Blackman, M., Krakauer, R., and Meade, B.: Suppressor T cells in the pathogenesis of hypogammaglobulinemia associated with thymoma. *Trans. Assoc. Amer. Phys.* **88**:120, 1976.

18. Dosch, H. M. and Gelfand, E. W.: *In vitro* antibody synthesis and suppression in humoral immunodeficiency states. *Clin. Res.* **24**:481A, 1976.
19. Jacobson, E. B., Herzenberg, L. A., Riblet, R., and Herzenberg, L. A.: Active suppression of immunoglobulin allotype synthesis. II. Transfer of suppressing factor with spleen cells. *J. Exp. Med.* **135**:1163, 1972.
20. Cruchaud, A., Laperrouza, C., and Megevand, R.: Agammaglobulinemia in monozygous twins: Therapeutic prospects. *In*: Immunologic Deficiency Diseases in Man (D. Bergsma and R. A. Good, eds) National Foundation Press, New York, 1968, p. 315.
21. Soothill, J. F., Hill, L. E., and Rowe, D. S.: A quantitative study of the immunoglobulins in the antibody deficiency syndrome. *In*: Immunologic Deficiency Diseases in Man (D. Bergsma and R. A. Good,) National Foundation Press, New York, 1968, p. 21.

DISCUSSION

Dr. YAMAMURA: In your experimental system of combination culture of lymphocytes from normal persons together with the patients', have you tested the genetic background of these persons? I mean, for such as HLA, and so on?

Dr. BLAESE: There is no requirement for HLA compatability for either suppression or help in any of the systems that we have looked at.

Dr. GOOD: In how many of your 14 cases of common variable immunodeficiency were you able to remove the T-cells, and provide either normal T-cells or get normal immunoglobulin production?

Dr. BLAESE: I think we have looked at perhaps 35 or 40 patients with common variable immunodeficiency, and probably 4 or 5 patients have responded.

Dr. GOOD: Irradiation is very effective in removing a suppressor influence in normals, and in a few cases in hypogammaglobulinemia. We have seen this same sort of thing in the patients with combined immunodefiency, where during reconstitution we will get a reconstitution of T-cells and then they can demonstrate suppressor effect. We have been able to eliminate that effect, or at least, with with massive doses of cyclophosphamide coupled with another marrow transplantation, we get a better adjustment of the population and eliminate the suppressor effect.

Dr. TADA: In the mice such cortisone sensitive cells may be LY-123+ cells, rather than LY-23+ cells. If that is the case, there are two populations of suppressor T-cells; one is cortisone insensitive, which has already been found in mouse systems, and another is the cortisone sensitive population, which may be the actual suppressor T-cells. These may accept the effect of other suppressor T-cells, and may be the suppressor of the suppressor, or the inducer of the suppressor. I think this hypothesis will make good sense in the whole picture of the suppressor phenomenon.

Pathogenesis of Antibody Deficiencies

M. D. Cooper, E. R. Pearl,[1] L. Moretta,[2] S. R. Webb,
A. J. Okos, L. B. Vogler,[3] and A. R. Lawton[4]

Now that more is known about the earlier stages in B-cell differentiation, it is possible to define blocks or arrests at several points during this development-al process which result in immunoglobulin deficiencies. The most frequent block is that in which circulating B lymphocytes are normally developed, but plasma cells and circulating immunoglobulins are missing.[2,3,26] That a spectrum of defects can lead to this phenotypic pattern has been revealed by studies in which terminal differentiation of B lymphocytes is induced in culture.[7,29,30] The use of pokeweed mitogen to induce B cell differentiation has been a par-ticularly useful study system, since T cells are required for B cell triggering and can also suppress the B cell response to this polyclonal mitogen[13,19b,29] Defini-tion of two distinct subpopulations of T cells, each of which has characteristic functions and distribution in the body, also promises to shed new light on the failure of terminal B-cell differentiation in certain immunodeficient patients. [15,18,19a] In this paper, we will briefly discuss these developments.

Early events in B-cell development

The first recognizable event is the appearance of lymphoid cells containing intracytoplasmic IgM.[6,24] These cells, called pre-B cells,[2,4,16] are found in the liver of human fetuses by 7–8 weeks of gestation, and are large lymphoid cells which divide rapidly and contain relatively small amounts of cytoplasmic IgM but no detectable surface immunoglobulin (sIg). They give rise to smaller non-dividing pre-B cells which contain a thin rim of cytoplasmic IgM and no

The Cellular Immunobiology Unit of the Tumor Institute, Departments of Pediatrics and Microbiology and The Comprehensive Cancer Center, University of Alabama in Birmingham, University Station, Birmingham, Alabama, U.S.A.
[1]Dr. Elliott R. Pearl is the recipient of NIH Fellowship 1 F32 AI05356.
[2]Dr. Lorenzo Moretta is on leave of absence from the University of Genoa, Italy.
[3]Dr. Larry B. Vogler is the recipient of NIH Fellowship 1 F32 CAO5776.
[4]Dr. Alexander R. Lawton is the recipient of NIH Research Career Development Award AI 70780.

detectable sIg. Both types of pre-B cells are found first in fetal liver and later mainly in the bone marrow. The smaller pre-B cells are sometimes found in peripheral tissues, but the larger ones normally are not.[6] Pre-B cells of all sizes lack receptors for aggregated IgG and C3 (Gathings et al., in press).

Pre-B cells appear to give rise to the small B lymphocytes which have easily detectable surface IgM.[20,25] The first B lymphocytes to appear during ontogeny are physiologically distinct from the B lymphocytes present in lymphoid tissues of mature animals. Persistent functional inhibition of immature B lymphocytes results from treatment with multivalent antigens, or with divalent anti-IgM antibodies.[17,23,27] During B lymphocyte maturation, Ia antigens, C3 receptors, Fc receptors and other classes of surface immunoglobulins are acquired[4,8,21] and B lymphocytes become responsive to antigens with the cooperation of helper T cells and macrophages.[12] Responsiveness to some of the polyclonal B cell mitogens appears very early in B lymphocyte development.

The general features of B lymphocyte proliferation to become memory B cells and B lymphocyte maturation into plasma cells are well known and will not be reviewed here. Suffice it to say that regulatory controls of this antigen- or mitogen-induced differentiation are exerted by helper and suppressor T cells, by specific antibody feedback control and probably by production of anti-idiotype antibodies.

Absence of bone marrow pre-B cells in patients with thymoma and immunodeficiency

We examined bone marrow samples from two men with spindle cell thymomas, panhypogammaglobulinemia and a virtual absence of circulating B lymphocytes[28] (unpublished observations). In contrast to normal individuals and other patients with hypogammaglobulinemia, pre-B cells were not detectable. Eosinophils were also missing in these individuals. We think that the simplest explanation for these findings is an acquired defect of stem cells which prevents development along B cell and eosinophilic lines. A more profound abnormality of stem cells could account for red-cell aplasia and aplastic anemia sometimes associated with thymoma. Later, we will present suggestive evidence that balanced maintenance of the T cell subpopulations may also be defective.

Block of B cell development in infantile or X-linked agammaglobulinemia

It has been shown through use of a variety of B lymphocyte markers that most boys with infantile agammaglobulinemia lack B lymphocytes in blood and peripheral lymphoid tissues.[3,10] We examined bone marrow from ten such patients, and pre-B cells containing cytoplasmic Ig were demonstrable in all[28] (unpublished observations). We looked for pre-B cells and sIg+ B lymphocytes in their blood and failed to find cells of either type. This is in accord with the fact that essentially all of their circulating mononuclear cells are identifiable as T cells or monocytes.

We conclude that these boys' pre-B cells fail to become normal B lymphocytes, because of an intrinsic defect or an abnormal environmental regulatory effect.

T cells are required for pokeweed mitogen-induced responses of B cells

Pokeweed mitogen (PWM) stimulates human B lymphocytes to proliferate and mature to plasma cells synthesizing and secreting all of the major classes of immunoglobulins.[29,30] B lymphocyte-enriched fractions depleted of T cells do not respond to PWM stimulation with either proliferation or maturation.[11,13] When T lymphocytes from normal individuals are added back to B lymphocytes before culture, the number of IgM-, IgG- and IgA-containing plasma cells increases in proportion to the number of T cells added. Allogeneic cells can help; the helper function resists irradiation, and preliminary evidence suggests that T cells activated by PWM release helper factors.

Analysis of arrested B lymphocyte differentiation in hypogammaglobulinemic patients

Many patients with hypogammaglobulinemia have normal numbers of B lymphocytes in their circulation and peripheral lymphoid tissues,[2,3,7,26,29,30] which fail to respond to antigens with normal plasma cell differentiation. Under certain culture conditions unfractionated peripheral blood lymphocytes from some of these patients are capable of completing plasma cell differentiation in response to PWM, whereas lymphocytes from other such patients lack this responsive capability.[7,29,30] We have begun to analyze the functional capabilities of T and B cells from the latter patients in the PWM response. Perhaps predictably, the clinical heterogeneity of the patients was reflected in the results obtained[3] (Keightley *et al.*, unpublished): (i) When cultured with normal allogeneic T cells, but not with autologous T cells, B lymphocytes from some of these patients respond to PWM stimulation with plasma cell differentiation. Conversely, some patients' T cells are only marginally capable of supporting plasma cell differentiation of normal B cells, suggesting that their helper T cells may be at fault. (ii) Waldmann *et al.* have described excessive suppressor T cell activity in agammaglobulinemic patients.[29] Our studies on a few such patients are consistent with this possibility, but in other phenotypically similar patients we find defective T-cell help *in vitro* without a demonstrable excess of suppressor activity. (iii) In other hypogammaglobulinemic patients with normal numbers of B lymphocytes, the T cells are capable of helping normal B cells but their B cells do not respond to PWM in the presence of autologous or normal allogeneic T cells. This suggests an inherent B cell defect. (iv) An even more intriguing situation has been observed in two individuals with the same phenotypic pattern of immunodeficiency; their T cells and B cells could cooperate with normal B or T cells, respectively, but no responses were seen in autologous combinations of T and B cells from the patients.

Definition of T-cell subpopulations in humans

While a considerable body of information exists with regard to rodent T cell subpopulations, comparable data on human T cells has been almost totally lacking until recently. Human T cells can now be subdivided into two distinct subpopulations[5,15,18a,18b,19]: those which carry receptors for the Fc portion of IgG (Tγ) and those capable of expressing *in vitro* a receptor for Fc of IgM (Tμ). Tγ and Tμ cells can be enumerated by rosetting T cells with bovine erythrocytes coated with rabbit antibodies of the IgG (for Tγ) or IgM (for Tμ) classes. By sequentially performing these two types of rosetting procedures in combination with density gradient centrifugation, Tγ and Tμ subpopulations can be isolated for further study.

The Tμ cells have less cytoplasm and smoother surfaces than Tγ cells, are the predominant T cell type in blood, tonsils and lymph nodes, respond better to PHA, and allogeneic cells, and can help B cells respond to PWM. In contrast, Tγ cells have extensive cytoplasm containing acidophilic granules and numerous mitochondria, have a villous surface, are the prevalent T cell type in the spleen, normally do not home to lymph nodes, respond poorly to PHA but well to concanavalin A, and do not help B cells respond to PWM; they can be activated via their Fc receptors to suppress the Tμ-cell help of B cell responses. Very few thymic cells have detectable receptors either for IgM or IgG, and a variable proportion of blood T cells lack these receptors (T "null").

Analysis of circulating T cell subpopulations in patients with various immunodeficiency diseases and autoimmune syndromes

We have enumerated the total numbers of T cells and the two subpopulations in patients with a variety of immunodeficiency diseases.[19] Reduction of the proportion of Tμ cells was observed in 10 of 28 patients with a spectrum of immunodeficiency diseases, and increased percentages of Tγ cells were seen in five patients. Imbalances in circulating Tμ and Tγ cells may sometimes be acquired, since only one of five boys with X-linked agammaglobulinemia (X-LA) had reduced numbers of Tμ cells and the same abnormality was observed in two adults who developed thymoma and immunodeficiency. Increased numbers of Tγ cells were also present in these three individuals, and excessive suppressor activity was demonstrated for T cells from the boy with X-LA who had reduced numbers of Tμ and increased numbers of Tγ cells. Continued thymus function may be needed for maintenance of the balance of T cell subpopulations; this is suggested by the results obtained in the two individuals with thymoma, one of whom had been thymectomized, by changes observed in a patient with thymic dysplasia and by reduction of Tμ cells in a young girl thymectomized for non-immunologic reasons. Reduction of the percentage of Tμ cells in three patients examined with SCID implies that an imbalance of T cell subpopulations may occur as an inherited disorder.

Tμ and Tγ cells were present in normal numbers in eight of nine patients with various autoimmune syndromes including chronic active hepatitis (4 patients), juvenile rheumatoid arthritis (1), Mickulicz's syndrome (1), Behcet's syndrome (1), dermatomyositis (1) and systemic lupus erythematosus (1). Several of these patients were receiving high doses of corticosteroids. One boy with chronic active hepatitis and chronic colitis had reduced numbers of Tμ cells. One out of eight IgA-deficient individuals examined had a low percentage of Tμ cells; this girl also had chronic active hepatitis.

These observations imply that an imbalance in T cell subpopulations may be important in the pathogenesis of some immunodeficiencies and possibly certain autoimmune syndromes.

SUMMARY AND CONCLUSIONS

Development of B cells in immunoglobulin-deficient patients can be arrested at several stages in differentiation and probably for a variety of reasons even when the block appears to be at the same level of B cell differentiation. Recognition of the pre-B stage in development of B cells has allowed us to show that infantile X-linked agammaglobulinemia reflects an arrest in B cell differentiation at this stage, whereas stem cell differentiation along B cell lines appears to be completely aborted in patients with thymoma and hypogammaglobulinemia. Further study of pre-B cells in the bone marrow of patients with X-LA may lead to detection of a molecular defect in these patients.

Many patients with antibody deficiency syndromes, especially those that are acquired, display arrested differentiation at a B lymphocyte level. *In vitro* analysis of their B lymphocyte response to PWM has revealed a variety of defects. Demonstration of the need for T cell help in this *in vitro* model system and in a similar assay[7] has been particularly valuable in analyzing arrested development of B lymphocytes. Either faulty T lymphocytes or B lymphocytes or collaboration between the two may be responsible for arrested development of B lymphocytes.

70 M. D. Cooper *et al.*

Two distinct subpopulations of human T cells have been identified and their functions partially defined. One can express receptors for IgM and can help B cells respond to PWM. The other has receptors for IgG and under certain conditions of activation can suppress the PWM response of a mixture of normal T and B cells. These T cell subpopulations may be present in abnormal proportions in patients with a variety of immunodeficiency diseases. Further analysis of these T cell subpopulations should lead to better definition of certain immunodeficiency diseases.

Acknowledgments

This research had been supported by Grants CA 16673, awarded by the National Cancer Institute, DHEW; AI 11502, awarded by the N.I.A.I.D., USPHS; 1–354, awarded by The National Foundation, March of Dimes; 5M01–RR32, awarded by National Institutes of Health; 5P01–HD00413 awarded by N.I.C.H.D.; 1 F32 AI05356, awarded by the N.I.A.I.D.; and 1 F32 CA05776, awarded by the National Cancer Institute.

REFERENCES

1. Balch, C. M., Dagg, M. K., and Cooper, M. D.: Cross-reactive T-cell antigens among mammalian species. *J. Immunol.* 117:447, 1976.
2. Cooper, M. D., Keightley, R. G., Wu, L. Y. F., and Lawton, A. R.: Developmental defects of T and B cell lines in humans. *Transplant Rev.* 16:51, 1973.
3. Cooper, M. D., Keightley, R. G., and Lawton, A. R. III: Defective T and B cells in primary immunodeficiencies. *In*: Membrane Receptors of Lymphocytes (M. Seligmann, J. L. Preud'homme, and F. M. Kourilsky, eds.). p. 431, North-Holland Publishing Co., Amsterdam, 1975.
4. Cooper, M. D., Kearney, J. F., Lawton, A. R., Abney, E. R., Parkhouse, R. M. E., Preud'homme, J. L., and Seligmann, M.: Generation of Ig class diversity in B cells: A discussion with emphasis on IgD development. *Ann. Inst. Pasteur* 127C:573, 1976.
5. Ferrarini, M., Moretta, L., Mingari, M. C., Tonda, P., and Pernis, B.: Receptor for IgM on T lymphocytes: Specificity for the pentameric Fc fragment. *Eur. J. Immunol.* 6:520, 1976.
6. Gathings, W. E., Cooper, M. D., Lawton, A. R., and Alfrod, C. A.: B cell ontogeny in humans. *Fed. Proc.* 35:393, 1976.
7. Geha, R. S., Schneeberger, E., Merler, E., and Rosen, F. S.: Heterogeneity of "acquired" or common variable panhypogammaglobulinemia. *N. Engl. J. Med.* 291:1, 1974.
8. Gelfand, M. C., Elfenbein, G. J., Frank, M. M., and Paul, W. E.: Ontogeny of B lymphocytes. II. Relative rates of appearance of lymphocytes bearing surface immunoglobulin and complement receptors. *J. Exp. Med.* 139:1128, 1974.
9. Gronowicz, E., Coutinho, A., and Möller, G.: Differentiation of B cells: Sequen-

tial appearance of responsiveness to polyclonal activators. *Scand. J. Immunol.* **3**:413, 1974.
10. Hayward, A. and Greaves, M.: Central failure of B lymphocyte induction in panhypogammaglobulinemia. *Clin. Immunol. Immunopathol.* **3**:461, 1975.
11. Janossy, G. and Greaves, M. F.: Functional analysis of murine and human B lymphocyte subsets. *Transplant Rev.* **24**:177, 1975.
12. Katz, D. H. and Benacerraf, B.: The regulatory influence of activated T cells on B cell responses to antigen. *Adv. Immunol.* **15**:1, 1972.
13. Keightley, R. G., Cooper, M. D., and Lawton, A. R.: The T cell dependence of B cell differentiation induced by pokeweed mitogen. *J. Immunol.* **117**: 1538, 1974.
14. La Fleur, L., Miller, R. G., and Phillips, R. A.: A quantitative assay for progenitors of bone marrow associated lymphocytes. *J. Exp. Med.* **135**:1363, 1972.
15. McConnell, I. and Hurd, C. M.: Lymphocyte receptors. II. Receptors for rabbit IgM on human T lymphocytes. *Immunology* **30**:385, 1976.
16. Melchers, F., von Boehmer, H., and Phillips, R. A.: B-lymphocyte subpopulations in the mouse. *Transplant Rev.* **25**:26, 1975.
17. Metcalf, E. S. and Klinman, N. R.: *In vitro* tolerance induction of neonatal murine B cells. *J. Exp. Med.* **143**:1327, 1976.
18a. Moretta, L., Ferrarini, M., Durante, M. L., and Mingari, M. C.: Expression of a receptor for IgM by human T cells. *Eur. J. Immunol.* **5**:565, 1975.
18b. Moretta, L., Ferrarini, M., Mingari, M. C., Moretta, A., and Webb, S. R.: Subpopulations of human T cells identified by receptors for immunoglobulins and mitogen responsiveness. *J. Immunol.* **117**: 2171, 1976.
19a. Moretta, L., Webb, S. R., Grossi, C. E., Lydyard, P. M., and Cooper, M. D.: Functional analysis of two subpopulations of human T cells and their distribution in immunodeficient patients. *Clin. Res.* **24**:448A, 1976.
19b. Moretta, L., Webb, S. R., Grossi, C.E., Lydyard, P. M. and Cooper, M.D.: Functional analysis of two human T-cell subpopulations: Help and suppression of B cell responses by T cells bearing receptors for IgM (T.M) or IgG (T.G). *J. Exp. Med.* **146**: 184, 1977
20. Osmond, D. G. and Nossal, G. J. V.: Differentiation of lymphocytes in mouse bone marrow. II. Kinetics of maturation and renewal of antiglobulin binding cells studied by double labelling. *Cell Immunol.* **13**:132, 1974.
21. Press, J. L., Klinman, N. R., Henry, C., Wolfsy, L., Delovitch, T., and McDevitt, H. O.: Ia antigens on B cells: Relationship to B cell precursor function and to surface immunoglobulins. *In*: Membrane Receptors of Lymphocytes (M. Seligmann, J. L. Preud' homme and F. M. Kourilsky, eds.). p. 247, North-Holland Publishing Co., Amsterdam, 1975.
22. Preud'homme, J. L. and Flandrin, G.: Identification by peroxidase staining of monocytes in surface immunofluorescence tests. *J. Immunol.* **113**:1650, 1974.
23. Raff, M. C., Owen, J. J. T., Cooper, M. D., Lawton, A. R., Megson, M., and Gathings, W. E.: Differences in susceptibility of mature and immature mouse B lymphocytes to anti-immunoglobulin-induced immunoglobulin suppression *in vitro*. Possible implications for B-cell tolerance to self. *J. Exp. Med.* **142**: 1052, 1975.

72	M. D. Cooper *et al.*

24. Raff, M. C., Megson, M., Owen, J. J. T., and Cooper, M. D.: Early production of intracellular IgM by B-lymphocyte precursors in mouse. *Nature* (Lond.) **259**:224, 1976.
25. Ryser, J. E. and Vassalli, P.: Mouse bone marrow lymphocytes and their differentiation. *J. Immunol.* **113**:719, 1974.
26. Seligmann, M., Preud'homme, J. L., and Brouet, J. C.: B and T cell markers in human proliferative blood diseases and primary immunodeficiencies with special reference to membrane immunoglobulins. *Transplant Rev.* **16**:85, 1973.
27. Sidman, C. L. and Unanue, E. R.: Receptor mediated inactivation of early B lymphocytes. *Nature* (Lond.) **257**:149, 1975.
28. Vogler, L. B., Pearl, E. R., Gathings, W. E., Lawton, A. R., and Cooper, M. D.: B-lymphocyte precursors in the bone marrow of patients with immunoglobulin (Ig) deficiency diseases. *Lancet* **ii**:376, 1976.
29. Waldmann, T. A., Durm, M., Broder, S., Blackman, M., Blaese, R. M., and Strober, W.: Role of suppressor T cells in pathogenesis of common variable hypogammaglobulinemia. *Lancet* **ii**:609, 1974.
30. Wu, L. Y. F., Lawton, A. R., and Cooper, M. D.: Differentiation capacity of cultured B lymphocytes from immunodeficient patients. *J. Clin. Invest.* **52**: 3180, 1973.

DISCUSSION

Dr. GOOD: What Hammerling has shown is that *ubiquitone*, which is a 74-amino acid, fully defined peptide with its active site in the terminal tridecapeptide, is capable of inducing precursors of B-cells to B-lymphocytes, and he has shown that this occurs in a series of steps, and that each of the steps depends upon the preceding one. The first thing that he can recognize is the induction of surface immunoglobulin, predominantly of IgM. Then, after a process that involves at least one proliferation, he can get to the Ia, and then to the C3 receptor, and finally the PC-1. Are these successive steps successions in your scheme of B-lymphocyte differentiations? Can you eliminate the precursor population in each step? Can you destroy that precursor cell present in the Bruton agamaglobulinemic patient's marrow with anti-immunoglobulin?

Dr. COOPER: I do not know, but in the mouse you cannot destroy the pre-B-cell in that way. If we take the mice that we render B-deprived by chronic treatment with anti-immunoglobulin, their bone marrows contain normal numbers of pre-B-cells that are capable of giving rise to normal B lymphocytes.

Dr. TADA: The I-region determinants are easily detected on suppressor T-cells, but not on helper T-cells. And it can be blocked by anti-Ia. Could you tell us something about the relationship of T-cells and Tμ-cells to, for example, MLC expression or any other HLA-linked expressions?

Dr. COOPER: Both can respond in MLC. Tμ cells seem to respond a bit better. Both can respond equally well to Con A. Tμ cells can respond to PHA at a high concentration only, and they respond very well: the Tγ respond poorly, but they respond to a wide range of PHA. We have not looked for expression of "Ia-like" or D-associated determinants before or after stimulatation of either T cell subpopulation.

Dr. GOOD: With respect to human T-lymphocytes, if you eliminate the HTLA positive cells, you can induce E-rosette forming cells; if you eliminate E-rosette forming cells, you can induce HTLA positive cells, but you cannot induce the CON-A and the PHA response, or the MLC. Now, what I would really like to know is whether the Tγ, or the Tμ relate to this sort of scheme, or whether it is a completely different scheme. It is very clear that this is a sequential differentiation in T cells.

Dr. AIUTI: In some patients with cell immunodeficiency, we saw that the E-rosette are decreased, but the Tμ and Tγ cells never reach the number of T cells. Have you any patients with these discrepancies in Tμ, Tγ, and the total number of T cells?

Dr. COOPER: Yes. In normals we find that 10 to 40% of the T cells are not enumerated as IgM binders, or IgG binders. We do not know what these null cells are; they may just have fewer receptors, or they may be precursors, or there could be some other explanation for them. In some of the patients, we find an excess of null T-cells, so we agree on that point.

Dr. YATA: We observe the increase of Tγ cells in atopic patients. We expect a decrease of IgE suppressors in these patients. If such Tγ cells are suppressor cells as you said, what would be the explanation for that?

Dr. COOPER: I cannot answer your question, but I can add one more complication to consider in trying to answer it.

The Tγ's, isolated by exclusion, rather than in a positive way, may not suppress, whereas from the same patient Tγ cells isolated by forming IgG rosettes may indeed have inhibitory effects on normal T and B collaboration in the pokeweed response. In the mouse system, several people have postulated that for T cells that bind IgG, binding of IgG antibodies may provide a stop-signal for a response to a particular antigen by the appropriate clone of T cells. If that were true, one would expect that the signal would not be given until the receptors for IgG were occupied; our data would be consistent with that idea.

Pokeweed Mitogen-Induced Peripheral Blood Lymphocyte Differentiation into Immunoglobulin Producing Cells in Humoral Immune Deficiency

Takashi Uchiyama, Kimitaka Sagawa and Kiyoshi Takatsuki

ABSTRACT

Pokeweed mitogen-induced peripheral blood lymphocyte differentiation was found to be dependent on T cells. Leukemic T cells from one out of three patients with adult T cell leukemia showed a marked suppressive effect on this B cell differentiation. Lymphocytes from sixteen patients with multiple myeloma had marked impairment of B cell differentiation in this system and co-culture experiments revealed the existence of cells with a suppressive effect in peripheral blood in these cases. But six patients with multiple myeloma and polyclonal hypogammaglobulinemia had no impaired B cell differentiation and these results may reflect the complexity of mechanisms underlying the humoral immune deficiency in multiple myeloma. Lymphocytes from a patient with Wiskott-Aldrich syndrome failed to mature into Ig producing cells. Lymphocytes from a patient with SLE and selective IgA deficiency were found to differentiate normally.

INTRODUCTION

Recently methods have been developed for analysis of cooperative interactions between T and B cells and macrophages in the immune system. Pokeweed mitogen (PWM) has been shown to trigger the terminal differentiation of B cells into immunoglobulin (Ig) producing cells in vitro[1] and a variety of immunodeficiency states underlying various human diseases has been studied with the experimental system using PWM.[2,3] We studied the capacity of the peripheral blood lymphocytes to differentiate into Ig producing cells in the

Department of Internal Medicine, Faculty of Medicine, Kyoto University, Kyoto, Japan

75

presence of PWM in order to analyze the factors responsible for the humoral immune deficiency in multiple myeloma, primary immune deficiencies and other related diseases and also studied the effect of leukemic T cells on normal B cell differentiation in this system.

MATERIALS AND METHODS

Cell cultures and immunofluorescence. One or two ml of 1.0×10^6/ml lymphocytes isolated from heparinized peripheral blood by Ficoll-sodium metrizoate gradient centrifugation and suspended in RPMI1640, supplemented with 20% fetal calf serum (Grand Island Biological Co., Lot A053119), kanamycin and an optimal dose of PWM (Grand Island Biological Co., Lot A045502) was cultured in a humid atmosphere of 5% CO_2 in air at 37°C for 7 days. Following 7 days' incubation the cells were washed and cytocentrifuge preparations were stained with monospecific FITC-conjugated antibodies to gamma, alpha, mu, kappa and lambda chains. The numbers of cells positive for intracytoplasmic immunoglobulin were enumerated.

Separation of T cells. The cells were separated by sheep red blood cell (SRBC) rosette centrifugation through Ficoll-sodium metrizoate gradient and lysis of attached SRBC by addition of 0.83% ammonium chloride solution.

Leukemic T cells and culture supernatants. Leukemic cells with T cell properties (SRBC rosette, sensitive to anti-thymocyte serum) from patients with adult type T cell leukemia were co-cultured with normal peripheral lymphocytes in the presence of PWM. Culture supernatants were obtained after 48 hours' culture of leukemic T cells at a cell concentration of 1.0×10^7/ml in RPMI medium with 20% fetal calf serum.

Normal controls and patients. Normal controls consisted of 10 healthy subjects whose ages ranged from 23 to 60 years. Twenty-two patients with multiple myeloma and related diseases consisted of nine with IgG, seven with IgA, one with IgD, one with Bence Jones protein and two with "non-secretory" type myeloma, one with primary macroglobulinemia and one with gamma chain disease. Serum immunoglobulin levels other than M-protein were lower than normal in all cases. Six patients were untreated and sixteen had received no therapy for at least two weeks before this study. An eighteen-month-old male with recurrent infections, thrombocytopenia, eczema and autoimmune hemolytic anemia (Wiskott-Aldrich syndrome), and a 29-year-old female with systemic lupus erythematosus (SLE) and selective IgA deficiency were also studied.

RESULTS AND DISCUSSION

Normals. In the peripheral blood lymphocytes from normal individuals, a marked increase in the number of blasts was seen on the fourth day and that of cytoplasmic Ig-containing cells on the fifth day (Fig. 1). On the seventh day, an average of 7.7% (3.6—11.9%) of the recovered cells was positive for IgG, 6.6% (2.4—11.4%) for IgA and 5.1% (range 3.0—8.8%) for IgM.

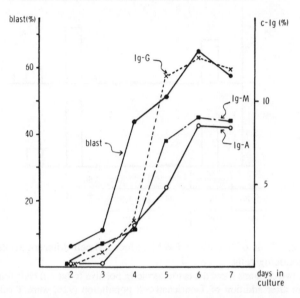

FIG. 1. Blastic transformation and the appearance of cytoplasmic Ig (c-Ig) positive cells in PWM-stimulated normal peripheral blood lymphocyte cultures.

T cell dependency. Results of culture studies after separation of peripheral blood lymphocytes into T cell-enriched and T cell-depleted cell populations are shown in Fig. 2. Cytoplasmic Ig positive cells were very scarce in the culture of the T cell-depleted population. But, if separated T cells were added again and cultured, an equal or greater number of Ig producing cells were found. These results indicate that B cell differentiation in this system is dependent on T cells.
Leukemic T cells. The effect of leukemic T cells from patients with adult T cell leukemia on PWM-induced B cell differentiation into Ig producing cells was studied. In brief, adult T cell leukemia is a leukemia characterized by lymphadenopathy, hepatosplenomegaly, frequent skin lesions, no mediastinal

T. Uchiyama *et al.*

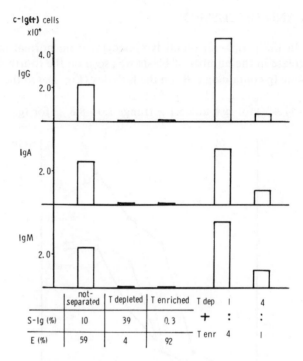

FIG. 2. Role of T cells in PWM-induced B cell differentiation into Ig producing cells.
Right two columns show the cytoplasmic Ig positive (c-Ig(+)) cells found in culture after addition of T-enriched cell population (92% were T cells) to T-depleted cell population (only 4% were T cells). At the start of culture T-enriched cell population occupied 4/5 of all cells in the left and 1/5 in the right column. S-Ig——surface immunoglobulin bearing cells, E——SRBC rosette forming cells.

mass and a subacute to chronic course with rapid terminal progression. And interestingly, most patients with this leukemia were born in Kyushu district, especially in Kagoshima Prefecture, the southern part of Japan. Leukemic cells are considered to have their origin perhaps in fairly differentiated T cells. The effect of co-cultured leukemic T cells and their culture supernatants on normal B cell differentiation induced by PWM is shown in Fig. 3. Leukemic T cells as well as their culture supernatant fluids from one case (U.S.) out of three were shown to have a suppressive effect on B cell differentiation. Waldmann and associates[5] found that leukemic T cells from a patient with Sézary syndrome had the remarkable property of reversing the inability of B

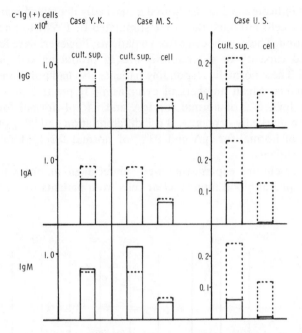

FIG. 3.   Effect of the leukemic T cells on PWM-induced B cell differentiation into Ig producing cells.
In the cases of Y.K. and M. S. one ml of 1.0×10^6/ml normal lymphocytes
were cultured with 0.1 ml of culture supernatant or equal numbers of
normal and leukemic T cells (0.5ml of 1.0×10^6/ml) were co-cultured. In
case U.S. also equal numbers (0.25ml of 1.0×10^6/ml) of normal and leukemic T cells were co-cultured. Note the marked suppression in case U.S.
---- predicted,—— observed value.

cells from a patient with hypogammaglobulinemia to develop into immunoglobulin secreting cells after stimulation *in vitro* with PWM. It seems likely that
the fairly well-differentiated leukemic T cells from patients with Sézary
syndrome and adult T cell leukemia may produce factors with an enhancing
or suppressive effect in the immune system as myeloma cells produce immunoglobulins. Thus the leukemic T cells from patient U.S. may have their origin
in normal precursors with suppressive function.
Multiple myeloma and related diseases.   Mean numbers of cytoplasmic Ig
positive cells found on the seventh day in cultures of lymphocytes from 22
patients with multiple myeloma were 32% of normal for IgG, 44% of normal
for IgA and 32% of normal for IgM. In these, lymphocytes from 16%

patients, as indicated in Fig. 4, showed a markedly depressed maturation into Ig producing cells although they were stimulated by PWM to undergo blastic transformation. The lymphocytes from 6 patients, however, were found to have no impaired capacity to differentiate into Ig producing cells under PWM stimulation. These normally responding patients also had polyclonal hypogammaglobulinemia. Mean numbers of cytoplasmic Ig positive cells were 7% of normal for IgG, 8% of normal for IgA and 8% of normal for IgM in 16 patients with markedly depressed B cell differentiation and 99% of normal for IgG, 141% of normal for IgA and 93% of normal for IgM in 6 normally responding patients.

Further, co-culture experiments were undertaken in order to determine whether peripheral blood mononuclear cells from patients with myeloma had

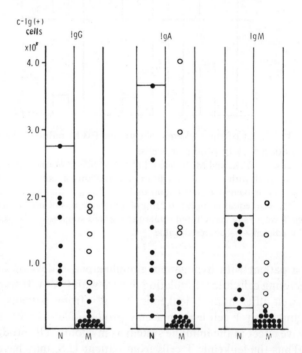

FIG. 4. PWM-induced immunoglobulin synthesis by peripheral blood lymphocytes from patients with multiple myeloma and related diseases.
Open circles in each right column show normally differentiated cases. N—normal, M—myeloma, c-Ig(+) cells—absolute numbers of cells positive for cytoplasmic immunoglobulin.

a suppressive or enhancing effect on normal PWM-induced B cell differentiation. The overall proportion of Ig producing cells found in co-culture of cells from pairs of normal individuals was greater than would have been expected from each culture (Fig. 5). The lymphocytes (including monocytes) from three patients with multiple myeloma suppressed B cell differentiation into Ig producing cells of normal lymphocytes (Fig. 6), whereas the plasma from the same patients and lymphocytes from a myeloma patient who normally responded to PWM and differentiated well did not (Fig. 7). These results strongly suggest that in the peripheral blood of most patients with multiple myeloma there exist cells with a suppressive effect on B cell differentiation in this system. Broder and his colleagues[6] reported similar results last year and demonstrated that the cells with a suppressive effect on normal B cell differentiation in multiple myeloma were the phagocytes. Marked impairment of PWM-induced lymphocyte differentiation, which is probably due to suppressor cells in the peripheral blood, may explain the decrease in the polyclonal immunoglobulins in most cases of multiple myeloma, but the results in the normally

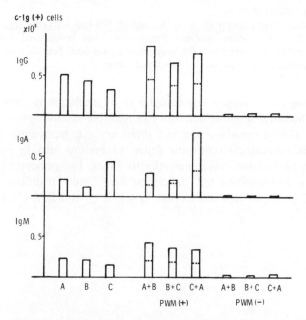

FIG. 5. PWM-induced lymphocyte differentiation into Ig producing cells in co-culture system of peripheral blood lymphocytes from three normal individuals (A, B, C).

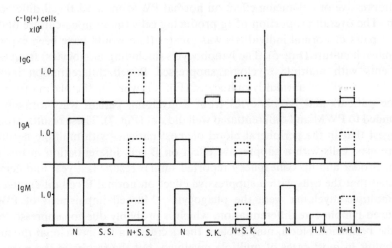

FIG. 6. Effect of peripheral blood mononuclear cells from patients with multiple myeloma on PWM-induced B cell differentiation of normal individuals.
These three patients (S. S., S. K. and H. N.) had markedly suppressed B cell differentiation. Normal lymphocytes were co-cultured with equal numbers of lymphocytes (including monocytes) from patients with multiple myeloma. N—normal, - - - -predicted value.

responding cases suggest the complexity of mechanisms responsible for the state of humoral immune deficiency in multiple myeloma.

Wiskott-Aldrich syndrome and IgA deficiency. Lymphocytes from a patient with Wiskott-Aldrich syndrome failed to mature into Ig producing cells, although they transformed normally to blasts. Lymphocytes from a patient with SLE and selective IgA deficiency were found to differentiate normally into IgG (5.2% of recovered cells), IgA (9.2%) and IgM (12.8%) producing cells.

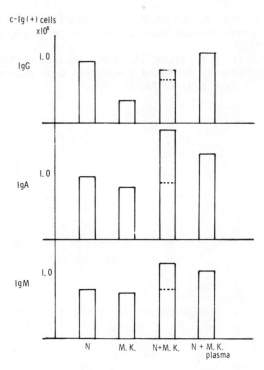

FIG. 7. Effect of peripheral blood mononuclear cells and plasma from a patient with multiple myeloma (M. K.) on PWM-induced normal lymphocyte differentiation into Ig producing cells. Lymphocytes from this patient differentiated normally into Ig producing cells.

REFERENCES

1. Greaves, M. F. and Roitt, I. M.: The effect of phytohemagglutinin and other lymphocyte mitogens on immunoglobulin synthesis by human peripheral blood lymphocytes *in vitro*. *Clin. Exp. Immunol.* **3**:393, 1968.
2. Wu, L. Y. F., Lawton, A. R., and Cooper, M. D.: Differentiation capacity of cultured B lymphocytes from immunodeficient patients. *J. Clin. Invest.* **52**: 3180, 1973.
3. Waldmann, T. A., Broder, S., Durm, M., *et al.*: Role of suppressor T cells in pathogenesis of common variable hypogammaglobulinemia. *Lancet* **2**:609, 1974.
4. Janossy, J. and Greaves, M. F.: Functional analysis of murine and human B lymphocyte subsets. *Transplant. Rev.* **24**: 177, 1975.

5. Lutzner, M.   Edelson   R., Schein, P., *et al*: Cutaneous T-cell lymphoma: The
   Sezary syndrome, mycosis fungoides, and related disorders. *Ann. Intern. Med.*
   83:534, 1975.
6. Broder, S., Humphrey, R., Durm, M., *et al.*: Impaired synthesis of polyclonal
   immunoglobulins by circulating lymphocytes from patients with multiple
   myeloma. *N. Engl. J. Med.* **293**:887, 1975.

Polymerized Flagellin as a Test Immunogen for an Evaluation of Immunological Functions in Immunodeficient States

Mutsuhiko MINAMI,* Tyoku MATUHASI,* and Kazuya YOSHINO**

ABSTRACT

POL was demonstrated to be an excellent test immunogen for evaluating the humoral antibody response in the following studies: i) Since the IgM response to POL is T cell-independent but the IgG response is T cell-dependent, the analysis of the response to POL could make it possible to evaluate T cell and B cell functions selectively; ii) natural anti-POL antibody titer is low in children; iii) after immunization with 10 μg of POL without adjuvant, good IgM and IgG responses were elicited in normal subjects; iv) no side effect was observed at all; v) the antibody response to POL was very low or was lacking in the patients with B cell deficiency.

INTRODUCTION

In immunodeficiency, it is important to evaluate the ability for humoral antibody response. For the evaluation, several kinds of vaccine have been employed as test immunogens.[1,2] However, an ideal test immunogen for this purpose should be pure and strong in immunogenicity and should not induce side effects. We considered that polymerized flagellin from *Salmonella adelaide* (POL) is one of the best test immunogens in man, because we have found i) the IgM response to POL is T cell-independent but the IgG response is T cell-dependent in mice; ii) naturally occurring antibody to POL is low in titer in children but both IgM and IgG antibody responses are high in immunized subjects; and iii) the antibody response to POL is very low in patients with B cell deficiency. In this paper, we will describe the outline of our experiments which lead us to the above conclusion.

*Department of Allergology, Institute of Medical Science, University of Tokyo, Tokyo, Japan
**Department of Pediatrics, Teikyo University School of Medicine, Tokyo, Japan

MATERIALS AND METHODS

Mice. Congenitally athymic nude mice on BALB/c background and their litter-mate mice were purchased from the Nippon Institute for Biological Science Co. The nude mice were the progeny of the 7th and 8th backcross generations. All mice were used at 5–8 weeks of age.

Human subjects. Healthy controls aged from 0 to 45 years and 4 patients with various immunodeficiencies were used.

Antigen. Polymerized flagellin (POL) was prepared from *Salmonella adelaide* by the method of Asakura *et al.*[3]

Serum antibody titration. Passive hemagglutination (PHA) tests were carried out on individual sera from mice or humans in microplate using antigen-coated erythrocytes. Sera were also tested for PHA activity after treatment with 0.1 M 2-mercaptoethanol (ME) for 2 hr at 37°C. 2-ME resistant PHA titers are considered to represent IgG activity.

POL was coated with erythrocytes using the chromic chloride method by incubating 2 ml of 10% suspension of erythrocytes with 100 μl of POL solution, 1 mg/ml in saline, and 100 μl of CrCl$_3$ 6H$_2$O solution, 1 mg/ml in saline, at room temperature for 20 min.[4] In the titration of anti-POL antibody, sheep erythrocytes were used for mouse sera and human group 0 erythrocytes for human sera. The erythrocytes coated with POL were washed three times with saline, resuspended to a final concentration of 1% in GVB (isotonic veronal-NaCl buffer, pH 7.4, 0.1% gelatine) and used in the PHA test.

RESULTS

The antibody response to POL in normal and nude mice. In order to examine whether the antibody response to POL is dependent on T cells or not, the antibody response to POL was explored in nude mice and their litter-mate mice. A group of 4 nude mice was injected intraperitoneally with 100 μg of POL in saline. Similarly, a group of 4 litter-mate mice (nu/+, +/+) was used as a control. At appropriate intervals after the injection, the mice were bled and the serum antibody titers were determined by the PHA test. As shown in Fig. 1, in the control mice, 100 μg of POL induced good IgM response, followed by significant IgG response. On the other hand, in nude mice, 100 μg of POL elicited high IgM response but no IgG response. The results indicate that the IgM response to POL can be induced in the absence of T cells but the IgG response requires the presence of T cells.

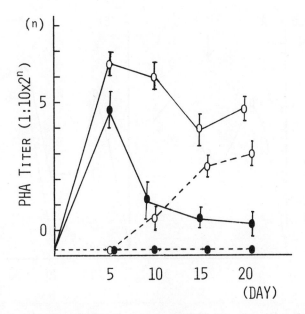

Fig. 1. Kinetics of antibody response to POL in nude mice and normal litter-mate mice.
Group of 4 litter-mate mice (○) and group of 4 nude mice (●) were immunized intraperitoneally with 100 μg of POL in saline. Total (—) and 2-ME resistant (---) PHA titers were determined on individual sera and represented as the mean of n values in $1:10 \times 2^n$ for each group of mice with standard deviation.

Restoration of the IgG response to POL with thymocytes in nude mice. The dependency of the IgG response to POL on T cells was further confirmed in the the following experiments in which the antibody response to POL was examined in nude mice given T cells.

The group of 4 nude mice were injected intravenously with 7.5×10^7 of thymocytes from their normal litter-mate mice. Immediately after the cell transfer, the nude mice were injected intraperitoneally with 100 μg of POL. Twenty days later the mice received a further 10 μg of POL intraperitoneally. As control mice, nude mice receiving no thymocytes were immunized with POL on the same schedule. At appropriate intervals after the primary and secondary challenge with POL, the mice were bled and the sera were tested for their anti-POL antibody activities. The results are depicted in Fig. 2.

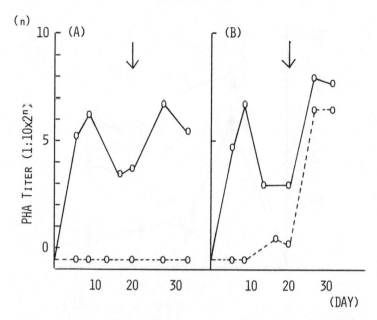

Fig. 2. Restoration of IgG response to POL in nude mice by injection of thymocytes.
Group of 4 nude mice (B) were injected intravenously with 7.5×10^7 thymocytes from litter-mate mice. The group of mice and control nude mice receiving no thymocytes (A) were immunized intraperitoneally with 100 μg of POL. Arrows indicate secondary challenge with 10 μg of POL 20 days after the primary immunization. Total (—) and 2-ME resistant (---) PHA titers were determined on individual sera and represented as the mean of n values in $1:10 \times 2^n$ for each group of mice.

Control mice produced a significant anti-POL response, but it consisted only of IgM response even after the secondary challenge. In contrast, the nude mice receiving thymocytes showed both IgM and IgG responses. Thus, it is established that the IgG response to POL requires the presence of T cells in mice. Moreover, in the nude mice given thymocytes, the IgG response was more remarkable after the secondary challenge. It seems to be a secondary response since the IgG response reached a maximum on day 6 after the challenge.

Further, these results suggested that, in the antibody response against POL, the absence of the IgG response shows a defect of T cell function and the absence of both IgM and IgG responses shows a defect of B cell function.

Naturally occurring antibody to POL in normal subjects.   Sera from 105 normal subjects aged from 0 to 45 years were assayed for natural antibody to POL by the PHA test. The results are shown in Table 1. The natural antibody to POL consisted of both IgM and IgG classes. In the sera from newborn babies and cord blood, only the IgG antibody was detected, which may have passed through the placenta. The natural antibody titers were lower in children than those in adults.

TABLE 1. Naturally occurring antibody to POL in normal subjects.

Age(years)	Anti-POL PHA Titer (Log$_2$)	
	Total	2-ME-resistant
Newborn Cord Blood	1.80 ± 2.03	1.43 ± 1.67
1–3	2.60 ± 1.90	1.00 ± 1.05
4–6	2.08 ± 2.39	0.83 ± 1.26
7–10	0.80 ± 1.31	0.70 ± 1.25
11–15	0.66 ± 1.11	0.18 ± 0.40
16–20	3.00 ± 2.82	2.33 ± 2.23
>20	4.14 ± 1.87	1.78 ± 1.67

Antibody response to POL in normal subjects and patients with immunodeficiency. We examined the antibody response to POL in normal subjects and patients with immunodeficiencies. Both normal subjects and patients were injected intradermally with 10 μg of POL in saline solution and they were bled and the serum anti-POL antibody titers were determined by the PHA test at appropriate intervals after the injection. The results are shown in Fig. 3.

In normal subjects, an IgM response to POL was clearly induced, followed by a significant IgG response. The anti-POL titers reached a plateau 2 wks after the injection (Fig. 3, A). No severe side effect was observed in any subject.

In a case of congenital sporadic agammagloublinemia, neither the IgM nor the IgG response to POL was observed after the immunization with POL (Fig. 3, B).

In a case of severe combined immunodeficiency, both IgM and IgG anti-POL antibodies were detected but in very small amounts after the immunization (Fig. 3, C).

Further, in a case of Wiskott-Aldrich syndrome, only poor IgM and IgG responses to POL were induced (Fig. 3, D).

In a case of reticulohistiocytosis, no response to POL was elicited. This patient was diagnosed as acquired combined immunodeficiency by absolute lymphopenia, low immunoglobulin levels in serum, negative delayed skin test to several antigens and decreased lymphocyte blastogenic response to phytohemagglutinin, concanavalin A and pokeweed mitogen (Fig. 3, E).

90 M. Minami *et al.*

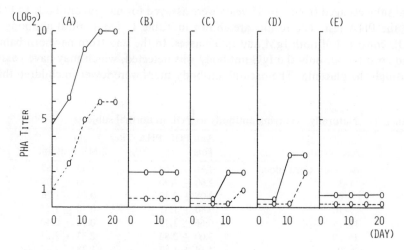

FIG. 3. Kinetics of antibody response to POL in normal subjects and in patients with immunodeficiency.
Normal subjects (A) were injected intradermally with 10 μg of POL in saline. Similarly, patients with congenital sporadic agammaglobulinemia (B), severe combined immunodeficiency (C), Wiskott-Aldrich syndrome (D) or reticulohistiocytosis (E) were injected with POL in the same way. Total (—) and 2-ME resistant (---) PHA titers were determined on individual sera and represented as log 2.

DISCUSSION

The purpose of this study is to examine whether POL is an excellent test immunogen to evaluate the capacity of immunological function in man. There are few reliable indices of the capacity of humoral antibody response in man. It is important to evaluate the capacity especially in immunodeficiency syndrome. In some studies, the malaria parasite,[5,6] plague vaccine[1] and yellow fever vaccine[2] were used as test immunogens. However, these studies are difficult to assess because of the complexity of these antigens.

In the present study, we used POL as a test immunogen. Before clincial application of POL, we examined the antibody response to POL in mice. When POL was injected into normal mice, the IgG response to POL was elicited, following the IgM response. However, in nude mice only the IgM response to POL was induced (Fig. 1). These results confirmed the previous observations by Langman et al.[7] and Huchet et al.[8] that anti-POL IgG response and anti-DNP IgG response against DNP-POL were dependent on T cells.

The T cell-dependency of anti-POL IgG response was more clearly proved by the restoration experiments in which nude mice were injected intravenously with their litter-mate thymocytes and then immunized twice with POL. These nude mice produced the IgG antibody to POL markedly after the secondary challenge. These results suggest that upon the injection of POL, the absence of the IgG response shows a defect in T cell function and the absence of the both IgM and IgG responses shows a defect in B cell function.

Before immunization of humans with POL, naturally occurring antibody to POL was examined in normal subjects. As shown in Table 1, natural antibody to POL consisted of both IgM and IgG classes and the titers are lower in children than those in adults. Rowley and Mackay reported that natural antibody to POL was detected in the sera from 86% of the healthy subjects and the titers ranged from 5 to 2560 (mean 26),[9] although all subjects they tested were adults.

After immunization with 10 μg of POL, good IgM and IgG antibody responses to POL were induced in normal subjects without side effect (Fig. 3, A). Thus, POL has strong immunogenicity against humans.

However, in the patients who were considered to have B cell deficiency with or without T cell deficiency, both IgM and IgG responses to POL decreased markedly (Fig. 3, B, C, D, E).

Considering the results mentioned above, POL is an excellent test immunogen to evaluate an ability for humoral antibody response.

Further application of POL to various immunodeficient patients may clarify the cellular mechanisms of the antibody response to POL in humans, making POL a more useful test immunogen.

REFERENCES

1. Adner, M. M., Ise, C., Schwab, R. S., Sherman, J. D., and Dameshek, W.: Immunologic studies of thymectomized and nonthymectomized patients with myasthenia gravis. Ann. N. Y. Acad. Sci. 135:536, 1966.
2. Levin, A. G., Cunningham, M. P., Steers, A. K., Miller, D. G., and Southam, C. M.: Production of 19S and 7S antibodies by cancer patients. Clin. Exp. Immunol. 7:839, 1970.
3. Asakura, S., Eguchi, G., and Iino, T.: Reconstitution of bacterial flagella in vitro. J. Mol. Biol. 10:41, 1964.
4. Langman, R. E.: The use of erythrocytes sensitized with flagellar antigens from Salmonella for the assay of antibody and antibody-forming cells. J. Immunol. Method. 2:59, 1972.

5. Tobie, J. E., Abele, D. C., Wolff, S. M., Contacos, P. G., and Evans, C. B.: Serum immunoglobulin levels in human malaria and their relationship to antibody production. *J. Immunol.* **97**:498, 1966.

6. Targett, G. A. T.: Antibody response to *Plasmodium falciparum* malaria, comparisons of immunoglobulin concentrations, antibody titers and the antigenicity of different a sexual forms of the parasite. *Clin. Exp. Immunol.* **7**:501, 1970.

7 Langman, R. E., Armstrong, W. D., and Diener, E.: Antigenic composition, not the degree of polymerization, determines the requirement for thymus-derived cells in immune responses to *Salmonella* flagellar proteins. *J. Immunol.* **113**:251, 1974.

8. Huchet, R. and Feldman, M.: Thymus-independent IgM and IgG responses in mice to flagellar antigens. *Int. Arch. Allergy.* **46**:600, 1974.

9. Rowley, M. J. and Mackay, I. R.: Measurement of antibody-producing capacity in man. I. The normal response to flagellin from *Salmonella adelaide. Clin. Exp. Immunol.* **5**:407, 1969.

Immunodeficiency in Human Disease with Special Consideration of Enzyme Disturbances

Robert A. Good and M. A. Hansen

ABSTRACT

It is beginning to be possible to link enzymes with syndromes of primary immunodeficiency. Severe combined immunodeficiency disease (SCID) has been associated with a deficiency of adenosine deaminase, nuclease phosphorylase and an apparent deficiency of adenosine deaminase associated with an inhibitor bound in the cell to adenosine deaminase. Correction of severe combined immunodeficiency using bone marrow transplantation has been effective in correcting three different forms of SCID, each of which is due to a separate genetically determined inborn error of metabolism. Bone marrow transplantation to correct SCID associated with an apparent deficiency of ADA corrects the deficiency of ADA in the leukocytes but not in the red blood cells of these patients producing a fascinating enzyme chimera at the cellular level. Fatal granulomatous disease of childhood is associated with enzymatic malfunctions of the leukocytes. The best current evidence still has not yielded a definition of the characteristic abnormality of the classical x-linked form of this disease originally described in my laboratory. Marsh et al. have shown that this disease is associated with an abnormality or deficiency of a membrane antigen which they have called Kx. We postulate that this defect is fundamental to the pathogenesis of CGD and is essential to the failure of phagocytosis to induce essential enzymatic processes that underly the deficiencies of generation of H_2O_2, O_2 superoxide necessary for the killing processes. Deficiencies of the Clr, Cls, Cl esterase inhibitor, C2, C4, C3, C3 inhibitor, C5, C6, C7 and C8 components of the complement system may produce deficiencies of enzymes essential to healthy and vigorous life. The association of deficiency of these components with susceptibility to infections, certain gram negative infections, lupus,

Memorial Sloan-Kettering Cancer Center, New York, New York, U. S. A.
The original work on which this report is based was aided by USPHS grants CA-05826, CA-08748, CA-17404, AI-11843 and NS-11457 from the National Institutes of Health; the National Foundation-March of Dimes; the Zelda Radow Weintraub Cancer Fund and the Judith Harris Selig Memorial Fund.

vasculitis, anaphylactoid purpura, dermatomyositis, and lupus-like syndrome has now been well documented. Means of cellular and macromolecular engineering to correct these enzyme-based immunodeficiencies will be described.

INTRODUCTION

The study of immunobiology has reaped the benefits of a close alliance between the clinic, where problems are posed, and the basic science laboratory, where answers have been sought and often found. Some notable names that have contributed significantly to our advancing knowledge through this mechanism are:

Jenner,[1] whose interpretation of the experiment of nature posed by the milkmaids resistant to smallpox launched immunology;

Pasteur,[2] whose major concern with all manner of sickness—sickness of beer, sickness of wine, cholera of chickens, anthrax, and hydrophobia—yielded the principles of etiology and the concept of attenuation;

Landsteiner,[3] who discovered agglutinins and agglutinogens and gave us the safe blood transfusions;

Von Pirquet and Schick,[4] who discovered in their classical study of serum sickness that immunity can produce injury and disease, as well as bring benefit to man;

Prausnitz and Kustner,[5] whose study of Prausnitz's sensitivity to boiled fish protein generated an understanding of and methods for analysis and treatment of atopic allergies;

Phillip Levine,[6] whose analysis of a single post partum transfusion reaction yielded the pathogenesis of erythroblastosis foetalis;

Kunkel,[7] whose studies of myeloma launched investigations culminating in a definition of the chemistry of antibodies;

Bing and Plum,[8] whose stuides of 11 cases of agranulocytosis linked plasma cells to globulin production;

Kolouch,[9] whose study of a single case of subacute bacterial endocarditis was the beginning of experimental analyses linking plasma cells to antibody production;

And Bruton,[10] whose discovery of agammaglobulinemia has lead to the dissection of the microbial universe into at least two separate components, and whose definition of roles played by antibodies and cell-mediated immunities in resistance to different infections has had far-reaching results.

All of these contributions were subsequent to the investigation of clinical issues which, upon laboratory analysis, yielded fundamental insights. This is a powerful approach that explains much of the past effectiveness of immunology and contributes much to its current vigor.

DEVELOPMENT AND FUNCTION OF THE LYMPHOID SYSTEM

Having very solid evidence, we now know that the immunological system develops as two main arms. There is the T arm, regulated by the thymus, with thymic-derived, thymic-dependent lymphocytes, and a B arm, derived from the as-yet-unknown human equivalent of the bursa of fabricius found in birds. These two separate arms have different jobs, the B arm being responsible for immunoglobulin and antibody secretion, the T arm serving as a long-lived immune memory and as a cell-mediated immune system. Both the T and the B cell systems address fundamental effector processes, such as inflammation, vascular reactivity, blood coagulation, and, above all, phagocytosis.[11]

In order for these two arms to develop, the primordial immune cells, all of which originate in the fetal yolk sac, undergo an odyssey that carries them to the fetal liver and eventually to the bone marrow, both primary hematopoietic organs. During these early travels, the primitive stem cells become capable of further differentiation and of finding their way to the central lymphoid organs. Committed hematopoietic cells then travel to the thymus or bursal equivalent where they undergo differentiative events necessary for the development of cellular characteristics which ultimately define their function.[12] The development of the lymphoid system is basically the same as for all the rest of the hematopoietic system, except that the inducing substances in the microchemical environment probably differ for each. (See Fig. 1 for a schematic drawing of lymphoid development.)

A most important recent finding about the immune system has been that the T and B arms can be shown to exert both positive and negative influences on one another. The helper influence of the T lymphocyte on the B lymphocyte, which is seen, for example, in the formation of antibody in reaction to a protein antigen such as sheep red blood cells (SRBC), is now well-documented and is beginning to be defined in molecular terms.[13] The work of Gershon and colleagues, on the other hand,[14,15] has helped us to identify a suppressor subpopulation among the T lymphocytes, and we are likewise now beginning to see suppressor influences in terms that will ultimately, I am sure, permit molecular definition.[16-21] While the two components, T and B, concept of the immune system, stated in simplest terms, is now somewhat outmoded, I think it is sufficiently flexible to serve as a point of departure for our present purposes.

96   R. A. Good and M. A. Hansen

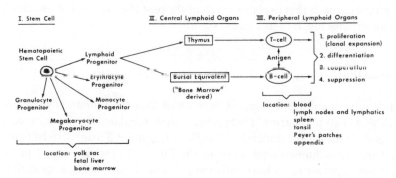

THE TWO COMPONENT SCHEME OF THE LYMPHOID SYSTEM

FIG. 1

When we talk about the T and B cells, we also need to talk about the T and B regions in lymphoid tissue. (See Figs. 2 and 3 for drawings of a stimulated lymph node where one can see areas specific for T and B cells.) B zones are classically found in the far cortical areas of the lymph node where germinal centers develop, and in the medullary cords where plasma cells develop. The deep cortical areas (or so-called paracortical regions) are thymus-dependent. These have been defined by Parrott et al.[22] for the mouse and by our own group for chickens[23] and humans.[24]

The cells in the peripheral lymphoid tissue and the circulation can now be defined both by surface marker methodology and by functional characteristics. Major markers of the T cells are the capacity to 1) form rosettes with SRBC; 2) respond to PHA and Con-A in a solution (although non-T cells will respond to these lectins when presented in a polymerized or nonsoluble form); 3) capacity to respond by proliferation to antigens against which those animals from which the cells are derived have already been immunized;[25] and 4) capacity to respond to allogeneic cells. T cells, furthermore, develop very early in their differentiation process cell surface antigens that permit us to define them in immunological terms. Antisera have also been prepared against human T lymphocytes, which are, after appropriate absorption, specific for T cells in tissues or in the peripheral blood.[13,26,27]

B cells, of course, are those which have on their surface readily demonstrable surface immunoglobulin. The basis for specificity in the B cells is found on the antigen combining site of the immunoglobulin molecule. This is probably true also of T cells. Whereas we know very much about the immunoglobulin molecule in humans and animals, the nature of the immunoglobulin or molecule containing this site on T cells is still enigmatic. There are five different classes of surface immunoglobulin on different subpopulations of B cells: IgM ac-

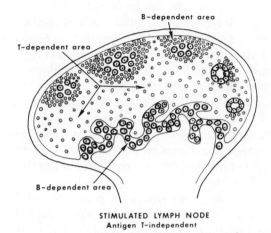

STIMULATED LYMPH NODE
Antigen T-independent

FIG. 2

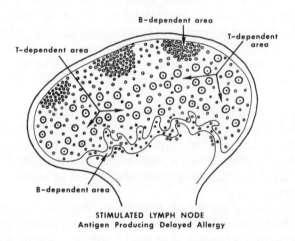

STIMULATED LYMPH NODE
Antigen Producing Delayed Allergy

FIG. 3

counts for the greater proportion of the cells with surface immunoglobulins; some also have IgM + IgD, but present also in blood and lymphoid tissue are B cells with surface IgG, IgE, and IgA, as well as IgD alone. B cells, or a major subpopulation of B cells, have also been identified through their predisposition for rosetting with mouse red blood cells. This rosetting technique is a tricky one, but it has yielded reproducible results in our laboratories in studies under the direction of Drs. Sudhir Gupta and Fred Siegal.[28-30] I believe this capacity to rosette with mouse cells can be considered a good marker for a major subpopulation of B lymphocytes. Other markers once used for B lymphocytes have not proved to be very useful. These include Fc receptors and C_3 receptors, which are also present on macrophages and other lymphocyte populations. Specific anti-B cell sera, however, have been developed.[13]

There is a third population of cells in which the cells look like lymphocytes and do not phagocytize. Many of the cells in this group are the so-called K cells, noted especially for their high avidity receptors for IgG molecules. The K cells can easily be demonstrated through a rosetting technique that employs a specific antisera against D antigens on human red blood cells. The reagent used to enumerate cells of this population is composed of Rh(D) red blood cells coated with Ripley serum. This represents an apparently monovalent anti-Rh(D) antiserum. K cells comprise a very significant proportion of the circulating lymphocytes. Like the B lymphocytes, K cells also have complement receptors, but they lack surface immunoglobulins and, as mentioned do not phagocytize particulate matter.[31]

Normally T lymphocytes comprise about 75% of circulating cells in the blood; B lymphocytes make up approximately 10% of the total lymphocyte population, and the third population, approximately 12–15%. Within this last group, K, or so-called killer cells, account for as many as 8–10% of circulating white blood cells. Functionally, K cells have aroused interest because they participate, in an as yet unknown way, in antibody-mediated cytotoxicity reactions.

Fully differentiated B lymphocytes are secretory lymphocytes—that is, their cytoplasm is full of immunoglobulin, which is easily demonstrated by fluorescent microscopy. These cells are capable of secreting the immunoglobulin. Mature B cells very often have the morphology of the classical Marshalko plasma cell. They derive from B lymphocytes that can be induced to differentiate in a variety of ways.[32]

Kishimoto and Ishizaka[33,43] have recently developed and described a most interesting method to stimulate rabbit B cells to become end-stage plasma cells. They have used a soluble factor derived from T cells that they are now defining. This factor stimulates B lymphocytes to proliferate and permits B cells to differentiate terminally to plasma cells after stimulation with anti-antibody against immunoglobulin. Another substance that induces terminal differentiation of B lymphocytes also induces B lymphocytes to first go through a proliferative phase, which Y.S. Choi, in our laboratory, has shown to be a necessary step in the differentiative process. After proliferation, B cells are known to go through a process of differentiation in which they develop a capacity for massive immunoglobulin synthesis and ultimately immunoglobulin secretion.

Upon this terminal differentiation, the cells become veritable immunoglobulin "pumper" cells.

DISORDERS OF THE IMMUNE SYSTEM

If one were to take out the thymus of the proper strain of rat or mouse during the neonatal period and couple this radical step with the implementation of either anti-T cell serum or irradiation, one could quite readily eliminate the animals' entire T cell population. The lymph nodes of such an animal have well-developed B zones, but essentially no T cells at all. The nude mouse provides another good experimental model of a B mouse (*i.e.* a mouse having only B cells—no T cells). Such mice are actually born with a congenital defect of thymus development and hence are grossly lacking in T cell populations. A mouse lacking a T cell system and living in a hostile environment, such as that encountered by the ordinary house mouse, begins to sicken, runts, and will die after a short time. If kept in a germ-free environment, however, these same animals grow and develop quite normally, a phenomenon which seems to indicate that the runting and wasting syndrome is, in large measure, a consequence of infections encountered in the nonsterile environment.

Mice, rabbits, and rats grossly deficient in T cells also develop later on in life extraordinary evidences of immunological excess. They are, for example, often troubled by autoimmune diseases, such as autoimmune hemolytic anemia, and by a progressive destructive disease of the kidney, by vasculitis and amyloidosis.[35] We can do immunological studies on animals which have been neonatally thymectomized, using a variety of techniques, all of which show that the cell-mediated responses in such animals are grossly defective. There is little or no response, for example, of their lymphocytes to PHA or Con-A stimulation, nor to grafted tissues nor to immunization that produces delayed allergy. Further, these B mice do not produce antibodies, especially of IgG class, to T-dependent antigens.[11] They do not reject allografts or other allogeneic tissue and have poorly developed T cell populations. They do, however, have B cell populations and are able to produce antibodies to T-independent antigens like pneumococcal polysaccharide. Additional tests on various strains of mice have shown that the thymus exercises an important function throughout the life span of the animal and that involution of the thymus, which normally occurs with aging, produces the basic immunodeficiency problems so often seen in the aging.[36,37]

An important step in the development of cellular engineering occurred when we studied correction of immunodeficiency associated with thymectomy. We learned that cell-mediated deficiency could be prevented in athymic animals simply by supplying them with a thymic transplant. We could not achieve reconstitution with thymuses in millipore chambers if the animals completely lacked T cells, because a crucial population of post-thymic T cells are absent. By contrast, one can correct the immunodeficiency of such animals by cellular engineering that involves giving syngeneic thymic lymphocytes to the deficient animals or by a transplantation of several thymuses. Indeed, with multiple thymic transplants, we found that we could even reverse the wasting and runting post-thymectomy syndrome commonly seen in the athymic animals.[11] Such transplantation of lymphoid cells yielded perfectly vigorous, long-lived survivors. We cannot at present reverse wasting and runting disease in athymic animals with any known thymic hormone, thymic extract, or even by using functionally active thymic tumors.[11,38,39] A normal thymic microenvironment seems to be essential for the development of fully competent T cells if the latter are completely absent or must develop from scratch. This could be simply a matter of thymic hormone concentration, and is an issue we are currently investigating with Gideon Goldstein.

Successful thymic transplantation in the mice lacking T cells gave us our first evidence that we could exercise a form of cellular engineering. Almost immediately this led us to try to reconstitute mice by transplanting across the major histocompatibility barriers, from young mice. When we transplanted a thymus containing thymic lymphocytes across the major histocompatibility barrier, we quickly found that such treatment would often kill the animals with a graft vs. host reaction (GVHR). In 1965, Edmund Yunis and colleagues discovered, however, that we could protect mice by transplanting T lymphocytes or thymuses from animals matched at the H2 major histocompatibility loci. Even though other histocompatibility differences existed, we could fully reconstruct the deficient immune system, reverse the wasting and runting process, and, best of all, not lose the animal to a fatal GVHR.[40] The degree of matching was the key. In subsequent experiments, however, we found that transplantation of small thymic anlagen from developing embryos could also be transplanted to correct immunodeficiency without producing GVHD.[11,41] To me, these studies represent the opening wedges that have yielded safe cellular engineering based on thymic, marrow, and fetal tissue transplantation by means that can avoid fatal graft vs. host reactions.

Just as immune disorders result from a lack of thymus or T lymphocytes, so do severe disorders arise from a lack of B lymphocytes. Classic examples of this phenomenon are patients with the Bruton type X-linked infantile agammaglobulinemia.[10] Such patients have virtually no B lymphocytes in the circulation,[11] their lymph nodes develop no germinal centers following antigenic stimulation, and no plasma cells are to be found.[42,43] These patients are fascinating because, as Cooper has recently found, even though they lack B cells and plasma cells, they do have in their bone marrow, although not in their circulation, an immunoglobulin producing cell which Cooper considers to be a precursor of the B cell line (personal communication). The B cell development seems to be arrested at a very early stage of differentiation. I have recently seen a patient in the wards of the Babies' Hospital in N. Y. who suffers from a variation of the Harrington-DiGeorge syndrome. Such patients are born without a thymus and therefore have extreme deficiencies of the cells in the deep cortical areas of the lymph node. While plasma cells and the far cortical B zone areas are quite welldeveloped, these patients generally also have poorly developed germinal centers. The failure of thymic development has been associated in the DiGeorge patients with the failure to properly develop the embryonic anlagen of the third and fourth pharyngeal pouches, and so the patients also commonly lack the parathyroid glands.[45]

The cell-mediated immune deficiencies which characterize the Digeorge syndrome patients have been corrected, and the lymph nodes and peripheral lymphoid system completely reconstructed by transplanting embryonic thymus into the subcutaneous tissue, just as we have done to correct this immunodeficiency in the nude mouse or the thymectomized mouse which lacks T cells. Often patients with the DiGeorge syndrome have in their circulation high numbers of B lymphocytes, the B population accounting for as many as 80–90 % of the circulating lymphoid cells. After embryonic thymus transplantation, full reconstitution has been observed in 6 of 7 patients. In these 6 patients the cell-mediated immunities have appeared and subsequently the B cell system has decreased to its normal level.[46] The DiGeorge syndrome, however, is a variable disease. It may be complete, incomplete, or, as in the case of the Harrington syndrome, it may result in no immunological deficit whatsoever. This variability makes it very hard to evaluate the results of thymus transplantation for the correction of T cell immunodeficiency.[11] We feel certain that thymic transplantation works to correct immunodeficiency in DiGeorge syndrome, and Aiuti et al.[47] have apparently corrected other forms of T cell immunodeficiency by thymus transplantation. Hong and coworkers have corrected at least one form of severe combined immunodeficiency by transplantation of cultured thymic epithelial cells.[48]

One can marvel that, in the nude mouse, in the neonatally thymectomized mouse, as well as in the DiGeorge patient, a small piece of transplanted embryonic thymus permits the development of a very beautiful thymic organ where once there was none. This new thymus reconstitutes the entire missing T cell immunological system. If, however, the transplanted anlagen differs from the host at a major histocompatibility barrier, rejection can occur once the host has been reconstituted. Hong now contends that culturing the thymus epithelium renders the transplant resistant to rejection,[48] as was orginally postulated by Summerlin et al.[49,50]

There are, in addition to the DiGeorge syndrome, other pure T cell abnormalities. One, described by Nezelof,[51] may not be a real entity but exists as such in the literature. Another T cell deficit has been associated with a deficiency of the enzyme nucleoside phosphorylase, and there are still others.[47] My personal view is that each immune deficient patient has to be considered as an entity unto himself. Each is an experiment of nature and most are unique or represent very small populations.

Some children are born without a T or a B cell immunity system. The tonsils of these children have no germinal centers, no lymphocytes, or plasma cells. The thymus, while present, is epithelial and very underdeveloped, having no cortex, no medulla, or Hassal's corpuscles. Lymph nodes and spleen may lack both B and T cells. Developmentally, these patients are thought to be hooked at an early stage, at which point both T and B systems are still one. The severe combined immunodeficiency diseases (SCID), however, are also very heterogeneous. Patients having these defects have varying genetic backgrounds, some being X-linked, some autosomal recessive, some appearing to be sporadic. A significant portion of SCID (about 10–20%) has occurred in conjunction with an adenosine deaminase (ADA) deficiency, or in some cases, with an apparent ADA deficiency which seems to be due to the presence of an inhibitor of ADA activity.[52,53] SCID has also frequently been associated with bony abnormalities and may be reflected in the short-limbed dwarfism defined by Gatti et al.[54]

The first indication that the terrible disease resulting from a combined immunodeficiency could be corrected through cellular engineering came eight years ago when we studied a little patient with the X-linked recessive form of the disease. This patient, who had virtually no T or B cells and therefore an extreme form of the disease, came from Connecticut to our hospital and laboratory in Minnesota. There had been 12 deaths in the family, obviously due to disease transmitted as an X-linked recessive trait and other family members had been shown to have lethal SCID.

By a line of reasoning derived from our work with experimental animals, we felt that if we could find a donor matched at the major histocompatibility system, we could correct this deficit. A matched sibling seemed ideal. We were not fortunate enough to have anyone in the family who was a perfect match at the major histocompatibility complex (MHC), but one of four sisters was found to be mismatched only at the HLA-A locus, HLA-D and -B being the same in the patient and his sister. Marrow taken from this sister completely reconstituted the patient's immune system. Because, however, of an additional ABO mismatch, and perhaps also partially due to the HLA-A mismatch, the transplant produced an iatrogenic immunologically-based aregenerative pancytopenia.

We therefore had an opportunity in the same patient to treat, for the first time successfully, an aplastic anemia by marrow transplantation, as well as to correct the SCID. Using the same donor, we completely changed the blood type of the patient, who remains today a fully vigorous child, to blood group 0 completely different from his own genetic blood group A. He is absolutely normal immunologically, with a normal hematopoietic system. All of the blood cells in his bone marrow are of the female karyotype, derived from the donor, and all of the cells in the peripheral blood which proliferate in response to stimulation are of female karyotype.[55,56]

Soon after this initial success, we corrected, by a series of bone marrow transplantations, the condition of a little girl with a combined immunodeficiency which was associated with an ADA deficiency. Our patient lacked ADA entirely; both parents had apparent half values of the enzyme, and a sister had normal values. Our patient and her sister were matched at the major histocompatibility loci, facilitating the transplantations. Today the girl remains an apparent chimera because her peripheral red blood cells still appear to lack the ADA, while all her lymphoid cells contain apparently normal amounts of the enzyme.[57] We have since cured another case of this form of SCID by marrow transplantation from a matched sibling donor, again creating the fascinating chimeric state.[58]

A third patient, with an as yet undefined enzymatic abnormality which also is an autosomal recessive trait, in conjunction with a combined immunodeficiency disease, came to us from the Babies' Hospital at Columbia. There was in this case no ADA deficiency or abnormality. A matched sibling donor, a sister, was available and this transplant could be accomplished very simply and almost like an outpatient procedure. It resulted in very prompt reconstruction of her entire immunological system without significant graft vs. host reaction. Today the patient remains absolutely normal and is completely well.

These children with transplanted bone marrow are surviving up to eight years following transplantation, and the procedure has now been done in many centers throughout the world. Table 1 contains our current best record of successful marrow transplants for combined immunodeficiency diseases. We have included all the various forms of the rare SCID cases, and the number fully corrected by marrow transplantation now reaches a total of 40 patients. We have yet to see, in the presence of an adequate match at the major histocompatibility complex, a GVHR to be fatal in patients with SCID. This fact becomes

TABLE 1.   Successful bone marrow transplantation for SCID

Minneapolis-NY	8	Bern-Geneva	1
London	5	Los Angeles	2
Boston	6	Detroit	1
Lyon	4	Ann Arbor	1
Paris	3	Cleveland	1
Copenhagen	2	Birmingham	1
Ulm	1	St. Louis	1
Leiden	2	Beirut	1

Total = 40

important later on in our discussion. GVHR often develops, but thus far it has not been fatal.

We have, however, too often seen a significant problem, now recognized and hopefully in most instances avoidable. It appears not to be wise to transplant patients while they have infections (e.g. pneumocystis carinii) which the patient, prior to transplantation, may be tolerating pretty well. If the patient receives a transplant before the infection has been cured, overwhelming, lethal amplification of the pneumonia can result as a consequence of the functions of the new immunological system as it interacts with the infectious agent. Tragic deaths have occurred from this process in several transplant centers after apparent full correction of the immunodeficiency disease.[11,57,59,60]

Another great problem with bone marrow transplantation has been, of course, that a matched sibling donor is not always available. When a MHC mismatched donor has been used to treat SCID, fatal GVH has been the rule. The development of our knowledge about the major histocompatibility complex has been growing apace. It is now known to be divided into four major systems, centered at the HLA-A, -B, -C, and -D loci, with the HLA-D locus seeming to be the most crucial of those thus far defined in successful matching for bone marrow transplantation.

The first breakthrough in the use of something other than a matched sibling donor came when we studied a pathologist's child in Copenhagen with Koch et al.[62] This particular child had no matched sibling, an older sibling having died previously of the SCID. We were, however, able to identify an uncle in the family who was matched at the D locus. This potential donor, however, showed a double haplotype mismatch at the A and B loci. Our experimental work with mice had suggested that matching at the D locus might be especially important in achieving a transplant without a lethal GVHR. The dilemma was that all of the children thus far transplanted with mismatched marrow had died of overwhelming GVHR.

After much discussion, we decided, because this was a fatal disease, to go ahead and to perform a transplant on the child with his uncle's partially matched marrow. It may have been a little more difficult to get this bone marrow transplant to take, but eventually the approach succeeded, and the child is now fully reconstructed and immunologically normal. Full development of the T cell system occurred, as did partial development of the B system, and this could be attributed to the donor cells. For a time a split chimerism was present in the B cell system, since some of the B cell functions in this interesting case seemed to be attributable to the recipient rather than to the donor. Since the child has received the transplant, he has recovered from a moderate GVHR and has been leading an active life, remaining free of significant disease. A subsequent child born to this family was found to be perfectly matched with the father at the D locus. This second child has been transplanted with his father's marrow and thus far seems to be developing a beautiful immune system.[63]

These, of course, are very rare cases, but they show that finding a relative who is matched at the D locus may permit bone marrow transplantation to correct SCID. One is not always able to find, to be sure, an uncle or a father that matches at the D locus. In Minneapolis we had earlier tried to transplant to a small child a haplotype-matched marrow taken from the father, but the child died of GVHR and infection.

After the move to New York, in the winter of 1972–73, one of the first SCID patients to come for treatment was a small baby for whom no matched donor was available within the family. Through a very extensive search that utilized computer systems and especially a donor panel set up in Denmark, we were able to find 10 people that were potentially matched with the patient at the B locus. Of those, three seemed by mixed leukocyte typing to be the best matches and one of them agreed to provide the necessary marrow. It is the long and short of a very long story to say that this little boy from Ohio has now been reconstructed immunologically at Memorial Hospital with the marrow of a woman from Copenhagen, identified by Svejgaard and his tissue typing colleagues at the Rigshospital in Copenhagen. Her marrow matched the patient's at the D and B loci, but was mismatched at the A locus.

It was necessary in this case, as in our original reconstruction of the immunological system, to switch the patient's blood type and entire hematopoietic system. Our patient lost several grafts and could not seem to get a marrow established until large doses of cyclophosphamide were given to insure engraftment. Today the child is reconstructed hematologically, and his immune function is near normal. He is still, however, bothered by an erythematous GVHR on his hands and elsewhere on his skin. This is a chronic scaling erythroderma which we have seen before in children transplanted even across minor histocompatibility barriers. We are hopeful that it will gradually subside and that we will have in this patient a full reconstruction, as well as an approach that can occasionally be used to treat patients with SCID.[64]

Sometimes, though, even a computerized search with available panels cannot find a suitable donor. However, SCID has been successfully treated in several centers with an early fetal liver transplantation.[65,66] The fetal liver, as you will recall, is a site for hematopoietic cell development. At the Sloan-Kettering Institute, Richard O'Reilly and Rajendra Pahwa have overseen fetal liver reconstruction of the immunological system on two occasions.[67]

The first patient was infected with a *Mycobacterium avium* that his immune system was unable to eliminate until after the successful fetal liver transplant. Now he has an immunological system with which he can address the organism, and he has developed delayed allergy to tuberculin. The second patient had SCID, and there was no donor either in the family or on the panels available to us. We know from experimental studies in mice that if stem cells are present in sufficient amounts and there are no postthymic T cells, it is possible to reconstruct such a patient with an early fetal liver. This has now been done and the patients are doing well. In at least one of these fetal liver transplants, the patient was shown to have marrow cells that responded effectively to thymic hormones. After reconstitution, the patient's T cell population could be shown to be of donor origin, and the B cell population of host origin, a fascinating form of chimerism.

Another disease that has, at least partially, been reconstructed immunologically is the Wiskott-Aldrich syndrome.[68] This is an immunodeficiency disease that has not yet been well defined. We do not know where the lesion is located or what cell system is involved in the deficiency. There seems to be a faulty presentation of antigens that may very well be due to abnormalities of the function of the monocyte-phagocyte system.

Eight years ago Bach's group in Wisconsin performed a transplant on a young boy with this disease, using marrow from a sister, and he continues to be chimeric still.[69] His hematopoietic abnormalities have not been corrected, e.g. his platelets are still abnormal, but he is living as a normal healthy child and seems to be immunologically reconstituted. This was another previously fatal disease which has been corrected, at least in part, by bone marrow transplantation.

From using bone marrow transplantation as a treatment for SCID and a regenerative anemia, we and many others have gone on to use it for correction of patients with aplastic anemia as well. The key here also is to use a matched sibling donor. Success with this therapy, of course, requires that the patient be prepared with large doses of cyclophosphamide with or without total body irradiation. From information based on cases using primarily the cyclophosphamide pretreatment reported from a large group in Seattle and from a registry we are conducting out of Milwaukee, one can show that marrow transplantation has been successful in curing aplastic anemia 50% of the time. It is the older patients, those over 20, who give us the most trouble. In the combined data of the Seattle group[70] and the Registry[71] series, it is shown that a patient under 20 was successfully transplanted more than 60% of the time. These observations may need reevaluation, because the numbers are limited, but it does seem that transplantation in younger children is easier. If we can solve several problems which we now can identify clearly, then we should be able, when a matched sibling donor is available, to correct aplastic anemia close to 90% of the time.

If in experimental animals you use irradiation or cyclophosphamide, or other cytotoxic agents, and then give marrow or lymphoid cells, even employing cells matched at the major histocompatibility complex, a GVHR is produced which may be fatal. This can occur even when the barrier being bridged is relatively minor. The irradiation and the cytotoxic agents couple their injurious consequences with the assault on the skin and bowel epithelium, which is initiated by the foreign lymphoid cells, to produce a very destructive disease. Eliminating from the hematopoietic cells being transplanted those that initiate a GVHR would permit us to salvage about 20% more of the patients with aplastic anemia than is now possible.

There are problems with infection. We are not good enough at controlling, preventing, or treating all infections, nor do we know how to handle the problems of actual rejection of the bone marrow. We have not developed an optimum protocol for immunosuppression. I think that each of these is an area in which we may soon make real progress, and I will say more about them later.

It has been reported[72] also that the disease I defined as the fatal chronic granulomatous syndrome of childhood can be corrected by bone marrow transplantation. In this disease the patient's cells can ingest certain bacteria, but cannot kill them. The basic enzymatic defect in patients with chronic granulomatous disease has not yet been defined. It has been attributed to an NADH oxidase deficiency, which we could not confirm. It has also been attributed to an abnormality of glucose-6-phosphate-dehydrogenase deficiency, which Holmes, Gatti, and myself[73,74] also found to exist only in stored cells. The defect has more recently been attributed to NADPH oxidase deficiency, which in our hands only showed up in the cells that are actively phagocytizing, as did the physiological anomaly which Holmes et al. originally described.[75] Finally, recent studies have proposed a defect of superoxide dismutase in this disease, which needs confirmation.[76] Most attractive to me is the idea that fatal granulomatous disease is one in which the leukocyte cell surface is abnormal, lacking the antigen Kx.[77] These patients, like those with aplastic anemia, must be prepared for bone marrow transplantation by a cyclophosphamide pretreatment.

Efforts to use the bone marrow transplant approach with leukemic patients have not yet been very encouraging. Both acute myeloleukemia and lymphoid leukemia have, however, been treated by bone marrow transplantation by Thomas' group in Seattle, but the leukemia sometimes recurs, and GVHR is a major obstacle. Fifteen to 20% long term survivors, however, have been obtained with otherwise highly lethal leukemia. This is the best anyone has been able to do so far, but it is just a beginning.[78,79] In addition to the recurrences of leukemia, the problems which plague treatment of aplastic anemia patients are also obstacles to the treatment of leukemia by marrow transplantation. These include, besides GVH disease, intercurrent infections, interstitial pneumonia, and graft rejection or failure.

Cyclic neutropenia in humans is an interesting disease that may one day be treated by bone marrow transplantation. In this disease process the neutrophils disappear every 21 days. We do not understand it very well as yet, but Malcolm Moore and his group at our institute, I believe, are progressing with this analysis. There is a nice experimental model of cyclic neutropenia to be found in the gray collie syndrome. Every 12 days, instead of every 21 days, as in man, neutrophils disappear from the circulating blood. These dogs with the gray collie anomaly are very easy to identify, even at birth, because of their coat color. The entire syndrome is transmitted as an autosomal recessive trait. If cells from a normal collie are given to an irradiated gray collie, the cyclic neutropenia is completely corrected. But it is much more intresting to note what happens if you give the normal irradiated collie matched bone marrow cells from the gray collie. Doing this, you produce cyclic neutropenia in the normal collie.[80] In other words, the disease resides right in the stem cells that are responsible for the development of the granulocyte-monocyte system.

We don't treat patients with cyclic neutropenia by bone marrow transplantation yet, because we are not good enough at bone marrow transplantation. However, when some of the present obstacles are cleared away, perhaps we will be able to help in the management of this otherwise difficult disease through marrow transplantation.

Major obstacles to the more widespread application of bone marrow transplantation and its therapeutic success include: 1) a need for definition of clinical indicators for the use of bone marrow transplantation as therapy; 2) the present requirement that a matched sibling donor be available; 3) resistance to engraftment. (Part of this is, of course, due to classic rejection mechanisms, but part of it may be quite another process which has been called allogeneic resistance by Cudkovich et al.[81] We think the number of cells used is absolutely crucial here); 4) the present inability to do away with GVH reactions. (This disease can now be specifically diagnosed, having its own pathological characteristics.[82] It has proven to be fatal to a significant proportion of patients receiving bone marrow transplantation for leukemia and aplastic anemia even when there has been an HLA matched donor); 5) infections, which often get out of control.

Fortunately, each of these obstacles is addressable, and I think we can do better than our present record. Leukemia patients have provided us with an additional problem to solve, that of a recurrence of the leukemic disease sometime after bone marrow transplantation. Such recurrence usually occurs in the cells of the recipient, but occasionally has been found in the cells of the donor.[83]

I am very optimistic about bone marrow transplantation because of what has transpired in the laboratory. We are able now in rats,[84] in mice,[85] and it looks as though, perhaps, in dogs, to transplant across the major histocompatibility barrier. To do this, we must get rid of all the lymphocytes, or all of the post-thymic T cells, in the hematopoietic resource that is chosen for the transplant. I say this on the basis of a large body of experimental data that I am not going to summarize in detail. Spleens, for example, taken from neonatally thymectomized mice and therefore spleens that are free of post-thymic T cells, can be used, as can early fetal liver from strains of mice which develop their T cell systems late.[86] Furthermore, we can precisely identify the number of cells which will correct fatal irradiation and the source of cells necessary to cross the major histocompatibility barrier. The trick is to avoid any post-thymic T lymphocytes in the hematopoietic resource and to give enough cells so that the fatal irradiation effects on hematopoietic cells are corrected before the lack of white cells kills the animal.

In some fascinating studies at Notre Dame, investigators have found that if donor and recipient are kept germ-free, bone marrow transplantation can be used to correct fatal irradiation across major histocompatibility barriers. Such transplants have already been used to cure and prevent the development of virus-based lymphomas.[87,88]

It has also been possible in the laboratory to pretreat marrow cells with an anti-T cell serum thus avoiding the GVHR even across major barriers. It is also absolutely necessary to avoid any damage to the hematopoietic stem cells. After proper serological specificity has been achieved by appropriate absorptions of antilymphocyte serum, the antiserum will not damage stem cells, but will prepare hematopoietic tissue so that it can be transplanted across major barriers, such as the AgB in the rat. This hematopoietic resource corrects fatal irradiation and produces long-lived, very vigorous animals whose cells are tolerant of the recipient and the donor.[84] This beginning is terribly important and may lead us to a much better approach to organ transplantation. If we can succeed in introducing a new hematopoietic system from any donor, we may then be able to stop the nonspecific immunosuppressive therapy which is currently necessary even for organ transplantation in humans. We should, if we can develop this approach, be able to do away with long-term treatment with cyclophosphamide and other carcinogenic and infection-producing reagents, such as 6MP, prednisone, actinomycin D, and antilymphocyte sera, in managing organ transplantation.

Indeed, it appears as though we are now well along the way toward the development of such antisera for human use. We desire an antiserum which will not damage stem cells but will, together with complement, eliminate all cells with thymic characteristics or post-thymic elements. We plan first to try bone marrow treated with such antisera on transplantation of leukemics and aplastic anemics, using matched sibling donors. If this should prove successful in avoiding completely the GVH reaction, we plan to go on to use the new technique to help us with the most difficult job of all—transplanting bone marrow pretreated in this way across major histocompatibility barriers without matching, or after incomplete matching. We believe that by this approach we can eliminate the GVHR that is such a problem to us now. Eventually every person might then have a chance to receive anyone else's marrow, should it be needed.

As we become more sophisticated in the use of cellular engineering our grasp of the possibilities inherent in macromolecular engineering is also growing apace. Allow me to give you a few examples. We now undertsand a great deal about T cell differentiation. Normally, pre-thymus cells are induced to become mature in the thymus under the influence of a trigger mechanism thought to be hormonal in nature. *In vitro* treatment of a pre-thymic cell, initially with a crude thymic extract and later with purified thymic substances, has been found to lead to T cell maturation.

Komuro and Boyse[89,90] have carried out a series of experiments using congenic mice in which Thy-1 was so induced. A molecule which can act in this induction process has now been identified. This molecule, called thymopoietin, has been purified and sequenced by Goldstein.[91] Goldstein and his colleagues found that its active site resides between the 29th and 42nd amino acid residues. Actually, a smaller octapeptide or pentapeptide, which also may be active, is something that can be synthesized. This has already been done for thymopoietin, and the synthesized product has shown differentiative activity. Thus we now have at least one substance from the thymus that is biologically active and has been fully defined.

Another substance, 74 amino acids in length, has been isolated by Goldstein *et al.* and defined by Schlesinger *et al.*[92,93] It is not characteristic of the thymus alone, but can be found in many other tissues as well. This has been called ubiquitin. Its terminal, hexadecapeptide, is the activity component. Goldstein and Schlesinger have synthesized part of this molecule, which has been found active in the differentiation of both T and B lymphocytes, whereas the thymic hormone seems largely to be active in the differentiation of T cells only, a relationship that reflects specificity imposed by receptors on the cell surface.

Identification and some understanding of the thymic hormone and ubiquitin have led to studies which have clearly established a succession of events (now defined by Shiku *et al.*[94] and Cantor, Shen, and Boyse[95,96,97]) by the appearance of different surface and functional markers in the T lymphocyte series), leading to a definition of at least two different T cell subpopulations. One of these is a helper population; the second comprises both killer and suppressor subpopulations. The groups differ from one another in the make-up of their LY surface alloantigens. (See Fig. 4). Helper cells are LY1+, LY2−, 3−; whereas the fully differentiated killer and suppressor cells are LY1−, LY2+, 3+. These alloantigens appear to be impeccable specific surface determinants of the two separate populations. It is interesting that there is a precursor for both populations which has LY 1, 2, 3 positivity that is TL negative and Thy 1-LY positive. As the cells become terminally differentiated, they may either lose or take on antigens that characterize their differentiative phase.

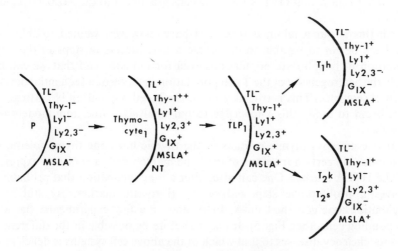

FIG. 4.   Differentiation antigens on the different developmental and functional stages of the mouse T lymphocyte.

Furthermore, one can show for B cell differentiation, as Hämmerling *et al.*[98] have done, that there is also a sequence of differentiation reflected in the development of cell surface characteristics, which can be induced, step-by-step, by the ubiquitin molecule. The first differentiative step to Fg producing cell is followed by a quantum proliferation and then development of IA antigenicity. Subsequently, in a series of developmental steps, the complement receptor, Fc receptor, and the plasma cell surface antigen PC1 appear as the cell develops machinery for massive immunoglobulin synthesis and secretion and becomes a pumper plasma cell. It is heartening to see that we are getting somewhere in defining these steps in B cell development and actually are able to analyze the successive relationships of the various steps in the sequence.

We have also made real progress for humans in defining the sequence of development for T cells. The first thing that seems to appear and on which the other steps depend is the human thymic lymphocyte antigen (HTLA). (See Fig. 5). Capacity to form E rosettes occurs during the second step, but not if HTLA positive cells have been eliminated. If, however, both of these are eliminated, one cannot induce differentiation to Con-A responsive cells or PHA responsive cells. Interestingly, if you induce differentiation to Con-A responsive cells and then eliminate the proliferating cells with bromodeoxyuridine (BUDR) and ultra violet light, you eliminate also the PHA responding cells and the phorbal myristate acetate (PMA) responding cells, but don't touch the MLC responders.[99,100,101] In experimental systems in mice, it has also been possible to show that GVHR inducing cells are linked to the MLC responding cells.

All this is but a minimal scheme. I have, however, wanted to show that we have begun to be able to define the actual successive steps in the differentiation of lymphocyte populations even for humans, and that we can now view the heterogeneity of the T cell population in terms of a sequential developmental sequence. This is true as well for the B cell population.[102] Already we can begin to apply this knowledge to our analysis of the immunodeficiency diseases.

If one employs thymic extracts or the thymic hormone thymopoietin, one can induce in certain fractions of the bone marrow cells a very nice expression of the HTLA marker. One can also, after a long incubation that probably involves a proliferative step, induce the E rosette marker. By still longer incubation, one gets the Con-A, PHA, and, in a few experiments, the MLC responding cells. (See Fig. 5). It may therefore be possible in the different immunodeficiency diseases to find which of the above cell systems is deficient and to determine whether or not it is possible to induce differentiation of a particular step.[103-114]

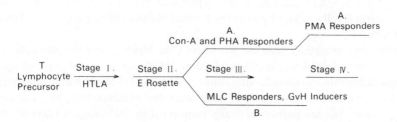

FIG. 5.   Stages of Differentiation of Human T Lymphocytes

While marrow cells of DiGeorge patients will go through the differentiation process, the marrow cells of certain patients with classical forms of SCID
have bone marrow that cannot be induced *in vitro* to develop either E rosettes
or HTLA markers.[115] These patients seem to lack a stem cell that is capable
of responding in a normal way to this sort of *in vitro* inductive influence. The
heterogeneity of SCID has also been defined using differentiation analyses.
Some SCID patients have bone marrow which will respond to form HTLA
phenotypes but cannot readily be induced to develop the E rosette phenotype.[116] This abnormality, like the classical one, is corrected by bone marrow
transplantation.[117] After transplantation, patients with SCID also have cells
which can be induced by a thymic extract to express functional T cell differentiation markers. These steps at first clearly involve transcription and translation, but not cell division. Later steps, however, require DNA synthesis and
probably also division of the cells.[118,119]

A fetal liver transplant which corrects the SCID will sometimes result in
development of peripheral blood cells which can respond to these inducing
effects, but it does not correct the marrow abnormality. This is a fascinating
phenomenon. It probably is explained by the fact that cells from a fetal liver
transplant do not home to the marrow in the normal way. Thus, even though
the abnormality leading to the disease is corrected, the abnormality of the bone
marrow remains. Perhaps the fetal liver cells have set up their stem cell colony in
the liver or spleen, where, I am sure, Dr. DeSousa would say it ought to be.[120]

Fred Siegal in our institute became excited by the tremendous suppressor
cell discovery of Tom Waldmann,[121] which followed up, for humans, the leads
of Gershon.[15,122] Waldmann showed that in common variable immunodeficiency, one part of the lymphoid system could exert an inhibitory influence on
the function of another part. Pokeweed mitogens, for example, cannot induce
peripheral blood cells taken from patients with agammaglobulinemia to differentiate into plasma cells. This suppressor influence operates through a T

lymphocyte. Furthermore, in some instances, lymphocyte cells taken from the peripheral blood of agammaglobulinemic patients were capable, when mixed with normal cells, of suppressing the normal plasma cell response to pokeweed mitogen.

This was intriguing because we knew that Mike Blaese,[123] working with bursectomized chickens, could produce an infectious, acquired form of agammaglobulinemia by transplanting suppressor cells of the bursectomized animals into normal chicks. Investigators have presented evidence that, in some cases, suppressor cells are pathogenetically important in the common variable form of immune deficiency.[121] The supressor cells, however, are also present in patients with the Bruton type agammaglobulinemia,[124] and in the thymoma agammaglobulinemia patients.[125]

Further, applying methods that Y. S. Choi and I developed at Minnesota,[126] in addition to working with different influences on lymphocyte proliferative responses, Stanley Schwartz and Lien Shou, at Sloan-Kettering, have been studying a variety of suppressor cells in both clinical and experimental situations.[127,128] One can study the suppression of immunoglobulin synthesis and secretion, the inhibition of mitogen proliferative responses, responses to common antigens, or to allogeneic cell stimulation. Following the lead of Rich and Pierce,[129] we have been able to induce human T cells to differentiate into suppressor cells by Con-A stimulation or even simply by incubation for two days.[130,131] We know that patients with Bruton's agammaglobulinemia suffer from a remarkable inhibition of immunoglobulin synthesis and secretion. Inhibition seems to occur at the initial point of synthesis in this disease. We do not know yet what is going on in molecular terms, but we now can be hard at work on the problem.

Max Cooper has shown[132] that it is also possible to define a subpopulation of T cells that have a helper capacity. These cells have receptors for IgM or mu chains on their surface. There is also a small population of T cells, a nonhelper variety, which have gamma receptors and which seem under some conditions to act as suppressor cells. We can thus now begin to separate T cell populations physically by these markers and investigate their different functions.

Kishimoto and Ralph[133] supplied our laboratory with one of its most recent findings in this area. Kishimoto came from Osaka University to work with Dr. Peter Ralph in investigating T cell lines and defined one of these as having helper and suppressor capabilities. They found that when pure B cells were stimulated by pokeweed mitogen, there was no proliferation and no differentiation into plasma cells. When pure B cells were, however, placed together with pokeweed mitogen in the presence of T mu cells, you did get proliferation and terminal differentiation of B cells. When pure B cells were, on the other hand, mixed with pokeweed mitogen and T gamma cells, proliferation of B cells occurred, but no final differentiation into plasma cells. In one experiment that Moretta et al.[134] carried out, it was possible to show that T gamma cells exerted a suppressor influence. This seems immensely complex, but as our understanding progresses, it will soon seem much simpler.

With all this new information concerning lymphocyte subclasses, one can see why it is now necessary to talk in terms of a network theory rather than only about T and B cell lines.[135] We must learn to contend with multiple subsets of T cells, multiple subsets of B cells, positive influences and negative influences as well. It rather looks, for the moment at least, that in our immunological game all cards in the deck, not just aces, are wild.

An extremely important aspect of immunobiology is the role played by complement.[136,137] This is an extraordinary biologic amplification system that has been well defined in molecular terms in recent studies which have not only yielded essential knowledge of the complement system in humans and animals, but have now defined diseases caused by deficiency of individual complement components.[137] It has, in fact, been possible to define inherited deficiencies of humans for each of the separate components of the complement cascade, with the exception of C9. It is also clear that illness and disease are associated with each of the specific component abnormalities or deficiencies.

Patients lacking the Cl esterase inhibitor have the well-defined Osler's syndrome. In this disease, painless non-pitting edema, which may be lethal if it affects the larynx, appears from time to time, often after minor trauma or even menstruation. Donaldson, Rosen and coworkers[138,139,140] have studied this disorder extensively and shown that the hereditary angioneurotic edema is due to inherited inability to form a normal inhibitor of the Cl esterase—the activated first component of complement. Pickering et al.[141] showed that attacks of the disease, and thus the major hazard of fatal laryngeal edema, can promptly be aborted by intravenous injection of fresh normal plasma which contains the Cl esterase inhibitor in large amounts. Such therapy is not hazardous and has been most helpful in management of this disease.

This treatment is now, however, probably obsolete because Frank et al.[142] have very recently shown that by treatment with anabolic steroids—the substituted androgens—one can in most of these patients induce the production of the inhibitor and prevent the dangerous attacks. This treatment seems to be able completely to prevent the life-threatening consequences of the immunologically based disorder.

In carrying out our marrow transplantation studies, Ballow et al.[143] found we could also correct deficits of Clq, which are often present in patients with SCID. C2 deficiency has been associated with all manner of interesting diseases, including glomerulonephritis, lupus-like syndromes, recurring infections, and anaphylactic purpura.[11,136,137,144,145] Interestingly, a few patients with C2 deficiency are normal, but most have serious disease problems. An approach allowing for correction of any particular deficiency would therefore be very worthwhile and would surely prevent serious disease in these patients.

In Minneapolis we discovered patients with a C1r deficiency[146,147] and in the first of these the deficiency caused destruction of the kidney.[147] We now know that a deficiency of any of the early components of complement is, in fact, often associated with kidney disease.[146] In a patient we studied with Pickering et al.[148] and Day,[145] we found that a kidney transplant corrected the complement abnormality, since cells in the transplanted organ were able to produce the missing complement component and correct the immunodeficiency disease.[11]

Miller, one of our colleagues working independently in Philadelphia, discovered that the Leiner's syndrome is often associated with an abnormality in phagocytosis of yeast particles. This he associated with an abnormality of C5 function.[149] The important point is that, in these cases, administration of appropriate plasma from normal donors allowed the patients to recover from an otherwise frequently fatal disease and to grow and develop normally. Through this sort of macromolecular therapy one could, in the neonatal period, get them over the life-threatening phase of their disease.[150,151]

Even the confusing transfer factor of Lawrence[152,153,154] seems to be effective in treating some of the most devastating diseases of humans.[155,156,157] One of the most dramatic influences has been in the treatment of some patients with chronic mucocutaneous candidiasis.[158,159,160,161] Approximately 50% of the patients with this disease, especially those with the granulomatous form, have benefited through treatment by transfer factor, an extract of leukocytes. DeSousa et al.[161] found that, while transfer factor did nothing to improve lymphocyte transformation to candida, it did have a positive effect on MIF production and on delayed skin test reactions. It also seemed to have an effect on antibody response (see Table 2).

Ballow et al.[162] and Dupont et al.[163] in our laboratory, and Griscelli in Paris,[164] have ascertained that transfer factor acts in an entirely nonspecific manner. We are, therefore, unable to accept the claim that there is real evidence of specificity associated with this little (2000D) molecule. Our view, I believe, makes transfer factor much more understandable and allows us to create experimental models which now ask the right question, i.e., does the transfer factor molecule enhance an antigen's capacity to produce delayed allergy? This is the kind of experiment we need in order to bring experimental studies in line with the clinical findings. One of the great problems with transfer factor

TABLE 2. Candida specific tests of immune function

Test	Before TF*	After TF
Lymphocyte transformation to candida	−	−
Migration inhibition factor production to candida	−	+
4 hour skin tests to candida	−	+
Anti-candida antibodies:		
IgG	high	falling
IgA	−	normal
IgM	low	normal

*TF = transfer factor
+ = positive
− = negative

HTLA: human thymic lymphocyte antigen
E Rosette: spontaneous rosette formation with sheep erythrocytes (ER)
Con-A: concanavalin A
PHA: phytohemagglutinin
PMA: phorbal myristate acetate
MLC: mixed lymphocyte culture
GvH: graft versus host

is that it has been thought that it acts only in humans and not in experimental animals. This I cannot accept, because everything about immunology that I have really understood holds for laboratory animals as well as for humans. In general, I do not take species differences in immunological processes very seriously, although I expect a few actually exist.

I would like to close with two interesting studies because I think that they too can be translated in very general terms. Lim et al.[165] have worked with the lepromatous form of leprosy and found that this disease features a general deficiency of cell-mediated immunity and deficiency in numbers of T lymphocytes. We found also that the disease process shows very early a selective defect in cellular immune response to antigens of the Lepra bacillus. By giving lepromatous patients, who have in their tissue macrophages large concentrations of the B leprae, a weekly intravenous injection of mismatched leukocytes, mismatched with them and with each of the donors used, we can produce a dramatic therapeutic response to the otherwise progressive infection.

In our initial study[165] we treated 6 patients with lepromatous leprosy in a form that could not be treated by conventional chemotherapy. The leukocyte infusion therapy, given to achieve an allogeneic influence and thus to activate the patients' macrophages, led to dramatic clinical, pathological, and bacteriological resolution of the lesions of lepromatous leprosy. Chemotherapy which had been impossible for these patients prior to the allogeneic cell therapy became possible after this treatment, and the reversal reactions were not seen. We then treated several patients with allogeneic leukocyte therapy before any chemotherapy was given, with similar results.[166,167]

Now why do I say that this accomplishment in a small number of patients is more generally exportable as such? Because it has been possible now in experimental systems to define T helper factors and to show, for example, that T helper substances of animals will even work for human lymphocytes,[168] and because this allogeneic factor is being defined in molecular terms. Thus the dramatic influences on clinical lepromatous leprosy seen with the cellular immunotherapy may soon be translated into therapy with a new biologically active drug. Such therapy is much needed and could perhaps replace not only the obtuse approach of giving injections of mismatched lymphocytes, but also the poor and hazardous drug therapies currently available for treatment of lepromatous leprosy.

The second interesting study focuses on the problems of aging and loss of immunological vigor. NZB and (NZB × NZW)Fl mice provide us with an excellent model for the study of waning immunological vigor with aging. It has been found that before these mice lose their immunological vigor they first lose a population of suppressor cells. Simply by cutting calories in half for the (NZB × NZW)Fl mice, we have been able to double their life span, whether measured as 50% longest survivors, 20% longest survivors 10% longest survivors, or very longest survivor.[169] With a low caloric intake, these animals are healthy little fellows.[134] Furthermore, we have found that a high fat diet accelerates development of autoimmune disease in NZB mice, whereas a lower fat, lower caloric intake delays this and prolongs life.[170,171]

In further studies with NZB mice, we showed that waning immunologic vigor could be forestalled by a low protein diet. This diet interfered also with development of autoimmunity, but it did not prolong life very much.[172] Thus immunodeficiency and autoimmunity that occur with aging in certain strains of mice can be dramatically manipulated by diet.

If we cannot be patient or persistent enough to manipulate the consequences of aging, loss of immunity, and diseases of aging by diet, perhaps there are alternatives. Michael Blaese told me just the other day how his colleagues approached the (NZB × NZW)Fl problem. They have taken lymphocytes from BALB/c mice and stimulated them with Con-A, as Pierce et al. have done[173] to produce soluble immune response suppressors (SIRS). When the supernatant was injected weekly into (NZB × NZW)Fl mice, one derived results similar to those obtained by Fernandes, Yunis and myself in our calorie-cutting experiments. The (NZB × NZW)Fl of Blaese are surviving longer and not developing the autoimmune diseases to which this strain is so prone as a consequence of aging.[174]

From studies of very rare diseases we are beginning to understand immunology well enough to begin to plan cellular and macromolecular engineering with much broader applications for the future. As a final gesture today I would like to make a few predictions. If we continue to maintain intense interaction between the clinic, as the source of our questions, and the very best and toughest of basic science, as the source of our answers, we are going to see a rapidly increased ability to address, treat, and prevent most of the diseases of aging. I believe we will even be able to deal with the problem of malignancy by immunologic approaches.

I feel absolutely certain now that we'll be able—from the immunological approach—to do a real job on cancer because Carey *et al.*[175] and Shiku *et al.*[176] have begun to define malignant melanoma with impeccable serology. These are true tumor specific antigens not found on fibroblasts, embryonic cells, or other cancer cells, but ones that are unique to melanomas and some of which are characteristic of the individual melanoma. This is an extraordinary beginning for human cancer serology.

Levine *et al.* with P. Hakamori, Levine and others with Forssman antigens, and Springer[177] with the Thompson Friedenreich antigen, or T antigen of the T, TN, M, N system of blood group antigens, have shown genetically illegitimate antigens to be present on cancer cells and not present on normal cells. If there are such antigens that one can address immunologically in cancer, then we should ultimately be able to use the immunological machinery, not only to treat the disease, but to develop early diagnoses and modes of immunoprophylaxis as well. Contributing to these achievements will be cellular and macromolecular engineering, as we have been considering them today. Indeed, the macromolecular engineering of immunostimulation is already well launched through major contributions by Lederer *et al.*,[178] Chedid *et al.*[179] and Azuma *et al.*[180]

I have covered much ground today, and I believe given you much to think about. I must make clear that what I have described is, of course, not my work, but is attributable to the splendid young immunologists and scientists with whom I am associated. The new things, which we cannot always reference properly because they are too new, represent their original work. These coworkers and colleagues are: Gabriel Fernandes, Soo Duk Lim, Yong Sung Choi, Genevieve Incefy, Maria DeSousa, Rajendra and Savita Pahwa, Sudhir Gupta, Fred and Marta Siegal, Bo Dupont, John Hansen, Stanley Schwartz, Richard O'Reilly and Katherine Pih. It is to them we must credit the original discoveries and analyses. They are, however, fortunate to be able to work at a time and in a place that fosters constant interaction between bedside and bench, a relationship that is essential to vigorous immunology. I believe this is a major reason why modern immunology is so dynamic.

I am absolutely convinced that we have much to look forward to in the decade ahead.

REFERENCES

1. Jenner, E.: An Inquiry into the Causes and Effects of the Variolae Vaccinae, a Disease Discovered in some of the Western Counties of England, particularly Gloucestershire and Known by the Name of the Cow Pox, Sampson Low, London, 1798.
2. Pasteur, L.: De l'attenuation du virus du cholera des poules, Comptes Rendus de L'Academie des Sciences 91:673, 1880.
3. Landsteiner, K.: Ueber Agglutinationserscheinungen normalen menschlichen Blutes, Wiener klinische Wochenschrift 14:1132, 1901.
4. Von Pirquet, C. and Schick, B.: Die Serumkrankheit, Franz Deuticke, Leipzig/ Wien, 1905.
5. Prausnitz, C. and Kustner, H.: Studien uber die Ueberempfindlichkeit, Centralbl Bakt. 86:160, 1921.
6. Levine, P., Katzin, E. M., and Burnham, L.: Isoimmunization in pregnancy: Its possible bearing on the etiology of erythroblastosis foetalis, J. Amer. Med. Assoc. 116:825, 1941.
7. Kunkel, H. G. Slater, R. J., and Good, R. A.: Relation between certain myeloma proteins and normal gammaglobulins, Proc. Soc. Exp. Biol. Med. 76:190, 1951.
8. Bing, J. and Plum, P.: Serum proteins in leukopenia, Acta Med. Scand. 92:415, 1937.
9. Kolouch, F., Jr.: Origin of bone marrow plasma cell associated with allergic and immune states in the rabbit, Proc. Soc. Exp. Biol. Med. 39:147, 1938.
10. Bruton, O. C.: Agammaglobulinemia, Pediatrics 9:722, 1952.
11. Good, R. A.: Immunodeficiency in developmental perspective, Harvey Lectures, Series 67, Academic Press, New York, 1973.
12. Good, R. A. and Gabrielsen, A. E.: The thymus and other lymphoid organs in the development of the immune system, In: Human Transplantation, (F. T. Rapaport and J. Dausset, eds.), Grune and Stratton, New York, 1968, pp. 526–564.
13. Greaves, M. F., Owen, J. J. T., and Raff, M. C.: T and B Lymphocytes: Origins, Properties and Roles in Immune Responses, Excerpta Medica Amsterdam, American Elsevier Publishing Co., Inc., New York, 1973.
14. Gershon, R. K. and Kondo, K: Cell interactions in the induction of tolerance: The role of thymic lymphocytes, Immunology 18: 723, 1970.
15. Gershon, R. K., Cohen, P., Hencin, R., and Liebhaber, S. A.: Suppressor T cells, J. Immunol. 108:586, 1972.

16. Rich, R. R. and Pierce, C. W.: Biological expressions of lymphocyte activation. II. Generation of a population of thymus-derived suppressor lymphocytes, *J. Exp. Med.* **137**:649, 1973.

17. Rich, R. R. and Rich, S. S.: Biological expressions of lymphocyte activation. IV. Concanavalin A-activated suppressor cells in mouse mixed lymphocyte reactions, *J. Immunol.* **114**:1112, 1975.

18. Gershon, R. K.: T cell regulation of immunity and tolerance, *in*: *Contemporary Topics in Immunobiology*, (M. D. Cooper and N.l L. Warner, eds.), Plenum Press, New York, 1974.

19. Pierce, C. W. and Kapp, J. A.: Regulation of immune responses by suppressor T cells, *In*: *Contemporary Topics in Immunobiology*, Vol. 5, (W. O. Weigle, ed.), Plenum Press, New York, 1976, p. 91.

20. Waldmann, T. A., Broder, S., Blaese, R. M., Durm, M., Blackman, M., and Strober, W.: Role of suppressor T cells in pathogenesis of common variable hypogammaglobulinemia, *Lancet* **2**:609, 1974.

21. Siegal, F. P., Siegal, M., and Good. R. A.: Suppression of B cell differentiation by leukocytes from hypogammaglobulinemic patients, *J. Clin. Invest.* **58**:109, 1976.

22. Parrott, D. M., DeSousa, M. A. B., and East, J.: Thymus-dependent areas in the lymphoid organs of neonatally thymectomized mice, *J. Exp. Med.* **123**:191, 1966.

23. Cooper, M. D., Peterson, R. D. A., South, M. A., and Good, R. A.: The functions of the thymus system and the bursa system in the chicken, *J. Exp. Med.* **123**:75, 1966.

24. Peterson, R. D. A., Cooper, M. D., and Good, R. A.: The pathogenesis of immunologic deficiency diseases, *Am. J. Med.* **38**:579, 1965.

25. Aiuti, F. and Wigzell, H.: A study on human T lymphocytes, their function and frequency in some diseases, *In*: *Microenvironmental Aspects of Immunity*, (B. D. Jankovic and B. Isakovic, eds.;, Plenum Press, New York, 1973, p. 307.

26. Touraine, J. L., Incefy, G. S., Touraine, F., Traeger, J., and Good, R. A.: Antilymphocyte antibodies: An approach to dissecting the heterogeneity of the immune system, *Postgrad. Med. J.* **52**(suppl 5):41, 1976.

27. Good, R. A., Incefy, G. S., and Touraine, J. L.: Human anti-T-cell cytotoxic sera as an approach to dissection of immunological systems, *Postgrad. Med. J.* **52**(suppl 5):35, 1976.

28. Gupta, S. and Grieco, M. H.: Letter: E rosette test, *Lancet* **2**:954, 1974.

29. Gupta, S., Good, R. A., and Siegal, F. P.: Rosette formation with mouse erythrocytes. II. A marker for human B and non T lymphocytes, *Clin. Exp. Immunol.* **25**:319, 1976.

30. Gupta, S., Good, R. A., and Siegal, F. P.: Rosette-formation with mouse erythrocytes. III. Studies in patients with primary immunodeficiency and lymphoproliferative disorders, *Clin. Exp. Immunol.* **26**: 204, 1976.

31. Froland, S. S. and Natvig, J. B.: Identification of three different lymphocyte populations by surface markers, *Transplant. Rev.* **16**: 114, 1973.

32. Cooper, M. D. and Lawton, A. R.,: The development of the immune system, *Sci. Am.* **231**:58, 1974.

33. Kishimoto, T. and Ishizaka, K.: Regulation of antibody response *in vitro*. IX. Induction of secondary anti-hapten IgG antibody response by antiimmunoglobulin and enhancing factor. *J. Immunol.* 114:585, 1975.

34. Kishimoto, T. and Ishizaka, K.: Immunologic and physicochemical properties of enhancing soluble factors for IgG and IgE antibody responses, *J. Immunol.* 114:1177, 1975.

35. Good, R. A. and Yunis, E. J.: Association of autoimmunity, immunodeficiency, and aging in man, rabbits and mice, *Fed. Proc.* 33:2040, 1974.

36. Sigel, M. M. and Good, R. A., eds.: *Tolerance, Autoimmunity and Aging*, American Lecture Series, No. 820, Charles C. Thomas, Springfield, Ill., 1972.

37. Makinodan, T., Good, R. A., and Kay, M. M. B.: Cellular basis of immunosenescence, *In*: *Immunology and Aging*, (T. Makinodan and E. J. Yunis, eds.), Plenum Press, New York. 1977, p. 9 (Comprehensive Immunology vol. 1).

38. Stutman, O., Yunis, E. J., Martinez, C., and Good, R. A.: Reversal of postthymectomy wasting disease in mice by multiple thymus grafts, *J. Immunol.* 98:79,

39. Stutman, O., Yunis, E. J., and Good, R. A.: Functional activity of a chemically induced thymic sarcoma, *Lancet* 1:1120, 1967.

40. Yunis, E. J., Hilgard, H. R., Martinez, C., and Good, R. A.: Studies on immunologic reconstitution of thymectomized mice, *J. Exp. Med.* 121:607, 1965.

41. Biggar, W. D., Stutman, O., and Good, R. A.: Morphological and functional studies of fetal thymus transplants in mice, *J. Exp. Med.* 135:793, 1972.

42. Good, R. A.: Absence of plasma cells from bone marrow and lymph nodes following antigenic stimulation in patients with agammaglobulinemia, *Revue d'Hematologie* 9:502, 1954.

43. Good, R. A.: Studies on agammaglobulinemia. II. Failure of plasma cell formation in the bone marrow and lymph nodes of patients with agammaglobulinemia, *J. Lab. Clin. Med.* 46:167, 1955.

44. Cooper, M. D., personal communication.

45. DiGeorge, A. M.: Congenital absence of the thymus and its immunologic consequences: Concurrence with congenital hypoparathyroidism, *In*: *Immunologic Deficiency Diseases in Man*, (D. Bergsma, ed.) Birth Defects, Original Article Series, The National Foundation-March of Dimes, White Plains, New York, Vol. IV., 1968, p.116.

46. Biggar, W. D., Park, B. H., Stutman, O., Gajl-Peczalska, K., and Good, R. A.: Fetal thymus transplantation: Experimental and clinical observation, *In*: *Immunodeficiency in Man and Animals*, (D. Bergsma, ed., R. A. Good, and J. Finstad, scientific eds.), Sinauer Associates, Inc., Sunderland, Mass., 1975, (Birth Defects, Original Article Series, Vol. XI., no. 1, 1975), p. 361.

47. Aiuti, F., Businco, L., and Gatti, R. A.: Reconstitution of T cell disorders following thymus transplantation, *In*: *Immunodeficiency in Man and Animals*, (D. Bergsma, ed., R. A. Good and J. Finstad, scientific eds.), Sinauer Associates, Inc., Sunderland, Mass., 1975, (Birth Defects, Original Article Series, Vol. XI., no. 1, 1975), p. 370.

48. Hong, R., Santosham, M., Schulte-Wissermann, H., Horowitz, S., Hsu, S. H., and Winkelstein, J. A.: Reconstitution of B and T lymphocyte function in

severe combined immunodeficiency disease following transplantation with thymic epithelium, *Lancet* (in press).

49. Summerlin, W. T., Miller, G. E., and Good, R. A.: Successful tissue and organ allotransplantation without immunosuppression. *J. Clin. Invest.* **52**:83a, 1973.

50. Summerlin, W. T., Brautbar, C., Faanes, R. B., Payne, R., Stutman, O., Hayflick, L., and Good, R. A.: Acceptance of phenotypically differing cultured skin in man and mice, *Transplant. Proc.* **5**:707, 1973.

51. Nezelof, C.: Thymic dysplasia with normal immunoglobulins and immunologic deficiency: pure alymphocytosis, *In: Immunologic Deficiency Diseases in Man*, (D. Bergsma, ed.), Birth Defects, Original Article Series, Vol. IV., The National Foundation-March of Dimes, New York, 1968, p. 104.

52. Trotta, P. P., Smithwick, E. M., and Balis, M. E.: A normal level of adenosine deaminase activity in the red cell lysates of carriers and patients with severe combined immunodeficiency disease, *Proc. Nat'l. Acad. Sci. USA* **73**:104, 1976.

53. Trotta, P. P., Smithwick, E. M., Good, R. A., and Balis, M. E.: Characterization of adenosine deaminase from red cell lysates of carriers and patients with severe combined immunodeficiency, *Fed. Proc.* **35**:1733, 1976, Abstract.

54. Gatti, R. A. Platt, N., Hong, R., Langer, L. O., Kay, H. E. M., and Good, R. A.: Hereditary lymphopenic agammaglobulinemia associated with a distinctive form of short-limbed dwarfism and ectodermal dysplasia, *J. Pediatr.* **75**:675, 1969.

55. Gatti, R. A., Meuwissen, H. J., Allen, H. D., Hong, R., and Good, R. A.: Immunologic reconstitution of sex-linked lymphopenic immunologic deficiency, *Lancet* **2**:1366, 1968.

56. Good, R. A.: Immunologic reconstitution: The achievement and its meaning, *Hospital Practice* **4**:41, 1969.

57. Biggar, W. D., Park, R. H., and Good, R. A.: Compatible bone marrow transplantation and immunologic reconstitution of combined immunodeficiency disease, *In: Immunodeficiency in Man and Animals*, (D. Bergsma, ed., R. A. Good, and J. Finstad, Scientific eds.), Sinauer Associates, Inc., Sunderland, Mass., 1975, (Birth Defects, Original Article Series, Vol. XI., no. 1, 1975), p. 385.

58. O'Reily, R. J., Everson, L. K., Emodi, G., Hansen, J., Smithwick, E. M., Grimes, E., Pahwa, S., Pahwa, R., Schwartz, S., Armstrong, D., Siegal, F. P., Gupta, S., Dupont, B., and Good, R. A.: Effects of exogenous interferon in cytomegalovirus infections complicating bone marrow transplantation, *Clin. Immunol. Immunopathol.* **6**:51, 1976.

59. Lawton, A. R., Bockman, D. E., and Cooper, M. D.: Treatment of autosomal recessive lymphopenic agammaglobulinemia by transplantation of matched allogeneic bone marrow, *Am. J. Med.* **54**:98, 1973.

60. Meuwissen, H. J., Rodey, G., McArthur, J., Pabst, H., Gatti, R., Chilgren, R., Hong, R., Frommel, D., Coifman, R., and Good, R. A.: Bone marrow transplantation: Therapeutic usefulness and complications, *Am. J. Med.* **51**:513, 1971.

61. L'Esperance, P., Hansen, J. A., Jersild, C., O'Reilly, R., Good, R. A., Thomsen,

M., Nielsen, L. S., Svejgaard, A., and Dupont, B.: Bone marrow donor selection among four unrelated locus-identical individuals, *Transplant. Proc.* 7:823, 1975.

62. Koch, C., Henriksen, K., Juhl, F., Andersen, V., Dupont, B., Ernest, P., Good, R. A., Hansen, G. S., Jensen, K., Killmann, S. A., Müller-Berat, N., Svejgaard, A., Thomsen, M., Wiik, A., and Faber, V.: Partial immunological reconstitution in a case of severe combined immunodeficiency by bone marrow transplantation from an HLA non-identical but MLC identical donor, *Lancet* 1:1146, 1973.

63. Faber, V., Svejgaard, A., Thomsen, M., Andersen, V., Astrup, L., Baek, L., Ernst, P., Henningsen, K, Juhl, F., Killmann, S. A., Koch, C., Müller-Berat, N., Permin, H., Philip, J., Platz, P., Jacobsen, R. K., Riewerts-Eriksen, K., Saxtrup, A., Hansen, G. S., Sorensen, H., Tvede, M., and Valerius, N. H.: A preliminary report of bone marrow transplantation from parent to child (both DW2 homozygous) *In*: Proceedings of the Third Workshop of the International Cooperative Group for Bone Marrow Transplantation in Man, Tarrytown, N. Y., 1976.

64. O'Reilly, R., Dupont, B., Pahwa, S., Grimes, E., Pahwa, R., Schwartz, S., Smithwick, E., Svejgaard, A., Jersild, C., Hansen, J., and Good, R. A.: Reconstitution of a child with severe combined immunodeficiency (SCID) and transplant-induced aplasia with marrow from an unrelated, HLA and ABO non-identical MLC compatible donor, *Clin. Res.* 24:482A, 1976. Abstract.

65. Keightley, R. G., Lawton, A. R., Cooper, M. D., and Yunis, E. J.: Successful fetal liver transplantation in a child with severe combined immunodeficiency disease, *Lancet* 2:850, 1975.

66. Buckley, R.: The current status of fetal liver transplantation in SCID, *In*: Proceedings of the Third Workshop of the International Cooperative Group for Bone Marrow Transplantation in Man, Tarrytown, N. Y., 1976.

67. O'Reilly, R. J, Pahwa, R., Pahwa, S., Schwartz, S., Smithwick, E. M., Dupont, B., and Good, R. A.: Fetal tissue transplantation in severe combined immunodeficiency, *In*: Proceedings of the Third Workshop of the International Cooperative Group for Bone Marrow Transplantation in Man, Tarrytown, N. Y., 1976.

68. Bach, F. H., Albertini, R. J., Joo, P., Anderson, J. J., and Bortin, M. M.: Bone marrow transplantation in a patient with Wiskott-Aldrich syndrome, *Lancet* 2:1364, 1968.

69. Meuwissen, H. J.: personal communication.

70. Thomas, E. D., Buckner, C. D., Cheever, M. A., Clift, R. A., Einstein, A. B., Fefer, A., Neiman, P. E., Sanders, J., Storb, R., and Weiden, P. .L: Marrow transplantation for leukemia and aplastic anemia, *Transplant. Proc.* (in press).

71. Advisory Committe of the Bone Marrow Transplant Registry: Bone marrow transplantation from donors with aplastic anemia: A report from the ACS/NIH Bone Marrow Transplant Registry; *JAMA* 236:1131, 1976.

72. The Westminster Hospital Bone-Marrow Transplant Team: Bone-marrow transplant from an unrelated donor for chronic granulomatous disease. *Lancet* 1:210, 1977.

73. Holmes, B., and Good, R. A.: Granulocytic disorders-qualitative abnormalities

of granulocytes. Chronic granulomatous disease, *In*: *Hematology*, (W. J. Williams, E. Beutler, A. J. Erslev, and R. W. Rundles, eds.), McGraw Hill, New York, 1972, pp. 664–670.

74. Gatti, R. A. and Good, R. A.: Lymphoreticular disorders-benign abnormalities of immunoglobulin synthesis. Immunologic deficiency diseases, *In*: *Hematology*, (W. J. Williams, E. Beutler, A. J. Erslev, and R. W. Rundles, eds.), McGraw Hill, New York, 1972, pp. 859–869.

75. Holmes, B., Sater, J., Park, B. H., Rodey, G. E., and Good, R. A.: Degranulation of leukocytes from patients with chronic granulomatous disease of childhood, *J. Clin. Invest.* **5**:232, 1972.

76. Johnston, R. B., Jr., Keale, B. B., Jr., Misra, H. P., Lehmeyer, J. E., Webb, L. S., Baehner, R. L., and Rajagopalan, K. V.: The role of superoxide anion generation in phagocytic bactericidal activity, *J. Clin. Invest.* **55**:1357, 1975.

77. Marsh, W. L., Öyen, R., Nichols, M. E., and Allen, F. H., Chronic granulomatous disease and the Kell blood groups, *Br. J. Haematol.* **29**:247, 1975.

78. Thomas, E. D., Storb, R., Clift, R. A., Fefer, A., Johnson, F. L., Neiman, P. E., Lerner, K. G., Glucksberg, H., and Buckner, C. D.: Bone marrow transplantation, *New Engl. J. Med.* **292**:832, 1975.

79. Thomas, E. D., Storb, R., Clift, R. A., Fefer, A., Johnson, F. L., Neiman, P. E., Lerner, K. G., Glucksberg, H., and Buckner, C. D.: Bone marrow transplantation, *New Engl. J. Med.* **292**:897, 1975.

80. Dale, D. C.: Bone marrow grafting in cyclic neutropenia in dogs, *Transplant Proc.* **8**:575, 1976.

81. Cudkovich, G.: Genetic control of resistance to allogeneic and xenogeneic bone marrow grafts in mice, *Transplant. Proc.* **7**:155, 1975.

82. Woodruff, J. M., Hansen, J. A., Good, R. A., Santos, G. W., and Slavin, R. E.: The pathology of the graft vs. host reaction (GVHR) in adults receiving bone marrow transplants, *Transplant. Proc.* **8**:675, 1976.

83. Thomas, E. D.: Bone marrow transplantation, *In*: *Clinical Immunobiology*, Vol. 2, (F. H. Bach and R. A. Good, eds.), Academic Press, New York, 1964, p. 2.

84. Müller-Rucholtz, W., Wottge, H. L. L., and Müller-Hermelink, H. K.: Bone marrow transplantation in rats across strong histocompatibility barriers by selective elimination of lymphoid cells in donor marrow, *Transplant. Proc.* **8**:537, 1976.

85. Tulunay, O., Good, R. A., and Yunis, E. J.: Protection of lethally irradiated mice with allogeneic fetal liver cells: Influence of irradiation dose on immunologic reconstitution, *Proc. Nat'l. Acad. Sci. USA* **72**:4100, 1975.

86. Yunis, E. J., Fernandes, G., Smith, J., and Good, R. A.: Long survival and immunological reconstitution following transplantation with syngeneic or allogeneic liver and neonatal spleen cells, *Transplant. Proc.* **8**:521, 1976,.

87. Pollard, M., Truitt, R. L., and Ashman, R. B.: Mouse leukemia and solid tumors treated with bone marrow grafting, *Transplant. Proc.* **8**:565, 1976.

88. Truitt, R. L. and Pollard, M.: Allogeneic bone marrow chimerism in germ free mice. IV. Therapy of "Hodgkin's-like" reticulum cell sarcoma in SJL mice, *Transplantation* **21**:12, 1976.

89. Komuro, K. and Boyse, E. A.: *In vitro* demonstration of thymic hormone in the mouse by conversion of precursor cells into lymphocytes, *Lancet* **1**:740, 1973.

126   R. A. Good and M. A. Hansen

90. Komuro, K. and Boyse, E. A.: Induction of T lymphocytes from precursor cells *in vitro* by a product of the thymus, *J. Exp. Med.* 138:479, 1973.
91. Goldstein, G.: The isolation of thymopoietin (thymin), *Ann. N.Y. Acad. Sci*, 249:177, 1975.
92. Goldstein, G., Scheid, M., and Hammerling, U.,: Isolation of a polypeptide that has lymphocyte-differentiating properties and is probably represented universally in living cells, *Proc. Nat'l. Acad. Sci. USA* 72:11, 1975.
93. Schlesinger, D. H., Goldstein, G., and Niall, H. D.: The complete amino acid sequence of ubiquitin, an adenylate cyclase stimulating polypeptide probably universal in living cells, *Biochemistry* 14:2214, 1975.
94. Shiku, H., Kisielow, P., Bean, M. A., Takahashi, T., Boyse, E. A., Oettgen, H., and Old, L. J.: Expression of T cell differentiation antigens on effector cells in cell-mediated cytotoxicity *in vitro*. Evidence for functional heterogeneity related to the surface phenotype of cells, *J. Exp. Med.* 141:227, 1975.
95. Cantor, H. and Boyse, E. A.: Functional subclasses of T lymphocytes bearing different Ly antigens. I. The generation of functionally distinct T cell subclasses is a differentiative process independent of antigen. *J. Exp. Med.* 141: 1376, 1975.
96. Cantor, H. and Boyse, E. A.: Functional subclasses of T lymphocytes bearing different Ly antigens. II. Cooperation between subclasses of Ly+ cells in the generation of killer activity, *J. Exp. Med.* 141:1390, 1975.
97. Cantor, H., Shen, F. W., and Boyse, E. A.: Separation of helper T cells from suppressor T cells expressing different Ly components. II. Activation by antigen: After immunization, antigen-specific suppressor and helper activities are mediated by distinct T cell subclasses. *J. Exp. Med.* 143:1391, 1976.
98. Hämmerling, U., Chin, A. F., and Abbott, J.: Ontogeny of murine B lymphocytes: Sequence of B cell differentiation from surface immunoglobulin-negative precursors to plasma cells. *Proc. Nat'l. Acad. Sci. USA* 73:2008, 1976.
99. Touraine, J. L., Touraine, F., Hadden, J. W., Hadden, E. M., and Good, R. A.: 5-Bromodeoxyuridine-light inactivation of human lymphocytes stimulated by mitogens and allogeneic cells: Evidence for distinct T lymphocyte subsets, *Int. Arch. Allergy Appl. Immunol.* 52:105, 1976.
100. Touraine, J. L., Hadden, J. W., Touraine, F., Hadden, E. M., Estensen, R., and Good, R. A.: Phorbol myristate acetate: A mitogen selective for a T lymphocyte subpopulation, *J. Exp. Med.* 145:460, 1977.
101. Touraine, J. L., Hadden, J. W. and Good, R. A.: Sequential stages of human T lymphocyte differentiation, *Proc. Nat'l. Acad. Sci. USA.* 74:3414, 1977.
102. Cooper, M. D. and Lawton, A. R., 3rd. The development of the immune system, *Sci. Am.* 231:58-72, 1974.
103. Touraine, J. L., Touraine, F., Kiszkiss, D. F., Choi, Y. S., and Good, R. A.: Heterologous specific antiserum for identification of human T lymphocytes. *Clin. Exp. Immunol.* 16:503, 1974.
104. Touraine, J. L., Incefy, G. S., Touraine, F., Rho, Y. M., and Good, R. A.: Differentiation of human bone marrow cells into T lymphocytes by *in vitro* incubation with thymic extracts, *Clin. Exp. Immunol.* 17:151, 1974.
105. Touraine, J. L., Incefy, G. S., Touraine, F., L'Esperance, P., Siegal, F. P., and

Good, R. A.: T-lymphocyte differentiation *in vitro* in primary immunodeficiency diseases, *Clin. Immunol. Immunopathol.* **3**:228, 1974.

106. Incefy, G. S., Touraine, J. L., Touraine, F., L'Esperance, P., Siegal, F. P., and Good, R. A.: *In vitro* studies on human T lymphocyte differentiation in primary immunodeficiency diseases. *Trans. Assoc. Am. Phys.* **87**:258, 1974.

107. Incefy, G. S., L'Esperance, P., and Good, R. A.: *In vitro* differentiation of human marrow cells into T lymphocytes by thymic extracts using the rosette technique. *Clin. Exp. Immunol.* **19**:475, 1975.

108. Touraine, J. L., Touraine, F., Incefy, G. S., and Good, R. A.: Effect of thymic factors on the differentiation of human marrow cells into T-lymphocytes *in vitro* in normals and patients with immunodeficiencies. *Ann. N.Y. Acad. Sci.* **249**:335, 1975.

109. Touraine, J. L., Kiszkiss, D. F., Choi, Y. S., and Good, R. A.: T-cells in immunodeficiencies as evaluated by an anti-human T-cell serum, *In*: *Immunodeficiency in Man and Animals* (D. Bergsma, ed., R. A. Good and J. Finstad, scientific eds.), Sinauer Associates, Sunderland, Mass., 1975, (Birth Defects, Original Article Series, Vol. XI., no. 1, 1975), p. 22.

110. Touraine, J. L., Touraine, F., Incefy, G. S., Goldstein, A. L., and Good, R. A.: Thymic factors and human T lymphocyte differentiation, *In*: *The Biological Activity of Thymic Hormones, Proceedings*, (D. W. van Bekkum, ed.), Kooyker Scientific Publications, Rotterdam, The Netherlands, 1975, p. 31.

111. Incefy, G. S., Boumsell, L., Touraine, J. L., L'Esperance, P., Smithwick, E., O'Reilly, R., and Good, R. A.: Enhancement of T-lymphocyte differentiation *in vitro* by thymic extracts after bone marrow transplantation in severe combined immunodeficiencies, *In*: *The Biological Activity of Thymic Hormones, Proceedings*, (D. W. van Bekkum, ed.), Kooyker Scientific Publications, Rotterdam, The Netherlands, 1975, p. 43.

112. Incefy, G. S., Boumsell, L., Touraine, J. L., L'Esperance, P., Smithwick, E., O'Reilly, R., and Good, R. A.: Enhancement of T lymphocyte differentiation *in vitro* by thymic extracts after bone marrow transplantation in severe combined immunodeficiencies, *Clin. Immunol. Immunopathol.* **4**:258, 1975.

113. Boumsell, L., Incefy, G. S., Bernard, A., Schwartz, S., Smithwick, E., and Good, R. A.: T lymphocyte differentiation *in vitro* in ataxia telangiectasia associated with lymphosarcoma. *J. Pediatr.* **87**:435, 1975.

114. Vogel, J. E., Incefy, G. S., and Good, R. A.: Differentiation of population of peripheral blood lymphocytes into cells bearing sheep erythrocyte receptors *in vitro* by human thymic extract. *Proc. Nat'l. Acad. Sci.* **72**:1175, 1975.

115. Incefy, G. S., Boumsell, L., Kagan, W., Goldstein, G., deSousa, M., Smithwick, E., O'Reilly, R., and Good, R. A.: Enhancement of T lymphocyte differentiation *in vitro* by thymic extracts and purified polypeptides in severe combined immunodeficiency diseases. *Trans. Assoc. Am. Phys.* **88**:135, 1975.

116. Incefy, G. S., Grimes, E., Kagan, W. A., Goldstein, G., Smithwick, E., O'Reilly, R., and Good, R. A.: Heterogeneity of stem cells in severe combined immunodeficiency, *Clin. Exp. Immunol.* **25**:462. 1976.

117. Incefy, G. S., Smithwick, E., O'Reilly, R., and Good, R. A.: *In vitro* differentiation of human marrow cells. The influence of bone marrow and fetal liver plus thymus transplantation of differentiable stem cell populations in SCID. *In*: Proceedings of The Third Workshop of The International Cooper-

ative Group for Bone Marrow Transplantation in Man, Tarrytown, N. Y. 1976.

118. Incefy, G. S. and Good, R. A.: The need for transcription and translation for differentiation of bone marrow cells by thymic factors in man. *In*: Fifth International Conference on Lymphatic Tissue and Germinal Centers in Immune Reactions, Tiberias, Israel, 1975. Immune Reactivity of Lymphocytes: *Development, Expression, and Control, Proceedings* (M. Feldman and A. Globerson, eds.), Plenum Press, New York, 1976, p. 41.

119. Incefy, G. S., Goldstein, G., and Good, R.. A: Studies on DNA, RNA and protein synthesis during human bone marrow cell differentiation induced *in vitro* by human thymic extracts and thymopoietin, (submitted for publication).

120. de Sousa, M., Yang, M., Lopez-Corrales, E., Tan, C., Hansen, J.A., Dupont, B. and Good, R.A.: Ecotaxis: the principle and its application to the study of Hodgkin's disease. *Clin. Exp. Immunol.* 27:143, 1977.

121. Waldmann, T. A., Durm, M., Broder, S., Blackman, M., Blaese, M., and Strober, W.: Role of suppressor T cells in pathogenesis of common variable hypogammaglobulinemia, *Lancet* 2:609, 1974.

122. Gershon, R. K.: T cell control of antibody production, Contemp. *Immunobiol.* 3:1, 1974.

123. Blaese, R. M., Weiden, P. L., Koski, I., and Dooley, N.: Infectious agammaglobulinemia: Transmission of immunodeficiency with grafts of agammaglobulinemic cells, *J. Exp. Med.* 140:1097, 1974.

124. Siegal, F. P., Siegal, M., and Good, R. A.: Suppression of B cell differentiation by leukocytes from hypogammaglobulinemic patients, *J. Clin. Invest.* 58: 109, 1976.

125. Waldmann, T. A., Broder, S., Urm, M., Blackman, M., Krakauer, R., and Meade, B.: The role of suppressor T cells in the pathogenesis of hypogammaglobulinemia with a thymoma, *Trans. Assoc. Am. Physicans*, 88:120, 1975.

126. Choi. Y. S., Biggar, W. D., and Good, R. A.: Biosynthesis and secretion of immunoglobulins by peripheral blood lymphocytes in severe hypogammaglobulinemia, *Lancet* 1:1149, 1972.

127. Shou, L., Schwartz, S. A., and Good, R. A.: Suppressor cell activity after concanavalin A treatment of lymphocytes from normal donors, *J. Exp. Med.* 143:1100, 1976.

128. Schwartz, S. A., Choi, Y. S., Shou, L., and Good, R. A.: Modulatory effects on immunoglobulin synthesis and secretion by lymphocytes from immunodeficient patients, *J. Clin. Invest.* 59:1176, 1977.

129. Rich, R. R. and Pierce, C. W.: Biological expressions of lymphocyte activation. II. Generation of population of thymus-derived suppressor lymphocytes, *J. Exp. Med.* 137:649, 1973.

130. Shou, L.: Immunoregulatory activities in human peripheral blood lymphocytes: A thesis presented to the faculty of the Graduate School of Cornell University for the degree of Doctor of Philosophy, November, 1976.

131. Schwartz, S. A., Shou, L., Good, R. A. and Choi, Y. S.: Suppression of immunoglobulin synthesis and secretion by peripheral blood lymphocytes

from normal donors, *Proc. Natl, Acad. Sci, USA.* **74**:2099, 1977.
132. Cooper, M. D.: personal communication.
133. Kishimoto, T., Ralph, P., and Good, R. A.: Stimulation of a human B lymphocyte line by anti-immunoglobulin and its concanavalin A induced suppression by a T cell line, *Clin. Exp. Immunol.* (in presss)
134. Moretta, L., Webb, S. R., Grossi, C. E., Lydyard, P. M., and Cooper, M. D.: Functional analysis of two subpopulations of human T cells and their distribution in immunodeficient patients, *Clin. Res. Abstract* **24**:448A, 1976.
135. Jerne, N. K.: Towards a network theory of the immune system, *Ann. Immunol.* (Paris) **125c**:373, 1974.
136. Müller-Eberhard, H. J.: Complement, *Ann. Rev. Biochem.* **44**:679, 1975.
137. Day, N.K., and Good, R.A., eds., *Biological Amplification Systems in Immunology*, Plenum Press, New York, (Comprehensive Immunology Vol. 2, 1977).
138. Donaldson, V. H. and Evans, R. R.: A biochemical abnormality in hereditary angioneurotic edema: Absence of serum inhibitor of C'1 esterase, *Am. J. Med.* **35**:37, 1963.
139. Donaldson, V. H. and Rosen, F. S.: Action of complement in hereditary angioneurotic edema: The role of C'1 esterase: *J. Clin. Invest.* **43**:2204, 1964.
140. Rosen, F. S., and Alper, C. A.: Disorders of the complement system, *in: Immunologic Disorders in Infants and Children*, (E. R. Stiehm and V. A. Fulginiti, eds.), W. B. Saunders, Co., Philadelphia, 1973, p. 289.
141. Pickering, R. J., Kelly, J. R., Good, R. A., and Gewurz, H.: Replacement therapy in hereditary angioedema: Successful treatment of two patients with fresh frozen plasma, *Lancet* **1**:326, 1969.
142. Frank, M. M., Gelfand, J. A., and Atkinson, J. P.: Hereditary angioedema: The clinical syndrome and its management, *Ann. Intern. Med.* **84**:580, 1976.
143. Ballow, M., Day, N. K., Biggar, W. D., Park, B. H., Yount, W. J., and Good, R. A.: Reconstitution of C1q following bone marrow transplantation in patients with severe combined immunodeficiency, *Clin. Immunol. Immunopathol.* **2**:28, 1973.
144. Day, N. K., Geiger, H., McLean, R., Michael, A., and Good, R. A.: C2 deficiency: Recognition of systemic lupus erythematosus, *J. Clin. Invest.* **52**:1601, 1973.
145. Day, N. K. and Good R. A.: Deficiencies of the complement system in man *in: Immunodeficiency in Man and Animals*, (D. Bergsma, ed., R. A. Good and J. Finstad, scientific eds.) Sinauer Associates, Sunderland, Mass., 1975, (Birth Defects, Original Article Series, Vol XI, no. 1, 1975), p. 306.
146. Pickering, R. J., Naff, G. B., Stroud, R. M., Good, R. A., and Gewurz, H.: Deficiency of C1r in human serum: Effects on the structure and function of macromolecular C1, *J. Exp. Med.* **141**:803, 1970.
147. Day, N. K., Geiger, H., Stroud, R., deBracco, M., Moncada, B., Windhorst, D., and Good, R. A.: C1r deficiency: An inborn error associated with cutaneous and renal disease, *J. Clin. Invest.* **51**:1102, 1972.
148. Pickering, R. J., Michael A. F., Herdman, R. C., Good, R. A., and Gewurz, H.: The complement system in chronic glomerulonephritis in three newly-associated aberrations, *J. Pediatr.* **78**:30, 1971.
149. Miller, M. E., Seals, J., Kaye, R., and Levitsky, L. C.: A familial plasma-

associated defect of phagocytosis: A new cause of recurrent bacterial infections, *Lancet* 1:60, 1968.

150. Miller, M. E. and Nilsson, U. R.: A familial deficiency of the phagocytosis-enhancing activity of serum related to a dysfunction of the fifth component of complement (C5), *New Engl. J. Med.* 282:354, 1970.

151. Miller, M. E. and Koblenzer, P. J.: Leiner's disease and deficiency of C5, *J. Pediatr.* 80:879, 1972.

152. Lawrence, H. S.: The transfer in humans of delayed skin sensitivity to streptococcal M substance and to tuberculin with disrupted leukocytes, *J. Clin. Invest.* 34:219, 1955.

153. Lawrence, H. S., Al-Askari, S., David, J. R., Franklin, E. C., and Zweiman, B.: Transfer of immunological information in humans with dialysates of leukocyte extracts, *Trans, Assoc. Amer. Physicians* 76:84, 1963.

154. Lawrence, H. S.: Transfer factor, *Adv. Immunol.* 11:195, 1969.

155. Levin, A. S., Spitler, L. E., and Fudenberg, H. H.: Transfer factor I. Methods of therapy, *in*: *Immunodeficiency in Man and Animals*, (D. Bergsma, ed., R. A. Good and J. Finstad, scientific eds.), Sinauer Associates, Sunderland, Mass., 1975, (Birth Defects, Original Article Series, Vol. XI., no. 1, 1975), p. 445.

156. Spitler, L. E., Levin, A. S., and Fudenberg, H. H.: Transfer factor II. Results of therapy, *in*: *Immunodeficiency in Man and Animals*, (D. Bergsma, ed., R. A. Good and J. Finstad, Scientific eds.), Sinauer Associates, Sunderland, Mass., 1975, (Birth Defects, Original Article Series, Vol. VI., on. 1, 1975), p. 449.

157. Rocklin, R. E.: Use of transfer factor in patients with depressed cellular immunity and chronic infection, *in*: *Immunodeficiency in Man and Animals*, (D. Bergsma, ed., R. A. Good and J. Finstad, scientific eds.), Sinauer Associates, Sunderland, Mass., 1975, (Birth Defects, Original Article Series, Vol. XI, no. 1, 1975) p. 431.

158. Schulkind, M. L., and Ayoub, E. M.: Transfer factor as an approach to the treatment of immune deficiency disease, *in*: *Immunodeficiency in Man and Animals*, (D. Bergsma, ed., R. A. Good and J. Finstad, scientific eds.,) Sinauer Associates, Sunderland, Mass., 1975, (Birth Defects, Original Article Series, Vol. XI, no. 1, 1975) p. 436.

159. Valdimarsson, H., Wood, C. B. S., Hobbs, J. R., and Holt, P. J. L.: Immunological features in a case of chronic granulomatous candidiasis and its treatment with transfer factor, *Clin. Exp. Immunol.* 11:151, 1972.

160. Jose, D. G.: Treatment of chronic mucocutaneous candidiasis by lymphocyte transfer factor, *Aust. N. Z. J. Med.* 5:318, 1975.

161. de Sousa, M., Cochran, R., Mackie, R., Parrott, D., and Arala-Chaves, M.: Chronic mucocutaneous candidiasis treated with transfer factor, *Br. J. Dermatol.* 94:79, 1976.

162. Ballow, M., Dupont, B., Hansen, J. A., and Good, R. A.: Transfer factor Therapy: Evidence for nonspecificity, *in*: *Immunodeficiency in Man and Animals*, (D. Bergsma, ed., R. A. Good and J. Finstad, scientific eds.), Sinauer Associates, Sunderland, Mass., 1975, (Birth Defects, Original Article Series, Vol XI., no. 1, 1975), p. 457.

163. Dupont, B., Ballow, M., Hansen, J. A., Quick, C., Yunis, E. J., and Good,

R. A.: Effect of transfer factor therapy on mixed lymphocyte culture reactivity, *Proc. Nat'l. Acad. Sci. USA* **71**:867, 1974.

164. Griscelli, C.: Transfer factor therapy in immunodeficiency, in: *Immunodeficiency in Man and Animals*, (D. Bergsma, ed., R. A. Good and J. Finstad, scientific eds.), Sinauer Associates, Sunderland, Mass., 1975, (Birth Defects, Original Article Series, Vol. XI., no. 1, 1975), p. 462.

165. Lim, S. D., Kiszkiss, D. F., Choi, Y. S., Gajl-Peczalska, K., and Good. R. A.: Immunodeficiency in leprosy, in: *Immunodeficiency In Man and Animals*, (D. Bergsma, ed., R. A. Good and J. Finstad, scientific eds.), Sinauer Associates, Sunderland, Mass., 1975, (Birth Defects, Original Article Series, Vol.XI., no.1, 1975), p. 244.

166. Lim, S. D., Fusaro, R. M., and Good, R. A.: Leprosy VI. The treatment of leprosy patients with intravenous infusions of leukocytes from normal persons, *Clin. Immunol. Immunopathol.* **1**:122, 1972.

167. Lim, S. D., Touraine, J. L., Storkan, M. A., Choi, Y. S., and Good, R. A.: Leprosy XI. Evaluation of thymus-derived lymphocytes by an antihuman T lymphocyte antiserum, *Int. J. Lepr.* **42**:260, 1974.

168. Taussig, M. J., Munro, A. J., and Luzzati, A. L.: I-Region gene products in cell cooperation, in: *The Role of Products of the Histocompatibility Gene Complex in Immune Responses*, (D. H. Katz and B. Benacerraf, eds.), Academic Press, Inc., New York, 1976.

169. Fernandes, G., Yunis, E. J., and Good, R. A.: Influence of diet on survival of mice, *Proc. Nat'l. Acad. Sci.* **73**:1279, 1976.

170. Fernandes, G., Yunis, E. J., Smith, J., and Good, R. A.: Dietary influence on breeding behaviour, hemolytic anemia, and longevity in NZB mice, *Proc. Soc. Exp. Biol. and Med.* **139**:1189, 1972.

171. Fernandes, G., Yunis, E. J., Jose, D. G., and Good, R. A.: Dietary influence on antinuclear antibodies and cell-mediated immunity in NZB mice, *Int. Arch. Allergy* **44**:770, 1973.

172. Fernandes, G., Yunis, E. J., and Good, R. A.: Influence of protein restriction on immune functions in NZB mice, *J. Immunol.* **116**:782, 1976.

173. Pierce, C. W., Tadakuma, T., Kühner, A. L., and David, J. R.: Characterization of a soluble immune response suppressor (SIRS) produced by concanavalin A-activated spleen cells, in: *The Role of Mitogens in Immunobiology*, (J. J. Oppenheim and D. L. Rosenstreich, eds.), Academic Press, New York, 1976.

174. Blaese, M.: personal communication.

175. Carey, T. E., Takahashi, T., Resnick, L. A., Oettgen, H. F., and Old, L. J.: Cell surface antigens of human malignant melanoma. I. Mixed hemadsorption assays for humoral immunity to cultured autologous melanoma cells, *Proc. Nat'l. Acad. Sci.* **73**:3278, 1976.

176. Shiku, H., Takahashi, T., Oettgen, H. F., and Old, L. J.: Cell surface antigens of human malignant melanoma. II. Serological typing with immune adherence assays and definition of two new surface antigens, *J. Exp. Med.* **144**:873, 1976.

177. Springer, G. F., Desai, P. R., and Banatwala, I.: Blood group MN antigens and precursors in normal and malignant human breast glandular tissue, *J. Nat'l. Cancer Inst.* **54**:335, 1975.

178. Lederer, E., Adam, A., Ciorbaru, R., Petit, J. F., and Wietzerbin, J.: Cell walls

132   R. A. Good and M. A. Hansen

of mycobacteria and related organisms: Chemistry and immunostimulant
properties, *Mol. Cell. Biochem.* **7**:87, 1975.
179. Chedid, L., Audibert, F., Lefrancier, P., Choay, J., and Lederer, E.: Modulation
of the immune response by a synthetic adjuvant and analogs, *Proc. Nat'l.
Acad. Sci. USA* **73**:2472, 1976.
180. Azuma, I., Kanetsuna, F., Taniyama, T., and Yamamura, Y.: Adjuvant activity
of mycobacterial fractions I Purification and *in vitro* adjuvant activity of
cell wall skeletons of Mycobacterium bovis BCG, Nocardia asteroides 131
and Corynebacterium diphtheriae PW8, *Biken J.* **181**:1, 1975.

DISCUSSION

Dr. SOOTHILL: The classification of immunodeficiency as T-cell and B-cell defects,
of course, was nonsense in any Mendelian inheritance, because enzymes are
controlled by single genes, not cells. The T- and the B-cell classifications have
been extraordinarily useful in focusing our attention on the genetics involved in
the control of differentiation, and it is very clear that we are now beginning to
be able to understand and analyse the cellular deficiencies in terms that may
make for better definitions of diseases. We have always wanted to get a genetic
definition, and after a genetic definition, then an enzymatic or a peptide definition; that is the direction in which one must go. But one must sometimes go
through cellular biology in order to get to the enzymes, as for example with the
fatal granulomatous disease.
Dr. TADA: The various deficiencies of this complement component are related to
the HLA complex. Is that really the linkage or association?
Dr. GOOD: I think it is the linkage. It is very clear in the mouse, and I think that
mice and man are very similar, that C4 or the SS-defined complement component
is actually controlled by genes that operate between the D and the K end of the
mouse major histocompatibility system. In man we have excellent evidence that
the controls of C2 and probably also C4 are closely associated with HLA-D.
This is also the part of the mouse major histocompatibility system that lies
between the K and the D end.

Differentiation of Thymus Epithelium in Nude Mice and Human Immunodeficiency

Norikazu TAMAOKI and Junichi HATA

ABSTRACT

The development of the thymus has at least two steps. The first step is the induction of thymocytes from precursor cells which requires the microenvironment formed by squamous epithelium. The glandular epithelium in nude mice seems to lack induction ability at this step. The second step is the development of mature T cells, probably under the influence of humoral factor(s), in addition to microenvironment. The latter step is likely to be related to development of secretory epithelial cells in the medulla.

Human thymic dysplasia is probably a defect in the first step of T cell development corresponding to that of nude mice. Thymic changes including abnormal Hassall's corpuscles and medullary epithelial cells are found in Down's syndrome and congenital biliary atresia. This type of abnormality results from a developmental disorder in late fetal life, probably related to intrauterine infection.

In the search for information on the role of the thymus in the development of T cells, thymic dysplasia in nude mice is considered to be a pertinent model for human immunodeficiency. The defect in nude mice exists at the level of the thymus as shown by experiments proving that immunological function can be reconstituted by host-type cells after thymus grafting.[1] Recent studies also indicate that the target of thymic function is not stem cells but committed prethymic cells, since weak θ-positive cells demonstrated by heteroantibody accumulate in the spleen of nude mice.[2]

We have examined the prenatal and postnatal thymus of both nude and normal mice by electron microscopy to find the relation of epithelial defect to the development of thymocytes. The findings on animals were compared with changes in the human thymus in various immunological disorders in childhood.

Department of Pathology, Tokai University School of Medicine, Isehara, Kanagawa, Japan

133

Electron microscopic findings of thymic anlage in nude mice

The mouse embryos were obtained by mating female BALB/c-*nu/nu* mice with male *nu/nu* or +/+ mice of the same genetical background. In this mating system, the littermates are genetically homogeneous and the possible effect of the maternal thymic humoral factor as well as transplacental migration of maternal T cells can be avoided.

The thymus of heterozygous (*nu*/+) normal mice at 13 and 15 days of gestation contains lymphoblasts with many ribosomes, several dense bodies and prominent nucleoli (Fig. 1). Epithelial cells in normal mice show many desmosomes and abundant tonofilaments indicating the differentiation towards squamous epithelial cells (Fig. 2).

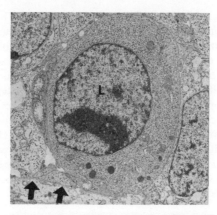

FIG. 1.   The thymus of a 15-day normal embryo (BALB/c-*nu*/+).
A lymphoblast (L) with large prominent nucleolus and cytoplasm containing many polysomes and several dense bodies is seen among epithelial cells with basement membrane (arrows).   ×6,600

On the other hand the thymus of homozygous (*nu/nu*) nude mice at 15 days of gestation consists of primitive epithelial cells with abundant glycogen and few desmosomes. After 18 days, the thymus in nude mice shows glandular lumina lined by epithelial cells with microvilli and becomes cystic after birth (Fig. 3).[3,4,5] Although very few in number, large lymphoblasts identical to those found in normal thymus are found among primitive thymic epithelial cells in nude mice from 15 days of gestation to the neonatal period (Fig. 4). It is likely that these lymphoblasts are prethymic cells migrating into rudimental thymus, since some lymphoblasts are crossing the basement menbrane of thymic epithelium (Fig. 5).

Large epithelial cells containing inclusions probably related to the secretion

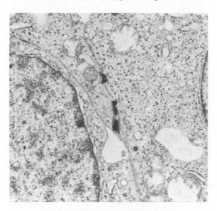

FIG. 2. Many desmosomes with tonofilaments are found in thymic epithelial cells of a 15-day normal embryo. ×13,000

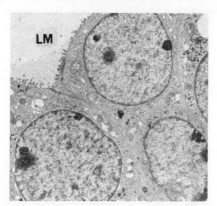

FIG. 3. The thymus of a 15-day nude embryo (BACB/c-*nu*/*nu*) consists of primitive epithelial cells with microvilli surrounding the lumen (LM). ×4,000

of thymic humoral factor do not appear until 18 days when thymic medulla begins to separate from the cortex in normal mice (Fig. 6). These secretory epithelial cells are lacking in nude mice.[4]

These findings indicate that the first step in the differentiation of thymocytes takes place around 13 days within the microenvironments formed by squamous epithelial cells. On the other hand, glandular epithelium in nude mice appears unable to induce thymocytes from precursor cells. Secretory epithelial cells in the thymic medulla appear to be related to the further maturation of T line-

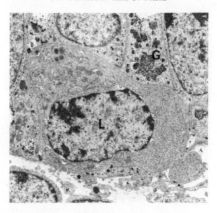

FIG. 4. A lymphoblast (L) identical with that in Fig. 1 in the thymic anlage of a 15-day nude embryo.
Epithelial cells contain abundant glycogen (G) and few desmosomes. ×6,600

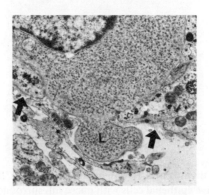

FIG. 5. A portion of cytoplasm of lymphoblast (L) is present outside of basement membrane (arrows), suggesting the migration of precursor cells into the thymic anlage of a 15-day nude embryo. ×10,000

age cells which takes place around and after birth both in and outside the thymus.

Thymus in human immunodeficiency

A histological survey on the thymuses of 211 children has revealed two types of epithelial changes. One is the well-established dysplastic thymus con-

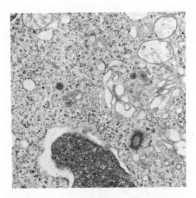

FIG. 6. An epithelial cell in the medulla of an 18-day normal embryo contains membrane-bound granules around Golgi apparatus suggesting secretory activity. ×30,000

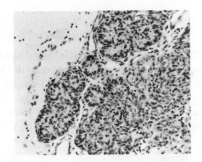

FIG. 7. The rudimentary thymus of severe combined immunodeficiency composed of epithelial cells showing acinous pattern. H & E. ×400

sisting of primitive epithelial cells sometimes arranged in an acinous pattern and devoid of Hassall's corpuscles and cortico-medullary distinction (Fig. 7). Judging from the morphological similarity, this type of thymic dysplasia could be interpreted as a human counterpart of that of nude mice, suggesting that the defect lies in the step from prethymic cells to thymocytes, probably due to insufficient epithelial development. However, the defect in B cells and/or in stem cells which almost inevitably accompanies severe combined immunodeficiency has not been demonstrated in nude mice.

The thymic change of the other type is found in Down's syndrome and congen-

138   N. Tamaoki and J. Hata

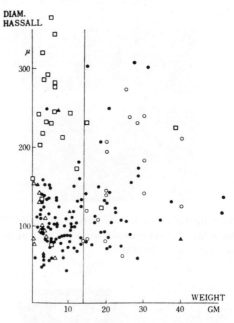

FIG. 8   The diameter of Hassall's corpuscles and weight of the thymus
in children. The diameter is significantly larger in Down's syndrome
than in other diseases, in cases with the thymus weighing under 14 gm.
Open square (□): Down's syndrome. Open triangle (△): 18 trisomy.
Solid triangle (▲): multiple malformation. Solid circle (●): congenital
heart disease. Open circle (○): accidental death.

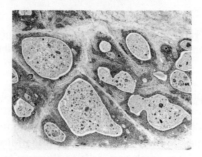

FIG. 9.   Cystic dilatation of Hassall's corpuscles seen in the thymus
of Down's syndrome. H & E. ×16

ital biliary atresia. The thymus in Down's syndrome shows severe involution
and significantly large Hassall's corpuscles compared with other diseases,

especially in the involuted thymus weighing under 14 gm[6] (Fig. 8 and Fig. 9). Immunologically, Down's syndrome is known to have an abnormal immunoglobulin level and susceptibility to infection. In congenital biliary atresia, the thymus shows marked hypoplasia or involution with fibrosis. In our study, Hassall's corpuscles were large and cystic in 9 cases and hypoplastic or absent in 11 out of 24 cases.[7] The changes seen in these two disorders are probably due to destructive processes in late fetal life after completion of thymic structure and may result in defective production of T cells. The etiology is likely to be related to viral infection *in utero*.

REFERENCES

1. Wortis, H. H., Nehlsen, S., and Owen, J. J.: Abnormal development of the thymus in "nude" mice. *J. Exp. Med.* **134**:681, 1971.
2. Loor, F. and Roelants, G. E.: High frequency of T lineage lymphocytes in nude mouse spleen. *Nature* **251**:229, 1974.
3. Cordier, A. C.: Ultrastructure of the thymus in "nude" mice. *J. Ultrast. Res.* **47**: 26, 1974.
4. Tamaoki, N. and Esaki, K.: Electron microscopic observation of the thymus and lymph nodes of the nude mouse. Proc. 1st International Workshop on Nude Mice. J. Rygaard and C. O. Povlsen, eds., Stuttgart, Gustav Fischer, 1974.
5. Groscurth, P. and Kistler, G.: Histogenese des Immunsystems der "nude" Maus IV Ultrastruktur der thymusanlage 12-und 13 tägiger Embryonen. *Beitr. Path.* **156**:359, 1975.
6. Tamaoki, N.: Pathology of the thymus in immunological disorders with special reference to autoimmune diseases. *Trans. Soc. Path. Jap.* **64**(suppl):74, 1974 (in Japanese).
7. Hata, J. and Shimizu, K.: Thymic changes in chromosomal abnormalities with special reference to Down's syndrome. *Saishin Igaku* **28**:1298, 1973 (in (Japanese).

DISCUSSION

Dr. LANDING: In a review of a large series of patients with biliary atresia, the thymus showed absence of Hassall's corpuscles in the same sort of manner that has just been shown. Clearly, something is going on in this disease which is deranging the thymic epithelial component, whatever bearing that has on the rest of the patient's immune system. The process appears to progress with time, which is not the same as saying whether or not it starts before birth. But biliary atresia may be telling, therefore, about acquired immunologic disorders. It is interesting, because it appears to be a pretty stereotyped, rigid disease, a pretty repetitive thing.

Dr. GOOD: Have you done any assays of the thymic humoral substance in the patients with biliary atresia using your nice nude mouse system?

Dr. TAMAOKI: No, I have not tested.

Dr. HITZIG: First, were these patients with biliary atresia and with severe diminishment of the Hassall's corpuscles well-nourished? And secondly, did you measure adenosine deaminase in these patients with biliary atresia?

Dr. TAMAOKI: The change of the thymus in congenital biliary atresia and Down's syndrome resembles the conditions caused by malnutrition or infection. In quantitative studies, however, the change of the Hassall's corpuscles in Down's syndrome and congenital biliary atresia appears far beyond the usual morphology of Hassall's corpuscles in various diseases, irrespective of immediate causes of death: cardiac failure, infection, death at operation or emanciation. For your second question, we did not check the ADA activity in biliary atresia.

Dr. COOPER: I am impressed that you can find any lymphoid cells in the thymus of the nude mouse, since the evidence seems to be very good. Those cells are of mesenchymal origin, at least in birds, and come there secondarily, and the data suggests that they are called there by some signal from the thymic epithelium. Then one wonders if many cells are what that traffic actually is. It could be that they come there, get some instructions even if they do not proliferate, turn around and leave, and that these are the cells which are detected by the Komuro-Boyese assay. The question being, when does commitment to T-cell differentiation begin? Some people argue that it happens before the cells come to the thymus, and some argue that they have to come to the thymus. Much of the evidence has been gained from study of the very mice that you are studying, the nude mice. Now, if cells do traffic through the thymus, it is possible that the data may need reinterpreting.

Dr. TAMAOKI: Judging from my experience on the development of nude mice, the first appearance of blastic cells, that might be coming from outside, is at about 15 days of gestation. In normal mice, thymocytes bearing θ and Ly-antigen appear in the 12th or 13th day of gestation. Reactivity in MLR and reactivity to Con A start to develop after 18 days or 19 days of gestation. In view of functional differentiation, I think that there are two steps. The first step begins in the normal thymus around 13 days and that requires a micro-environment composed of squamous cells. The second step requires secretion by epithelial cells starting about 18 days of gestation. Dr. Auerbach's group has substantiated that cultured anlagen of nude thymus develops lymphocytes. It appears that there exist pre-thymic cells in the anlagen of nude mice, but they cannot proliferate under such circumstances.

Dr. GOOD: We cannot recognise any mesenchymal cells in the anlagen for the thymus from 11- or 12-day-old animals. That is a critical time, however, because it is a time when these cells must come, for the first time, into the thymus. But there is no question that what looks like implants of epithelial thymus developed in the nude mouse. I do not think this answers the critical question as to whether any of these cells can come from epithelial sources, but we think that is extremely unlikely now.

Immunopathological Findings of Tonsils in Primary Immunodeficiency

T. KAWAI,* K. KAWANO,** AND H. SAITO***

ABSTRACT

The tonsils belong to the immune organs, and it is now certain that they function as one of the peripheral immune organs which is capable of producing antibodies locally. However, the exact biological functions are not fully understood. Fourteen cases of primary immunodeficiency were available for immunopathological study of the palatine tonsils. As a general tendency, hypoplastic findings in the lymphoid tissue of the tonsils are parallel to those seen in the peripheral lymph nodes, and the more deficient the cell-mediated immune system, the smaller the size of the palatine tonsils. In an adult case of Bruton-type agammaglobulinemia, the biopsied palatine tonsils show an almost normal lymphoid structure, showing hyperplastic germinal centers. In an infantile case of congenital agammaglobulinemia, however, marked hypoplasia of the tonsils is recognized. The possibility that the tonsils act as one of the central immune organs cannot be ruled out, particularly in the fetal and/or neonatal stages.

There have been many hypotheses on the biological functions of the tonsils. However, it is no doubt today that the tonsils belong to the immune organs. Their immunological functions have been investigated only recently, and there are many points to be investigated further.

Primary immunodeficiency is the condition where the immune response fails to appear without being due to any recognizable disease, and they are considered to be extremely important as "experiments of nature" in order to investigate immune mechanisms in the living body.

---

*Department of Clinical Pathology, Jichi Medical School, Tochigi, Japan
**Department of Clinical Pathology, Nihon University School of Medicine, Tokyo, Japan
***Department of Oto-rhino-laryngology, Nihon University School of Medicine, Tokyo, Japan

Development and histological characteristics of the tonsils
    The tonsils develop from the third and fourth pharyngeal pouches, as does
the thymus. They grow gradually in the fetal and neonatal periods and increase
in size rapidly after three or four years of age. However, they gradually involute
after puberty, similar to the thymic involution.
    The ovoid masses of lymphoid tissue are embedded in the lamina propria
of the mucous membrane, and the epithelium is of the stratified squamous non-
keratinizing type and dips deeply into the underlying lymphoid tissue to form
10 to 20 little gland-like pits (primary crypts).[1] Their lining epithelium further
extends out into the adjacent lymphoid tissue to form many secondary or smaller crypts, their entire surface area being said to cover as much as 259 cm².
Many efferent lymphatics are present, although few afferent lymphatics are
recognized. The tonsils are histologically quite similar to other lymphoid structures, although the germinal centers are comparatively large. The mantle zone
of lymphocytes surrounds each germinal center, being composed of heavy
lymphocytic infiltration. The lymphoid tissue in the tonsils is mostly arranged
close to the epithelium, and many small lymphocytes are known to invade
through and extend even outside the epithelial layer (Figs. 1, 2). In addition to
lymphocytes there are many plasma cells in this tissue.

Site of immunoglobulin production in the palatine tonsils
    The site of immunoglobulin production in the palatine tonsils includes the
mantle zone of the follicular structure, the epithelial basement membrane and

Abbreviations: LC-lymphocyte, HC-Hassall's corpuscle, FS-follicular structure and ger-
          minal center, PC-paracortical lymphocytic infiltration, PL-plasma cell,
          I.D.-immunodeficiency.
Grading of the histological findings:
    (0)—none or extremely scanty
    (1)—follicle-like structure or glandular structure
    (2)—follicular structure of abortive Hassall's corpuscle
    (3)—germinal center or cystic dilatation of Hassall's corpuscle
    (4)—normal, numerous

around the blood vessels of the medullary area.[2] IgG and IgM are localized in
the mantle zone, while IgG, IgA and IgE are localized in the epithelial basement
membrane. All the classes of the immunoglobulins are localized in the medullary area. By using fluorescent antibody techniques, since they are quite different from the thymic lymphoid tissue, many IgG- and IgA-producing cells
are identified through both the epithelial and lymphoid tissues of the tonsils,
the IgA-producing cells being more predominant. A large amount of IgA is

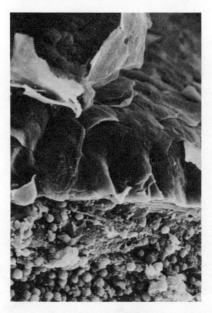

FIG. 1.   A scanning electron microgram of the palatine tonsil.
The upper portion of the photograph shows the surface epithelium of
stratified squamous cell type, while the lower portion indicates the cut
surface of the tonsil showing many cellular components, mostly lymphocytes.

stained in and outside the epithelium, indicating the existence of secretory IgA.
Interestingly, also, the tonsils are the lymphoid tissue that carry the most abundant IgE-producing cells.

The ratio between IgG and IgA levels in the tonsil tissue (IgG/IgA) is 3.5 to
4.0, being significantly lower than that in the serum. The relative concentration of IgA in the tonsil tissue is much larger in patients with habitual angina
than that in ordinary tonsilar hypertrophy.[3]

Immunological characteristics of the tonsilar lymphocytes
The lymphocytes in the tonsils can be similarly analyzed by using various
surface markers. It has been reported that the sheep erythrocyte rosette-form-
ing cells occupy approximately 20% (13 − 43%) of the lymphocytes eluted
from the palatine tonsils, while about 60% (54 − 72%) are stained positively
for the surface immunoglobulins.[4,5] All classes of immunoglobulins could be
identified on the lymphocyte surface, IgD being unexpectedly large at about
10%.[6] The surface IgA was identified as having no secretory component.[7]

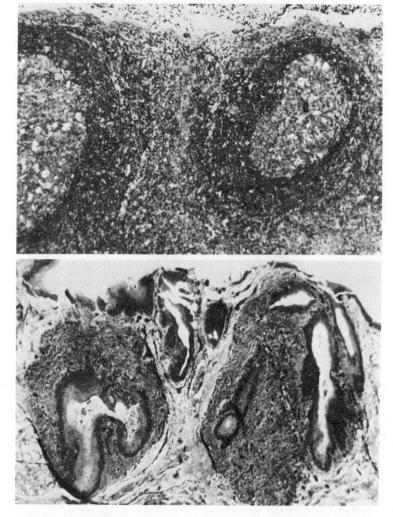

FIG. 2.   Microphotographs of the normal and hypoplastic palatine tonsils.

The upper photograph shows the normal palatine tonsil, representing large germinal centers (G) surrounded by dense mantle zone of the lymphocytes. The surface is lined by the squamous epithelium, through which many small lymphocytes are seen to exude out. The lower photograph indicates the markedly hypoplastic tonsil taken from a 7 m.o. female infant who suffered from severe combined immunodeficiency. No follicular structure is seen and crypts are extremely prominent due to marked depletion of the lymphoid components.

TABLE 1.   Clinical and histopathological findings in the cases with primary immuno-deficiency diseases studied

Case No.	Clinical Data (Institutions)	Thymus (LC) (HC)		Lymph Nodes (FS) (PC) (PL)			Tonsils (FS) (LC) (PL)		
1	DiGeorge syndrome, 4 m.o., F. Died of pneumonia (Tokyo Univ.)	agenesis (0)	(0)	hypoplastic (4)	(1)	(4)	atrophic (4)	(2)	(3)
2	Dysgammaglobulinemia, 2 y.o., F. (IgG 0, IgA ↓, IgM ↑) Died of pneumonia (Kyushu Univ.)	normal (19 g) (4)	(4)	almost normal (3) (3)		(3)	almost normal (3)	(4)	(2–3)
3	Ataxia-telangiectasia, 11 y.o., F. Died of pneumonia (Kyushu Univ.)	hypopl. (1)	(2)	hypoplastic (3) (1)		(4)	atrophic (3)	(1–2)	(4)
4	Agammaglobulinemia (Bruton ?) 10 m.o., M. Died of peritonitis (Kyushu Univ.)	normal (18 g) (2)	(3)	hypoplastic (2) (3)		(2)	hypoplastic (3)	(1–2)	(2)
5	I.D. with nomral serum Ig, 11 m.o., F. (Fuchu Hosp.)	fetal (3 g) (2–3)	(2)	hypoplastic (3) (2–3)		(2)	hypoplastic (2–3)	(2–3)	(2)
6	Swiss type I.D., 19 m.o., F. Died of chr. granulomatous pneumonitis. (Wakayama Univ.)	not found		hypoplastic (2) (1)		(1)	atrophic (0)	(1)	(1)
7	Swiss type I.D., 5 m.o., M. (Nat'l Child Hosp.)	fetal (0)	(0)	hypoplastic (0) (1)			atrophic (0)	(0)	(0)
8	Swiss type I.D., 5 m.o., M. (Nat'l Child Hosp.)	not available		not available			atrophic (0)	(0)	(0)
9	Thymic alymphoplasia, 3 m.o., M. (Nat'l Child Hosp.)	fetal (0.8 g)		not available			atrophic (0)	(0)	(0)
10	Severe combined I.D., 7 m.o., F. with M-Proteins Died of penumonia (Nihon Univ.)	fetal (2 g) (0)	(1)	hypoplastic (0) (1)		(4)	atrophic (0)	(1)	(4)
11	Thymic alymphoplasia with hyper-IgE, 5 m.o., F. Died of giant cell pneumonitis (Nihon Univ.)	fetal (2 g) (0)	(0–1)	hypoplastic (3) (1)		(1)	atrophic (3)	(1–2)	(1)
13	Agammaglobulinemia, Bruton-type 12 y.o., M. (Kumamoto Univ.)	normal (4)	(4)	not biopsied			atrophic (0)	(1)	(1)
17	Agammaglobulinemia in adult F. Normal cell-mediated immunity (Nat'l Tokyo 2nd Hosp.)	not examined		not examined			normal (4)	(4)	(1)
18	Swiss type I.D. (Gunma Univ.)	fetal (0)	(1)	atrophic (0) (0–1)		(0)	atrophic (0)	(0)	(0)

T cells in the tonsils respond to phytohemagglutinin (PHA), and B cells do not by themselves; however, B cells may respond very weakly if they are mixed with T cells. Both T cells and B cells in the tonsils may respond to pokeweed mitogen, although B cells may not respond as much as the splenic B cells. No apparent response is recognized against lipopolysaccharide for the tonsilar B cells.[8]

Through *in vitro* culture of the tonsilar lymphocytes, they were recognized to produce anti-hapten antibodies (anti-dinitrophenylated keyhole limpet hemocyanin, antitrinitrophenylated horse erythrocyte) with the helper function of T cells.[9] Also confirmed in experimental rabbits was the existence of plaque-forming cells (antibody-forming cells) in the tonsils. Therefore, it is certain that the tonsils are capable of producing humoral antibodies locally.

Through mixed lymphocyte culture was found allogeneic recognition among the tonsilar lymphocytes eluted from different individuals. In addition, the tonsilar lymphocytes were recognized to induce cell-mediated cytotoxicity, basically by T cells and not by B cells.[9]

Pathological findings for the tonsils in primary immunodeficiency

Pathological findings for the palatine tonsils in primary immunodeficiency are summarized in Table 1.[10] A total of 14 cases were available for study, including 2 Bruton-type cases (congenital form and adult form), 1 primary hypogammaglobulinemia, 1 dysgammaglobulinemia, 1 DiGeorge type, 2 Nezelof type, 1 ataxia-telangiectasia, and 5 severe combined immunodeficiency. In general, the following conclusions may be possible: Hypoplastic findings in the lymphoid tissue of the tonsils are parallel to those seen in the peripheral lymph nodes, and the more deficient the cell-mediated immune system the smaller the size of the palatine tonsils. Considering that the tonsils are capable of producing humoral antibodies and of inducing cell-mediated immunity, as previously described, the tonsils certainly function as one of the peripheral immune organs, but seem to be closely influenced by the thymus.

In two cases of the Bruton-type agammaglobulinemia, entirely different findings are recognized in the tonsils. In an adult case, the biopsied palatine tonsils show an almost normal lymphoid structure, although the hyperplastic germinal centers are seen without immunopathological evidence of producing immunoglobulins. In an infantile case, marked hypoplasia of the tonsilar lymphoid tissue was confirmed on autopsy, although the thymus has been found to be normal. More cases of the Bruton-type agammaglobulinemia must be examined before any conclusion is made. However, if the tonsils might function also as one of the central immune organs, particularly in the fetal and/or neonatal periods, they seem to be related more closely to the humoral antibody response, probably bursa-equivalent.

The tonsil tissue is widely distributed in the nasal and pharyngeal regions, and a condition which is entirely deficient in tonsil tissue is impossible to produce either surgically or experimentally. Therefore, it is still uncertain if one can assume that the tonsils play any role as a central immune organ.

REFERENCES

1. Fioretti, A.: Die Gaumenmandel. George Thieme Verlag, Stuttgart 1961.
2. Hamashima, Y.: Immunohistopathology. Igaku-Shoin, Ltd, Tokyo, 1976.
3. Saito, H., Ohki, T., and Kawai, T.: Immunoglobulins of human palatine tonsil tissue. *Jap. J. Tonsil* **11**:90, 1972 (in Japanese).
4. Watanabe, T., Yoshizaki, K., Yagura, T., and Yamamura, Y.: *In vitro* antibody formation by human tonsil lymphocytes. *J. Immunol.* **113**:608, 1974.
5. Ishii, Y., Koshiba, H., Ueno, H., Maeyama, I., Takemi, T., Ishibashi, F., and Kikuchi, K.: Characterization of human B lymphocyte-specific antigens. *J. Immunol.* **114**:466, 1975.
6. van Boxel, J. A., Paul, W. E., Terry, W. D., and Green, I.: Communications. IgD-bearing human lymphocytes. *J. Immunol.* **109**:648, 1972.
7. Platts-Mills, T. A. E. and Ishizaka, K.: IgG and IgA diphtheria antitoxin responses from human tonsil lymphocytes. *J. Immunol.* **114**:1058, 1975.
8. Greaves, M., Janossy, G., and Doenhoff, M.: Selective triggering of human T and B lymphocytes *in vitro* by polyclonal mitogens. *J. Exp. Med.* **140**:1, 1974.
9. Yoshizaki, K. and Watanabe, T.: Immunological functions of human tonsil lymphocytes, *Clin. Immunol.* **7**:467, 1975. (in Japanese)
10. Kawai, T. and Kawano, K.: Immunopathology of primary immunodeficiency disease. *Acta. path. Jap.* **23**:887, 1973.

DISCUSSION

Dr. KAWAI: We have experienced a marked eosinophile infiltration in the thymus and also lymphoid tissues in some cases of severe T-cell deficiency. Severe peripheral eosinophilia is suggestive of thymic disfunction. So I was wondering if you have the same feeling, or any evidence for this?

Dr. GOOD: When I see eosinophilia associated with T-cell deficiency, the thing that I worry about is graft-versus-host reaction. You will have the cells in the blood, you will see the infiltrations in many sites including the thymus, and in the thymus they are in the medullary portion.

Dr. AIUTI: We could demonstrate no synthesis of immunoglobulin by circulating lymphocytes in common variable hypogammaglobulinemia by the tonsils and bone marrow. We were also able to demonstrate in one of the patients very few plasma cells, and very little synthesis by the bone marrow, while B-lymphocytes were absent in the peripheral blood lymphocytes and also in the tonsils. We cultured peripheral blood lymphocytes from a Bruton-type patient. After one month we could demonstrate that 10 % of the cells had IgM on the cell surface and also IgM in the cytoplasm. So this could mean that perhaps a few B cells which we could not detect by immunofluorescence are present also in the peripheral blood, and that they came from the marrow.

Dr. COOPER: My thinking on it has been that in Bruton's agammaglobulinemia, there are a few B-lymphocytes that are formed, and those have been seen by people in various places. The ones that they have must be normal, because they have the capacity to go on and differentiate into plasma cells; and many people have seen varying levels of immunoglobulins in patients who clearly had X-linked agammaglobulinemia with a marked deficiency of B-lymphocytes in their circulation, and when looked for, in the lymph nodes as well.

I would like to ask you more about your patient, MM, with the marked restriction of heterogeneity of IgM, IgG and IgA.

Dr. KAWAI: This is a 7-month-old female who was admitted to the hospital with convulsions, and eventually died of septicemia in a few months. The T-cell function was really deficient.

We were struck by the most unusual findings of immunoelectrophoretic analysis of the immunoglobulins. IgA and IgM were of monoclonal nature. And, the IgA level was greater than normal for the patient's age. IgG was present in a very minute amount.

Dr. GOOD: Dr. Hong had a very similar experience with a patient that I took care of, and in this instance both parents contributed a rare genotype on the heavy chain and the patient ended up with a very profound hypogammaglobulinemia with monoclonal type of immunoglobulin, and he had the Gm factors that were defined. Both of the parents had contributed this rare component. It looked as though in that instance it was a genetic abnormality of what you would say was a recessive type, which was involving the structure of genes of the immunoglobulin.

Chronic Progressive Panencephalitis in Hypogammaglobulinemia*

Michael A. MEDICI, Benjamin M. KAGAN,
John H. MENKES, and Richard A. GATTI

ABSTRACT

Chronic progressive panencephalitis is recognized as a consequence of hypogammaglobulinemia in a small group of patients adequately controlled by antibiotic and gammaglobulin replacement therapy. We are aware of at least 15 such cases; only one is female. The four year course of our patient includes progressive mental and neurologic deterioration beginning at age 10 years as recurrent episodes of aseptic meningoencephalitis with CSF mononuclear pleocytosis and elevated protein. Later, pneumoencephalography, carotid angiography and computerized axial tomography revealed progressive generalized brain atrophy. Brain biopsy demonstrated neuronal degeneration, gliosis and perivascular lymphocytic infiltrates. We have tried unsuccessfully to isolate an etiologic agent on numerous occasions, specifically attempting to identify enteroviruses and slow viruses. Plasma from ABO compatible family members was not able to alter the course of his encephalitis. Immunostimulation with *Corynebacterium parvum* and Levamisole begun late in the course of his disease has not been successful in arresting or reversing his mental and neurologic deterioration. His HLA type B7, DW2 is associated with abberant viral syndromes, especially with rubeola, for which he was vaccinated at age 6 years. The other cases whose HLA types are known to us are also HLA-B7. It is suggested that vigorous immunotherapy and antiviral agents be used early in the course of recurrent aseptic meningitis to prevent the development of this progressive and fatal encephalitis.

Hypogammaglobulinemia may be congenital or acquired. Initially, infections with encapsulated micro-organisms were a primary cause for concern. Advances in antibiotic therapy and gammaglobulin replacement have dramat-

Department of Pediatrics, Cedars-Sinai Medical Center, Los Angeles, California, U.S.A.
*This work was supported in part by the Amie Karen Cancer Fund for Children.

150   M. A. Medici *et al.*

ically improved the survival and prognosis of these patients. With increased survival, other sequelae of this disorder are becoming apparent. The Disseminated vaccinia, viral hepatitis, generalized cytomegalic viral diseases and problems with polio virus Type I have also been noted in these patients, although the thymic dependent system appears intact, as evaluated by present methods. Recently, it has become increasingly evident that a small group of patients with hypogammaglobulinemia develop chronic progressive panencephalitis. We are aware of at least 15 such cases and we report the following case history as one well-studied prototype of this increasingly frequent association for comparison with several previous isolated reports.

CASE REPORT

The patient, a 14-year-old male of Scandinavian descent, was essentially well until 18 months of age. He then began to sleep more than normal and had recurrent upper respiratory tract infections every 2–4 months associated with high fevers. At two years, a subcutaneous nodule developed at the lateral aspect of the right knee. Later that year, he developed swelling of the hands and wrists, with involvement of the ankle and feet at age three years. The polyarthritis and subcutaneous nodules responded to aspirin and physical therapy. At four years of age, biopsy of one of these nodules revealed chronic inflammatory cells, but no plasma cells. A lymph node biopsy showed enlarged follicles, but no germinal centers; bone marrow examination revealed the absence of plasma cells and his serum was devoid of immunoglobulin. Synovial punch biopsy of the left knee revealed several cells staining for IgG and IgM by immunofluorescence in the synovium and IgG, A and M in the synovial fluid. *In vitro* lymphocyte stimulation with phytohemagglutinin (PHA) was normal. Mumps and DNCB skin test responses were intact. At four years of age, the patient developed *Pseudomonas* osteomyelitis. Gammaglobulin replacement therapy was added to the antibiotic regime with complete remission of his polyarthritis. For further details see *Am. J. Med.* **48**:40–49, 1970.

The patient did well on gammaglobulin therapy until the age of ten when he began to have recurrent headaches, fever, irritability and lethargy. Lumbar puncture revealed pleocytosis (up to 62 white blood cells, predominantly lymphocytes) with normal glucose and protein. Bacterial cultures of the cerebrospinal fluid (CSF) were negative on three occasions. The following month he was reevaluated because of recurrent headaches. Sinus radiography demonstrated chronic sinusitis. CSF examination revealed continued mononuclear pleocytosis and elevated protein levels (45–102 mg/dl). The EEG pattern of diffuse slow wave activity was consistent with diffuse encephalitis. Brain scan demonstrated increased uptake bilaterally in the posterior parietal area. Gammaglobulin replacement therapy was increased to 15 cc. every two weeks. History revealed that he had received a rubeola live-virus vaccination at the age of six.

These episodes of "aseptic meningoencephalitis" recurred over the next year with persistent CSF mononuclear pleocytosis and elevated protein levels. He was again evaluated with EEG and brain scan which remained abnormal. Bilateral carotid angiograms failed to reveal any mass lesions. After discharge, he had recurrent episodes of emotional lability with loss of memory, inability to concentrate, slurring of speech and resting tremors of the hands.

Because of continuous frontal headaches, intermittent disorientation, ataxia, resting tremors and left-sided weakness, the patient was evaluated further the following year (age 13). At this time, the deep-tendon reflexes were hyperactive and the skull was tender to percussion. Although the EEG improved from previous studies, the brain scan again revealed extensive bilateral abnormalities. Cerebral angiography demonstrated mild to moderate enlargement of the lateral ventricles and displacement of the surface vessels away from the inner table of the skull. Pneumoencephalogram revealed mild ventricular dilatation with air seen in the subarachnoid space over the convexities of the brain. Brain biopsy was performed twenty-five months after onset of the CNS symptoms. Histologically, there were chronic perivascular lymphocytic infiltrates, considerable neuronal degeneration, gliosis and reactive astrocytosis. Electron microscopy failed to reveal intracellular inclusions. Viral, fungal and bacterial (aerobic and anaerobic) cultures were negative. The patient was placed on prophylactic antibiotic therapy.

The mental confusion, ataxia, dysarthria and hyperreflexia were progressive. Aggressive steroid therapy was instituted in an attempt to reverse the chronic progressive panencephalitis. On 60 mg. Prednisone daily, transient mental improvement was noted. Progressive paresis of cranial nerve VI developed and a cyclic pattern of CNS exacerbations, every 8–10 weeks, became evident. EEG demonstrated diffuse encephalopathy with deterioration from previous studies. Three years after the onset, the progressive deterioration of CNS function continued with increased tremor, dysmetria, expressive and receptive aphasia as well as pathologic reflexes. Computerized axial tomography (CAT) was consistent with generalized severe cerebral atrophy. Recent brain scans and CAT scans revealed increased cerebral atrophy. Numerous recent attempts to isolate normal or slow viruses from the CSF as well as from blood, naso-pharynx and stool have been unsuccessful at Sloan-Kettering and Duke University laboratories.

Immunological studies repeatedly demonstrate normal circulating T-cell

numbers with normal PHA and mixed leukocyte culture (MLC) responses.
In vitro, he has normal T-cell helper function with no demonstrable abnormal
T cell suppressor activity. Although he has no serum immunoglobulins and no
membrane immunoglobulin positive cells are demonstrable by immunofluorescence, normal numbers of EA and EAC cells are present. *In vitro*, pokeweed
mitogen stimulates his lymphocytes to synthesize and to secrete immunoglobulin. A B-cell cytotoxic factor has been demonstrated intermittently in the
patient's serum in the presence of rabbit complement. Anti-μ, α, or γ antibody
specificities were not demonstrable by inhibition of hemagglutination or by fluorescent labelling of his serum using normal cells. His serum was cytotoxic at one
point to lymphocytes from 8 of 15 patients with chronic lymphocytic leukemia
(CLL) and 9 of 15 samples of normal peripheral blood. Anti-δ antibody specificity was not demonstrable either by the Ouchterlony technique with a reference IgD line or in the presence of a serum with a known low level of IgD. The
patient's own IgD level was determined to be 7 μg/dl (2μg-40 mg/dl. normal values). Preliminary evidence also sugests that his macrophage population (adherent layer) may repress the expression of surface markers on normal peripheral blood lymphocytes when incubated *in vitro* for 12–14 days.

Therapeutic attempts to date have not been successful in arresting or reversing his chronic progressive panencephalitis. Since he can synthesize and secrete
immunoglobulin *in vitro* when stimulated by pokeweed mitogen, we have attempted to duplicate this stimulation *in vivo* by *Corynebacterium parvum* and
Levamisole. *C. parvum* was given at 2.5 mg/M² for seven doses, IV or subcutaneously at 7–14 day intervals. Although his cyclic CNS exacerbations were
transiently decreased in severity and remission somewhat prolonged during *C.
parvum* administration, there was no significant change in lymphocyte markers
or serum globulin status. Levamisole, a drug with reported immunostimulatory
and antiviral potential, was administered at 2.5 mg/kg/day for 2 days at weekly
intervals. Significantly increased irritability and tremor precluded continuation
of this drug after two weekly cycles. Currently, the patient is receiving weekly
plasma transfusion from ABO compatible family members in an attempt to
provide specific antibody to the unknown etiologic agent of his encephalitis.
He is currently being considered for bone marrow transplanation from his
ABO/HLA/MLC matched healthy sister.

DISCUSSION

Progress in antibiotic and gammaglobulin replacement therapy has allowed
adequate control of most of the infectious complications of hypogammaglob-

ulinemia. With prolonged survival, an additional consequence of the under-lying disease in a small group of these patients has become apparent. This sub-set develops a chronic progressive panencephalitis.

Although the frequency of this complication is not yet known, we are aware of at least 15 such cases, not including cases of acute viral encephalitis,[1,2] the meningoencephalitis follow-ing vaccination with live polio vaccine[3,4,5] and the encephalitis described in patients with T-cell deficiencies.[6,7,8]

The first major study of hypogammaglobulinemia was a ten-year prospective study by the Medical Research Council of the United Kingdom.[9,10] Three (1.7%) of the 176 patients on long-term gammaglobulin replacement therapy (Table 1) had a progressive pattern of neurological deterioration with ataxia, spasticity and optic atrophy. Adenovirus 9 was isolated from one of these cases (111M) while the other cases had a history of Herpes/varicella exposure predat-ing the onset of neurological symptoms. Although the etiologic agent is not reported, the possibility of a slow virus infection was raised. Webster[11] and Buckley[12] described other patients with hypogammaglobulinemia and chronic encephalitis associated with ECHO type viruses isolated from the cere-bro-spinal fluid (CSF). Several patients[1] are reported to have been infected by two viruses which might have synergistic effects. Detailed case reports[13,14,15,16] of this chronic panencephalitis document a progressive neurological deteriora-tion which uniformly leads to death from two to four years after the onset of CNS symptoms. It is intriguing to note that although the etiologic agent could not be cultured from the CSF, all but one were reported to have been previous-ly exposed to rubeola, naturally or by vaccination, between the ages of 4–6 years of age. In one report, Hanissian et al.[13] were able to demonstrate intracellu-lar measles antigen by immunofluorescence techniques in brain biopsy cultures.

These patients present the clinical picture of meningoencephalitis: head-ache, lethargy and irritability. Bacterial and viral cultures were usually nega-tive and after several investigations, the CSF revealed mononuclear pleocytosis and elevated protein levels with normal glucose. All but one of the patients are male. The female, three years old at diagnosis of hypogammaglobulinemia, developed a meningoencephalitis with CSF pleocytosis and elevated protein. Although the symptoms resolved in six weeks, the patient shed ECHO 30 virus for five months.[17] Subsequently this patient developed a progressive panenceph-alitis and the CSF is again positive for ECHO 30. It is curious to note that although these patients could not normally synthesize antibody, the CSF con-tained normal or elevated amounts of IgG or IgM antibody in four of the five cases (Table 2). To date, no analysis of the specificity of this immunoglobulin has been reported.

The patients' mental and physical deterioration progressed and ataxia, dys-

TABLE 1. Chronic progressive panencephalitis in hypogammaglobulinemia from MRC report (1969/1971) 176 patients

Case	111M	119m	236m
Sex	Male	Male	Male
Age of IgG replacement	8 mos.	6 mos.	6 1/2 yrs.
Viral exposure age	?	chickenpox 1 1/2 yrs.	Herpes Zoster 1 1/2 yrs.
Age of onset of encephalitis	8 yrs.	3 1/2 yrs.	11 3/4 yrs.
CSF: pleocytosis	mononuclear	?	?
protein	69 mg%	?	?
virus isolated	Adenovirus 9	?	?
Duration of CNS symptoms	2 mos.	3 yrs. +	4 yrs. +
Outcome	Expired	deteriorating	deteriorating

TABLE 2. Chronic progressive panencephalitis in hypogammaglobulinemia

Reference:	Hanissian et al.[13]	White et al.[14]	Lyon et al.[15]	Lord et al.[16]	Patient
	1972	1972	1972	1973	1973
Sex	Male	Male	Male	Male	Male
Age Dx. of hypogammaglob.	1 yr.	19 mos.	2 1/2 yrs.	12 yrs.	4 yrs.
Viral Exposure age	Rubeola 5 yrs.		Rubeola 4 yrs.	Rubeola 5 yrs.	Rubeola 6 yrs.
Age onset of encephalitis	5 1/2 yrs.	7 1/2 yrs.	7 yrs.	16 yrs.	10 yrs.
CSF: pleocytosis	?	80% mononuclear	30–90 WBC	3–7 lymphs	11–60 WBC up to 76% lymphs
protein	52 mg/dl	42–90 mg/dl	156 mg.	23–68 mg/dl	45–105 mg/dl
globulin	IgG 140 mg/dl	IgG 3.4 mg/dl	0	IgM 16 mg/dl	IgG 3.7 mg/dl; IgM 0
bact/virus	no	no	no	no	no
Clinical status: headache/lethargy dysarthria/ataxia	++	++?	++		++
seizure	myoclonic	+←	no	focal motor	no
↓mentation	+→	++←	++←	+?	++←
reflexes					
EEGs	slow wave burst	slow wave burst	diffuse slow dysrhythmia	no	slow wave burst
Brain: atrophy	++	++	++	++	++
gliosis	+	+	+	+	+
perivascular infiltrate	intracytoplasmic fluorescence +for measles	none	tubular inclusions endothelial cells	none	none
intracellular inclusion	hyperimmunoglobulin	–	no	–	
Therapy	–	–	no	–	Prednisone C. parvum Levamisole plasma 4+ yrs.
Duration of CNS symptoms	2 1/2 yrs.	3 yrs.	3+ yrs.	2 yrs.	
Outcome	expired	expired	deteriorating	expired	deteriorating

156   M. A. Medici *et al.*

arthria and pathologic reflexes developed. EEG revealed abnormal slow wave patterns and cerebral atrophy was demonstrable by pneumoencephalogram, carotid arteriogram or by computerized axial tomography. Brain biopsy revealed neuronal degeneration, reactive gliosis and perivascular infiltration. Typically, there was no evidence of intranuclear or intracytoplasmic inclusions in the nerve cells, although one case[13] revealed positive cytoplasmic fluorescence using labelled measles antibody.

Therapeutic intervention to date has been uniformly unsuccessful. Continuous prophylactic or repeated courses of antibiotics have not been useful in arresting or reversing the cerebral pathology. Administration of specific hyperimmune globulin to the putative etiologic agent was reported in several cases[11,13] without significant changes in the progressively deteriorating mental, neurologic and physical status of the patient. Theoretically, providing the specific antibody against the etiologic agent should be beneficial. However, the lack of success may be related to one of several factors. In most cases, the etiologic agent is not known and the specific antibody cannot be provided. In an attempt to overcome this difficulty, it was our hope that the patient might be intermittently shedding a virus which might immunize close family members. We, therefore, administered plasma from ABO compatible family members, but without significant amelioration of symptoms. On the other hand, such specific antibodies might not be effective if they cannot cross the blood brain barrier. In an attempt to provide local antibody, we tried to stimulate antibody synthesis with immunostimulants. Both *C. parvum* and Levamisole were unsuccessful in duplicating *in vivo* the *in vitro* immunoglobulin synthesis and secretion stimulated by pokeweed mitogen.

A third possible explanation for the therapeutic failure is that the patient may not be able to respond immunologically to the virus. Four of the five cases with sufficiently detailed histories (Table 2) were found to have been exposed to rubeola between 4–6 years of age. The age of exposure to rubeola may have some effect on the type of viral host interaction that takes place.[18] Rubeola is a neurotropic virus particularly associated with chronic progressive neurological degeneration in subacute sclerosing panencephalitis (SSPE) and multiple sclerosis (MS). There is also rapidly mounting evidence that the HLA type of the patient may predispose him to aberrant viral syndromes. Several studies have shown an increased correlation of HLA-A3, B7 and DW2 (LD-7a) with multiple sclerosis[19,20,21] and with a more malignant course of the disease. HLA-A3, B7 has also been reported in patients with a rubella virus SSPE-like disease.[22] Production of high titer specific antibody both in the serum and in the CSF significantly aids in the diagnosis of the etiologic agents in these cases. Our patient is HLA-A28,24,B5,7, DW2,4. Two other patients with chronic panencephalitis and hypogammaglobulinemia known to us and followed by Dr. Buckley at Duke University are HLA-B7.[23] Thus, all the patients with this syndrome whose HLA type is known to us are HLA-B7 and probably DW2. It may well be, therefore, that there is a lacunar deficiency which might predispose to a progressive viral encephalitis by an agent similar to rubeola virus. If this association of HLA-B7, DW2 and chronic progressive panencephalitis in patients with hypogammaglobulinemia persists, aggressive antiviral therapy may be effective if initiated early in the course of aseptic meningo encephalitis before permanent damage is produced. Immunological approaches such as interferon and transfer factor or vigorous antiviral chemotherapeutic agents may arrest the disease before it becomes progressive. Agents such as isoprinosine have been shown to be effective in some cases of SSPE with arrest of the disease and even reversal of some of the CNS dysfunction.[24,25] Mononuclear pleocytosis and elevated CNS protein are found early in the course when the mental status of the patient is salvageable. These may be adequate indications for aggressive therapy early in the course of recurrent aseptic meningoencephalitis in an effort to prevent this chronic progressive disease and to date fatal encephalitis.

Acknowledgements
We wish to thank Doctors G. Geraldo and C. Wilfert for special viral studies, Doctors N. Abdou and R. Walford for cytotoxic assays, Dr. D. Heiner for IgD studies and Doctors R. Seeger and R. Stevens for *in vitro* antibody production studies in our patient.

REFERENCES

1. Linneman, C. C., May, D. B., Schubert, W. K., Caraway, C. T., and Schiff, G. M.: Fatal viral encephalitis in children with X-linked hypogammaglobulinemia. *Am. J. Dis. Child.* **126**:100–103, 1973.
2. Ziegler, J. B. and Penny, R.: Fatal Echo 30 virus infection and amyloidosis in X-linked hypogammaglobulinemia. *Clin. Immunol. Immunopathol.* **3**:347–352, 1975.
3. Chang, T-W., Weinstein, L., and MacMahon, H. E.: Paralytic poliomyelitis in a child with hypogammaglobulinemia: Probable implication of Type 1 vaccine strain. *Pediatrics*, **37**:630–636, 1966.
4. Riker, J. B., Brandt, C. D., Chandra, R., Arrobio, J. O., and Nakano, J. H.: Vaccine-associated poliomyelitis in a child with thymic abnormality. *Pediatrics* **48**:923–929, 1971.
5. Verhaart, W. J. C.: Polio-encephalopathy or masked encephalitis in familial hypogammaglobulinemia. *J. Neuropathol. Exp. Neurol.* **20**:380–385, 1961.
6. Dayan, A.D.: Combined immunodeficiency and chronic encephalitis. *Lancet* **1**:1178–1179, 1971.

7. Dayan, A.D.: Chronic encephalitis in children with severe immunodeficiency. *Acta Neuropathol.* **19**:234–241, 1971.
8. Bensch, J., Berg, T., Hazberg, B., Johansson, S. G. O., and Skoog, W.: Congenital immunological defect with early progressive brain disorder. *Lancet* **1**: 1070, 1971.
9. Medical Research Council Working Party: Hypogammaglobulinemia in the United Kingdom. *Lancet* **1**:163 168, 1969.
10. Medical Research Council Working Party: *Hypogammaglobulinemia in the United Kingdom.* Medical Research Council Special Report Series No. 310, London, 1971.
11. Webster, A. D. B. and Good, R. A.: Primary immunodeficiency. *Prog. in Immunol. II*, **5**:361–365, 1974.
12. Buckley, R., *et al.* Lancet (submitted for publication).
13. Hanissian, A. S., Jabbour, J. T., Lamereus, S., Garcia, H. J., and Horta-Barbosa, L.: Subacute encephalitis and hypogammaglobulinemia. *Amer. J. Dis. Child.* **123**:151–155, 1972.
14. White, H. H., Kepes, J. H., Kirkpatrick, C. H., and Schimke, R. N.: Subacute encephalitis and congenital hypogammaglobulinemia. *Arch. Neurol.* **26**: 359–365, 1972.
15. Lyon, G., Griscelli, C., and Lebon, P.: Endothelial intracisternal tubular inclusions in a case of chronic encephalitis associated with immunological deficiency. *Neuropadiatrie* **3**:459–469, 1972.
16. Lord, R. A., Goldblum, R. M., Forman, P. M., Dupree, E., Storey, W. D., and Goldman, A. S.: Cerebrospinal fluid IgM in the absence of serum IgM in combined immunodeficiency. *Lancet* **11**:528–29, 1973.
17. Whisnant, J. K., Treadwell, E. L., Mohanakumar, T., Wilfert, C. M., and Buckley, R. H.: Prolonged CNS viral infection with Echo 30 in an agammglobulinemic child with intact cell-mediated immunity. *Ped. Res.* **9**:336, 1975.
18, Alter, M. and Cendrowski, W.: Multiple sclerosis and childhood infection. *Neurology* **26**:201–204, 1976.
19. Bertrams, J. and Kuwert, E.: HLA antigen frequencies in multiple sclerosis. Significant increase of HLA-A3, HLA-A10 and W5 and decrease of HLA-A12. *Eur. Neurol.* **7**:74–80, 1972.
20. Naito, S., Namerow, N., Mickey, M. R., and Terasaki, P. I.: Multiple sclerosis: Association with HLA-A3. *Tissue Antigens* **2**:1–4, 1972.
21. Jersild, C., Fog, T., Hansen, G. S., Thomsen, M., Svejgaard, A., and Dupont, B.: Histocompatibility determinants in multiple sclerosis, with special reference to clinical course. *Lancet* **11**:1221–1224, 1973.
22. Weil, M. L., Itabashi, H. H., Cremer, N. E., Oshior, L. S., Lennette, E. H., Carnay, L.: Chronic progressive panencephalitis due to Rubella virus simulating subacute sclerosing panencephalitis. *New Engl. Med.* **292**:994–998, 1975.
23. Buckley, R. H.: personal communication.
24. Mattson, R. H.: Subacute sclerosing panencephalitis recovery associated with isoprinosine therapy: Report of a case. *Neurology* **24**:383, 1974.
25. Huttenlocher, P. R.: Isoprinosine therapy in subacute sclerosing panencephalitis. *Neurology* **26**:364, 1976.

DISCUSSION

Dr. SOOTHILL: The most important viral brain damage is cytomegalovirus infection, because it affects 1 % of our population, so we have started treating these patients with transfer factor or leukocyte extract, and we have turned off the virus excretion briefly in three of them, and we are now looking for more long-term effects.

Now, Webster used transfer factor prepared from an infected mother, an immunized mother, in the ECHO virus patient you have quoted him as working on, and that produced no effect there. It is an intriguing thought that the mother might have had the same HLA leukocyte as the patient.

Dr. GATTI: We transplanted a thymus into a T-deficient patient with very high levels of Epstein-Barr virus titers, and within a few weeks after the take and the reconstitution of the T-cell system, the Epstein-Barr virus titers dropped precipitously. And this was repeated again in another patient. As you know, recently there have been reports that in children with congenital rubella syndrome, after ten years, they suddenly developed a chronic encephalitis.

Also among the patients that Colin Barry surveyed in his autopsy study, were a number of patients with congenital rubella who were pulled out of the study because they looked like immunodeficiency, and at least some of them do not develop congenital rubella syndrome because they are immunodeficient. Of course one can argue from the other standpoint too, and that is that they look like they are immunodeficient because they have a chronic viral infection.

Dr. GOOD: I think patients with the antibody deficiency syndrome, or the Bruton type of immunodeficiency if you will, do have problems with virus infections. I mean, this is not a unique thing for the central nervous system virus. They have had, of course, the progressive fatal liver disease, and although many patients with immunodeficiency are able to tolerate both the hepatitis B virus and, apparently, the hepatitis A virus quite well, they may be chronically infected. We have also seen polio to be more frequent in these patients, not just in the patients with T-cell deficiency. So I think that the rule of thumb that the B-cell system is primarily for defense against the encapsulated bacterial pathogens is really relative. These patients do have greater susceptibility. I think the possibility that you raise, that they have a combination of that immunodeficiency and the B7 HLA which makes them susceptible to something that is ubiquitous in the environment that we have not yet defined, perhaps related to the measles virus responsible for multiple sclerosis, is a good possibility. We have looked at the SSPE patients, however we do not find any predominant HLA haplotype, or HLA determinant, or D determinant.

Dr. COOPER: Michael Ulston has described that antibodies will cap the measles virus antigens as they are being budded from the cell and will strip those antigens, or virions, and cause them to be intercytosed and the cells will remain healthy as long as the antibodies are present. As soon as the antibodies are removed, and this stripping phenomenon, or stripping mechanism, is eliminated, then the cells are destroyed by the viruses which rapidly grow back. In the central nervous system, lacking antibody producing cells, and lacking the ability to get antibodies efficiently through the blood-brain barrier from passive sources, it may be that this important mechanism of defense against viruses comes into play and then renders the brain or the central nervous system especially vulnerable. If that is correct reasoning, then it is going to be difficult to repair it with anything that has to do with levelling up cellular immunity; it is almost going to have to be an attack on the virus.

Dr. GATTI: There is no doubt that we can muster a very good, let us call it, intra-cerebral-spinal system immunologic response, as shown in the MS patients, where they develop very high levels of IgG. I do not think all of that is coming across the blood-brain barrier, because the levels are higher than what they are in the serum—you would have to have an active transport mechanism. The problem with these patients is that they do not have the capacity to respond. What is most frustrating in this particular patient to us, is that we know we can induce him to make immunoglobulin *in vitro*, but we cannot do it *in vivo*.

Dr. HITZIG: I think there are more cases where one at least has the impression that they were healthy children and after a virus infection they remained infected or they had other problems with cell-mediated immunity. For instance, mucocutaneous candidiasis. We have three such cases after measles, or measles vaccination, or Herpes infection, rubella infection, and so on. Epstein-Barr virus seems to be such an agent. Now in these cases it is sometimes impossible to prove that they had normal reactions before this infection, and it is very well possible that they just got this chronic virus infection because they were, from the beginning, immunodeficient.

II. ETIOLOGICAL SIGNIFICANCE OF IMMUNO-DEFICIENCY AND ITS IMPLICATIONS FOR PATHOGENESIS OF HUMAN DISEASE

Lymphocytotoxic Antibodies to B Cells in a Patient with Hypogammaglobulinemia and Ulcerative Colitis

T. Tursz, J. L. Preud'homme, and M. Seligmann

ABSTRACT

A young woman developed serious bronchopulmonary infections and severe ulcerative colitis. Serum Ig levels varied between 2 and 5 mg/ml for IgG, 0.3 and 0.7 mg/ml for IgM, 0.1 and 0.15 mg/ml for IgA. Antibody formation was impaired for some antigens. *In vivo* delayed hypersensitivity reactions and *in vitro* response of circulating lymphocytes to mitogens and allogeneic cells were normal. Lymphocyte counts varied between 600 and 1000 per mm^3 with 0.5–1 % of B cells and 98–99 % of T cells.

Antilymphocyte antibodies were detected by direct immunofluorescence and by microlymphocytotoxicity with increased reactivity at $+4°C$. These antibodies belonged to the IgM class and were polyclonal. Studies performed with various normal lymphocyte subpopulations, with several lymphoblastoid cell lines and with lymphocytes from immunodeficiency patients showed that these antibodies reacted with B cells and practically not at all with T cells. The corresponding antigen(s) is distinct from membrane bound immunoglobulins and is presumably not an alloantigen of the LA-like series since B cells from all tested normal individuals with various H-LA phenotypes were reactive.

Cells from various lymphoproliferative disorders were tested. T derived and non-T, non-B leukemic cells did not react with the antibody. Malignant cells from B-derived lymphomas and prolymphocytic leukemias were reactive. The incidence of positivity of the leukemic cells in patients with common B chronic lymphocytic leukemia was surprisingly low (1/3 of the patients). This lack of reactivity of CLL cells from many patients may be related to the expression of the corresponding antigen only at certain stages of B cell maturation.

The pathogenic role of the anti B cell antibodies in the genesis of the patient's hypogammaglobulinemia was demonstrated by the effect of massive plasmaphereses which were followed by a dramatic and transitory increase

Laboratory of Immunochemistry and Immunopathology (INSERM U108), Research Institute on Blood Diseases, Hôpital Saint-Louis, Paris, France.

of B cell figures, whereas the antibodies, no more detectable at the end of plasmapheresis, rose progressively back to the initial titer.

Whereas most primary immunodeficiency syndromes appear to result from an arrest in the differentiation capabilities of immunologically competent cells, autoantibodies to circulating B lymphocytes may be incriminated in the pathogenesis of some cases of hypogammaglobulinemia.

Data on the occurrence of anti-lymphocyte antibodies in immunodeficiency (ID) patients are very scarce. A complement dependent lymphocytotoxic factor was demonstrated in the serum of a young boy with low serum IgM, impaired cellular immunity, absent immunologic memory and episodic lymphopenia.[1] In another boy with recurrent infections and deficiency of both cellular and humoral immunity, a high titer IgM antibody or IgG was found and was thought to be responsible for a non H-LA-associated lymphocytotoxicity which was blocked by IgG.[2]

Lymphocytotoxins have recently been reported in a variety of human diseases, including systemic lupus erythematosus and inflammatory bowel diseases.[3-5] These lymphocytotoxic antibodies usually show no specificity for B or T lymphocyte subpopulations and their physiologic or pathogenic role in the disease process remains unclear.

We have found in the serum of a patient with hypogammaglobulinemia and ulcerative colitis an anti-lymphocyte antibody with clear specificity for B lymphocytes. This antibody belonged to the IgM class and was shown to play a role in the pathogenesis of the hypogammaglobulinemia.

CASE REPORT

Patient D.S. is a Portuguese woman born in 1943. She was entirely well until 1970 when she developed recurrent bronchitis and diarrhea. In 1972 she was found to have a moderately enlarged spleen, bronchiectasia and ulcerative colitis. In 1975 she had very serious bronchopulmonary infections with cardiac failure and severe ulcerative colitis leading to total colectomy. The family clinical history was not contributive.

Serum immunoglobulin (Ig) levels were repeatedly measured and varied between 2 and 5 mg/ml for IgG, 0.3 and 0.7 mg/ml for IgM and 0.1 and 0.15 mg/ml for IgA. The level of anti-B isohemagglutinins was normal, no antipoliomyelitis antibodies were found, the titers of antibodies to tetanus toxoid remained low after challenge, whereas the patient responded normally to stimulation by diphtheria toxoid. Some plasma cells containing IgA, IgM or IgG were found in the jejunal mucosa and germinal centers were present in the mesenteric lymph nodes. The level of serum total hemolytic complement was normal.

The patient was unresponsive to intradermal injections of streptokinase-streptodornase and tuberculin but the intradermal reaction to candidin was positive and she showed a normal response after sensitization to dinitrochlorobenzene. Her peripheral blood lymphocytes (PBLs) responded normally to *in vitro* stimulation by phytohemagglutinin, pokeweed mitogen and allogeneic cells.

Blood lymphocytes count varied between 600 and 1000 per mm^3. Repeated studies of surface Ig (S.Ig), of aggregated IgG binding and of E rosettes, according to published methods,[6] showed values of 0.5–1 % for B cells and 98–99 % for T lymphocytes, without any lymphocytes unidentified by these surface markers.

The discrepancy between these extremely low figures for circulating B lymphocytes and the fair but relatively moderate hypogammaglobulinemia led us to look for anti-B cell antibodies in this patient.

CHARACTERIZATION AND B CELL SPECIFICITY OF THE ANTI-LYMPHOCYTE ANTIBODIES

Using a microcytotoxicity technique,[7] serum D.S. was shown to kill 15–30% of PBLs from all 57 normal individuals tested. The serum titer reached 1/128. The lymphocytotoxic activity was detectable at 37°C and at room temperature but was increased at 4°C. An ammonium sulfate precipitate obtained from serum D.S. was coupled to fluorescein and used in direct immunofluorescence tests. This conjugate stained 10–25% of normal PBLs.

The percentage of reactive lymphocytes in normal human blood by both microcytotoxicity and direct immunofluorescence was on the same order of magnitude as figures for B cells. Table 1 shows the correlation between the number of lymphocytes stained by D.S. antibody in immunofluorescence tests and the number of B cells in various normal lymphocyte subpopulations.

Double labeling of normal peripheral blood lymphocytes with fluorescein-coupled D.S. antibody and a mixture of anti-μ and anti-λ antiserum conjugated to rhodamine showed that the vast majority, though not all, of the D.S. reactive lymphocytes bore S.Ig. Similarly, the vast majority of D.S. positive cells did not form E rosettes although 1 % of the E rosetting cells in peripheral blood (but none in tonsils) reacted with D.S. conjugate. Peripheral blood

TABLE 1.   Percentage of normal lymphocytes stained by conjugated D. S. antibody compared to usual lymphocyte markers

Lymphocyte population	Experiment number	D.S. conjugate	S.Ig	Aggregated IgG	E rosettes
PBLs					
Unfractionated	1	13	13	15	68
	2	11	11	16	64
	3	24	18		
	4	13	12		
T enriched*	1	0.5	1		
	2	0.5	0.5		
B enriched**	1	74	72		
	2	65	65		
Tonsil	1	39	45		53
	2	46	52		47
Thymus	1	0	0		98

*After passage through nylon wool column.
**After depletion of E rosetting cells by Ficoll centrifugation.

lymphocytes from three patients with sex-linked or variable immunodeficiencies and no detectable B cells were not stained by D.S. antibody. Several lymphoblastoid cell lines were tested by direct immunofluorescence. The T derived line Molt 4 was negative whereas the line 1022 which forms E rosettes and expresses IgG Fc and C3 receptors was positive. The two classical B lymphoblastoid lines Daudi and Raji were heavily labeled and D.S. antibody could be absorbed on Raji cells.

The pure IgG fraction obtained from the patient's serum by diethylaminoethyl cellulose chromatography and conjugated to fluorescein yielded negative results. The anti-lymphocyte antibody was shown to belong to the IgM class. Indeed, in indirect immunofluorescence tests performed with D.S. serum after capping of S.Ig on target lymphocytes, it was revealed by specific anti-μ conjugates and not by antisera to the other heavy chain classes. That the IgM antibody possesses both light chain types was demonstrated by the following indirect immunofluorescence experiment: D.S. antibody bound to B lymphocytes which bore only γ chains and were devoid of light chains (proliferating lymphocytes from a patient with γ heavy chain disease) was labeled by both anti-μ and anti-λ conjugated antisera. Thus D.S. antibody was characterized as polyclonal IgM molecules.

That D.S. antibody did not react with S.Ig on B cells was demonstrated by the positive reaction with Raji cells (which do not produce S.Ig) and by experiments showing independent capping of the antigen(s) stained by fluoresceinated D.S. antibody and of S.Ig revealed by anti-δ and anti-μ rhodamine conjugates on normal and leukemic lymphocytes.

Since B cells from all tested normal individuals of both sexes with various H-LA phenotypes were shown to react with serum D.S., the corresponding B cell antigen(s) is presumably not an alloantigen of the LA-like series. This does not, however, exclude the fact that D.S. antibody reacts with the "constant" moiety of the la molecule.

D.S. ANTIGEN(S) IN LYMPHOPROLIFERATIVE DISORDERS

Table 2 shows that T-derived leukemic cells and non-T, non-B acute lymphoblastic leukemia cells tested so far lacked D.S. antigen(s). Proliferating B cells from 3 patients with poorly differentiated lymphocytic lymphoma, 2 patients with γ heavy chain disease and one with acute lymphoblastic leukemia with Burkitt cells were reactive with serum D.S. In contrast to these results and to the fact that almost all B lymphocytes in the blood from all normal individuals reacted with D.S. antibody, the incidence of cases with reactive proliferating cells among patients with B CLL was surprisingly low (one third of cases of common B CLL). In some of the negative B CLL patients the absence of the antigen(s) combining with serum D.S. was confirmed by the fact that these B CLL cells, similarly to T-derived leukemic cells, were unable to absorb out the antibodies. It should be noted that the presence or absence

TABLE 2. D. S. antigen(s) in lymphoproliferative diseases (direct immunofluorescence and/or microcytotoxicity)

	B or T nature	Number tested	Number reactive with D.S. antibody
B CLL			
common	B	33	11
prolymphocytic	B	4	4
with serum monoclonal Ig	B	4	3
Poorly differentiated lymphocytic lymphoma	B	3	3
γ heavy chain disease	B	2	2
Acute leukemia with Burkitt cells	B	1	1
T CLL	T	7	0
Acute lymphoblastic leukemia	T	1	0
	non-T, non-B	4	0

168   T. Tursz *et al.*

of the antigen(s) reacting with serum D.S. roughly paralleled the intensity of the S.Ig fluorescence pattern: Whereas in all B CLL cases where serum D.S. yielded negative results the leukemic cells faintly stained for S.Ig, CLL cells with high density S.Ig reacted with D.S. antibody. The latter included 4 of 4 cases of prolymphocytic leukemia and 3 of 4 cases of CLL with a monoclonal Ig serum spike which likely reflects some degree of persistent maturation of the B cell clone.[6] The lack of D.S. antigen(s) on the cells from two-thirds of patients with common B CLL can probably not be explained on the basis of the arising of these leukemic clones from a D.S. negative B cell subset since such a subset accounts for less than 5% of normal B peripheral blood lymphocytes. Whether this negative finding is related to the neoplastic nature of the CLL cells or to the various levels in the differentiation pathway of the B cell line where proliferating clones from individual CLL patients appear to be blocked[6] is presently unknown. It is worth noting that the antigen(s) reacting with serum D.S. is expressed on only a small proportion of S.Ig bearing B blast cells induced by pokeweed mitogen stimulation on the 4th day of culture and is no longer detectable on the 7th day. Thus D.S. antigen(s) is possibly expressed at certain stages of B cell maturation only.

PATHOGENICITY OF D.S. ANTIBODY

The effects of plasmapheresis strongly suggest the pathogenic role of the anti-B cell antibody in the genesis of hypogammaglobulinemia in patient D.S. Two consecutive plasmaphereses were achieved using a continuous flow blood cell separator, the first for 6 hours with a pulled out plasma volume of more than twice the patient's plasma volume, the second for 4 hours only. Figure 1 shows that the first plasmapheresis was followed by a dramatic and transitory increase in B cell figures which reached 5% on the second day and normal percentages on the third day, whereas the antibody which was no longer detectable at the end of plasmapheresis rose progressively back to the initial titer after 6 days. Similar but less striking effects were observed after the second plasmapheresis.

REACTIVITY WITH OTHER TISSUES

D.S. anti-lymphocytic antibody did not react with human erythrocytes of various subgroups. A positive reaction with human fibroblasts was noted by direct immunofluorescence and cytotoxicity and adsorption of serum D.S.

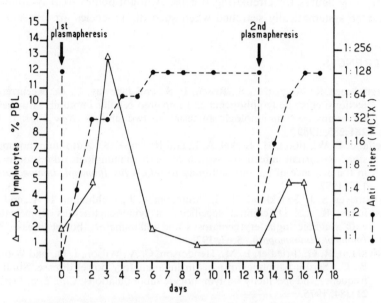

FIG. 1. Effects of plasmaphereses on the titers of anti-B cell antibodies and on the percentage of B lymphocytes in the blood.

on fibroblasts abolished its reactivity with B cells. D.S. conjugate gave a bright staining of colonic epithelium whereas the goblet cells and surface mucous were unstained. The fluorescence pattern was therefore distinct from that typically observed in ulcerative colitis.[8] The specificity of this reaction with colonic mucosa is currently under study.

CONCLUDING REMARKS

Whereas most primary immunodeficiency syndromes appear to result from an arrest in the differentiation capabilities of immunologically competent cells at various stages,[9] autoantibodies to circulating B lymphocytes may be incriminated in the pathogenesis of some hypogammaglobulinemias. Since in such cases those B cells which escape the nocivity of these antibodies are presumably able to differentiate normally, it is not suprising that in patient D.S. the impairment of humoral immunity was relatively moderate and that lymph node germinal centers and intestinal plasma cells were found, in contrast

170   T. Tursz *et al.*

to very low figures for circulating B cells. Autoantibodies to B lymphocytes
should be systematically searched when such discrepancies are observed.

Kretschmer, R., August, C. S., Rosen, F. S., and Janeway, C. A.: Recurrent in
   fections, episodic lymphopenia and impaired cellular immunity. Further observations on "immunologic amnesia" in two siblings. *New Engl. J. Med.*
   281:285, 1969.
2. Gelfand, E. W., Borel, H., Berkel, A. L, and Rosen, F. S.: Auto-immunosuppres-
   sion: Recurrent infections associated with immunologic unresponsiveness
   in the presence of an auto-antibody to IgG. *Clin. Immunol. Immunopath.* **1**:
   155, 1972.
3. Korsmeyer, S. J., Strickland, R. G., Ammann, A. J., Waldmann, T. A., and Williams, R. C.: Differential specificity of lymphocytotoxins from patients
   with systemic lupus erythematosus and inflammatory bowel disease. *Clin.
   Immunol. Immunopath.* **5**:67, 1976.
4. Strickland, R. G., Friedler, E. M., Henderson, C. A., Wilson, I. D., and Williams,
   R. C.: Serum lymphocytotoxins in inflammatory bowel disease. Studies of
   frequency and specificity for lymphocyte subpopulations. *Clin. Exp. Immunol.*
   21:384, 1975.
5. Winchester, R. J., Winfield, J. B., Siegal, F., Wernet, P., Bentwich, Z., and Kunkel, H. G.: Analyses of lymphocytes from patients with rheumatoid arthritis
   and systemic lupus erythematosus. Occurrence of interfering cold-reactive
   antilymphocyte antibodies. *J. Clin. Invest.* **54**:1082, 1974.
6. Seligmann, M., Preud'homme, J. L., and Brouet, J. C.: B and T cell markers in
   human proliferative blood diseases and primary immunodeficiencies, with
   special reference to membrane bound immunoglobulins. *Transpl. Reviews*
   16:85, 1973.
7. Terasaki, P. I., Terasaki, A. C., and Clelland, J. D.: Microdroplet assay of human
   serum cytotoxins. *Nature* **206**:998, 1964.
8. Lagercrantz, R., Hammarstrom, S., Perlmann, P., and Gustafsson, B. E.: Immunological studies in ulcerative colitis. III. Incidence of antibodies to colon-
   antigen in ulcerative colitis and other gastrointestinal diseases. *Clin. Exp.
   Immunol.* **1**:263, 1966.
9. Cooper, M. D. and Seligmann, M.: B and T lymphocytes in lymphoproliferative
   and immunodeficiency diseases. *In*: B and T cells in immune recognition
   (F. Loor and G. E. Roelants, eds), John Wiley and Sons Ltd, London, 1967
   (in press).

Dr. COOPER: The quick repair of the B-lymphocytes after you plasma-pheresis your
   patient suggest that these are being formed very rapidly from cells which lacked

the antigen to which the antibody was directed. It might be interesting to look and see if the reservoir of pre-B-cells in the bone marrow is present in excess. It is interesting that in mice treated with anti-μ antibodies and thus depleted of B-cells, there may be a compensatory increase in the frequency of pre-B-cells. One would expect, perhaps, that there would be lymphokinesis such as erythropoietin, and that these might be produced in excess and that could contribute to the rapid return when you study kinetics after plasma pheresis.

Dr. GATTI: I would like to know how this antibody, in your opinion, does not shut itself off. If this is an antibody against these B-cells, why does the patient continue to make antibodies? Do you think that the cells which are being killed, are being killed after a stage where they would be synthesizing this IgM? And also, how does this compare to the antibody that Abdou describes in the anti-μ in the patients with aquired hypo-immunogammaglobulinemia?

Dr. SELIGMANN: This antibody does not react with surface immunoglobulins. So it has nothing to do with this Abdou-type of antibody. Now to your first question, I am afraid I cannot presently answer. But you can see here, in this patient, there were intestine plasma cells there, and I think that is important. There were three classes. The enterologists are very excited because they find IgA plasma cells only in the duodenum of this patient and not in the colon, whereas they have IgG and IgM plasma cells everywhere, and the level of serum IgA, as you can see, is only 1.

Role of Immunodeficiency in Neurological Diseases

Yoshigoro Kuroiwa* and Ryoichi Mori**

1. INTRODUCTION

Immunodeficiency is involved in a wide variety of the problems encountered in clinical medicine. However, most of the cases reported so for have been rare congenital types of immunodeficiency. Immunodeficiency also can be seen in various disease sequelae. In this paper, immunodeficiency as an etiological or pathogenetical factor in disease will be discussed. We will also mention the dysimmune state, e.g. plasma cell dyscrasia connected with neurovisceral disorders.

Pathogenetically, immunodeficiency might be related to all kinds of infectious diseases, acute infections or tuberculous infections. However, in this paper we will mainly discuss the so-called slow infections.

Table 1 shows our classification of various neurological diseases in terms of immunodeficiency. They can be classified in terms of primary and secondary immunodeficiency. The dysimmune state in connection with neurological diseases is also included here. Ataxia telangiectasia is representative of the primary group. Of the secondary one, progressive multifocal leucoencephalopathy (PML) is representative. Among the "possible" group, those diseases in which immunodeficiency is only hypothesized to play a part, we have included multiple sclerosis (MS), subacute sclerosing panencephalitis (SSPE), and others.

As the dysimmune state, plasma cell dyscrasis with neurovisceral involvement has been noted recently in Japan.

---

* Department of Neurology, Neurological Institute, Faculty of Medicine, Kyushu University, Fukuoka, Japan
** Department of Microbiology, Faculty of Medicine, Kyushu University, Fukuoka, Japan

2. PRIMARY IMMUNODEFICIENCY

Ataxia telangiectasia. This is a well-known congenital error in metabolism with IgA deficiency and thymic hypolasia. These T and B cell hypofunctions result in recurrent infections as well as cerebellar degeneration. It has yet to be clarified whether the cellular degeneration is caused directly by the infection or by metabolic deviation.

TABLE 1. Immunodeficiency or dysimmune state in neurological diseases

1. PRIMARY
   Ataxia telangiectasia
2. SECONDARY
   Progressive multifocal leucoencephalopathy (PML)
3. POSSIBLE
   Multiple sclerosis (MS)
   SSPE
   Creutzfeldt-Jakob disease
4. DYSIMMUNE STATE
   Plasma cell dyscrasia

3. SECONDARY IMMUNODEFICIENCY

Slow virus diseases (Table 2) have been documented in the neurological diseases.[1] Most of them are rare, slowly progressive degenerative processes, which can be separated into the conventional and unconventional groups. Conventional slow virus diseases are slow latent infections caused by conventional viruses, such as measles (SSPE), papova (PML), Russian spring-summer encephalitis virus[2] (RSSE virus) (chronic encephalitis), and rubella virus[3] (SSPE).

Some of these conventional viruses cause both acute and slow infections (measles, rubella, RSSE), while slow infections are very rare compared with acute infections. Why only selected individuals are affected by slow infections should be thoroughly studied from the viewpoint of immunodeficiency.

Among the unconventional slow virus infections, Kuru from New Guinea and Creutzfeldt-Jakob disease are known in humans. In animals, transmissible mink encephalopathy and scrapie are well known.

Progressive multifocal leucoencephalopathy (PML). This disease was first named by Aström[4] *et al.* in 1958 while working on the progressive demyelination of the brains found in Hodgkin's disease or lymphatic leukemia. Their insight united the demyelinating disease with different severe diseases in

TABLE 2.   Slow virus infections

A. CONVENTIONAL VIRUSES
PML ....Papova
SSPE ....Measles (var.)
Russian Spring Summer Encephalitis
B. UNCONVENTIONAL VIRUSES
Kuru   (New Guinea)
Creutzfeldt-Jakob Disease
Animal
Scrapie (Sheep, goats)
Transmissible Mink Encephalopathy

a single entity. Later, papova-virus-like inclusions were demonstrated pathologically by ZuRein *et al.* (1965), and after that virus isolation was accomplished (Padgett *et al.*, 1971).[5,6]

Since Aström's work, more than 100 cases have been reported in the literature, and in PML various underlying diseases have been noted (Table 3). Among these lymphoproliferative or myeloproliferative diseases, sarcoma, granuloma, sarcoidosis and others have been reported.

TABLE 3.   PML-Underlying diseases

Lymph. leukemia	16%
Lymph. sarcoma	10
Hodgkin	21
Myel. leukemia	6
Sarcoidosis	5
Carcinomatosis	4
Malig. lymphoma	2
Reticulosarcoma	2
Multiple myeloma	2

81 cases (100%)

PML case report (Kyushu Univ. Hospital) (Kuroiwa et al.).

A 46-year-old man six months before admission suffered from blurred vision, milliary skin rash, and slowly progressing mental deterioration. On admission, skin rash and mental deterioration were major symptoms, with both Gerstmann's and Balint syndromes. Minor cranial nerve signs and dysarthria were noted; generalized paralysis developed and the patient died in two months. The premortem diagnosis was PML. A CBC revealed chronic lymphatic leukemia, and a fresh brain autopsy was done. Pathology revealed typical PML demyelinating lesions in the cerebral white matter. Virus particles were isolated from the fresh brain and various virological and immunological tests were performed.[7] The following PML virus was shown: 40–45 mμ in diameter, with 72 dextratype capsomeres, different serologically from any known papova group (SV 40, human papilloma, and polyoma viruses) verified by the microagglutination technique.

Using isolated PML virion from the fresh brain, antibodies in sera from various diseases were studied by the microagglutination technique. In addition to this case of PML, other non-PML cases such as Hodgkin's disease, leukemia, and papilloma frequently showed positive antibodies (Table 4). Although we did not find any antibody in the normal control (4 cases), Padgett reported 70% of normal individuals have positive antibody to JC virus. This suggests that PML viruses are more widespread than the rare cases of PML. Immunological tests in our case showed poor response of antibody formation to vaccination of Japanese B encephalitis as well as negative Tuberculine test (namely both B and T cell functions were deficient). Imano et al. (1976) reported a remarkable T cell decrease in his case of PML, whereas B cells increased.

TABLE 4.   Immunological tests of PML virus and serum (Amako, KUH)

A.	PML serum (this case)
	Positive with PML virus (this case)
	Negative with other Papova viruses
	(SV40, h. papilloma, polyoma v.)
B.	PML virus (this case)
	Positive with sera of papilloma (3/7)
	Hodgkin (2/2)
	Lymph. leukemia (2/4)
	Negative in normal control (0/4)

Such hypoimmune states which are due to underlying diseases might provide an explanation for the rare manifestations of PML in connection with common virus infections.

4. POSSIBLE GROUP

Subacute sclerosing panencephalitis. Whether SSPE might be related to immunodeficiency of any kind or not is an interesting problem. There are many studies on this subject. However, the studies on the existence of immunodeficiency are not consistent. One case we studied recently immunologically revealed cellular and humoral immune responses by LMI test and lymphocyte blastogenesis. The rarity of SSPE, in contrast to common acute measles infection, might be explained by a variation of the virus (SSPE variant of measles virus), *e.g.* Niigata I strain, a defective virus without budding formation. Whether a virus factor or individual factors might be important in the pathogenesis of SSPE should be studied further.

Multiple sclerosis (MS). MS is an important neurological disease, *e.g.* demyelinating encephalomyelitis, with some inflammatory nature in the acute stage. The etiological agent for such inflammation is unknown, but the unique geographical distribution of this disease might be related to its etiology. Japan and Asia are known to be low risk areas. The prevalence rates of MS are beautifully correlated with latitude, suggesting that the exogenous etiological factors are universally distributed along the lines of latitude. However, even in the high risk areas, only one out of 2,000, or 50 per 100,000, roughly speaking, are affected (Table 5). What could be another factor? Individual factors might be genetic or immunological ones. As to Japanese MS,[8] exogenous factors seem to be reduced to about one tenth of Caucasian MS, compared with the same latitude. Such racially related factors could be genetic ones. The age of onset of MS in low and high risk areas are surprisingly similar with the mean age of onset of about 30 years. If only exogenous viral factors were responsible, different ages of onset would appear in low and high risk areas. Thus other age dependent individual factors should be considered.

As to genetic factor HLA studies have indicated certain possibilities; HLA−A3, −B7, and −LD7a are considered to be prevalent in MS cases. There has been an attempt to explain the rarity of MS in Japan by the low incidence of these genes. In order to test the HLA theory, we have studied Japanese MS cases,[9] and no relationship was seen with A3 and B7. However, further studies are now being done.

Lymphocytotoxicity of MS lymphocytes. The cellular immunity of MS to basic

TABLE 5.   Multiple sclerosis

1. High risk area over 50/100,000 popul.
Japan   2–4/100,000
2. Geographical factor-latitude
(universal)
3. Why selected person affected?
—Individual factors
a. HL-A 3, 7 (Naito, Terasaki, Jersild)
LD 7a
g. Immunodeficiency to viruses?
Utermohlen *et al.* (MIF)
Mori & Kuroiwa (Cytotoxicity of lymphocyte)

proteins, measles antigens, etc., has been studied. However, no consistent results have been obtained as to the pathogenesis of MS.

Since Imagawa and Meulen slow infection by paramyxovirus remains an important problem in MS. We have studied lymphocyte toxicity to measles virus-infected HeLa cells by direct observation with time-lapsed cinematography.[10] Normal lymphocytes killed a considerable number of the measles infected HeLa cells during the course of 30 hrs. However, MS lymphocytes killed fewer cells as shown by the cell growth index, and this weaker cytotoxicity of MS lymphocytes vs. normal ones is significant (Fig. 1.). Similar data was observed by Utermohlen et al.[11] by the MIT method; however, our data might interpret the pathogenesis of MS more directly.

CELL GROWTH INDEX OF MS AND NON-MS

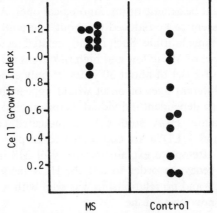

FIG. 1.   Cell growth index of MS and non-MS (from Mori et al.)
Cytotoxic activity of peripheral blood lymphocytes against HeLa cells
persistently infected with measles virus: Neurology 26 (6 part 2): 78, 1976

Whether this hypoimmune state (cellular-immunity) associated with MS might be a factor which allows a slow infection of some viruses to MS cases or not is another important question.

5. DYSGLOBULINEMIC STATE WITH NEUROVISCERAL IN-VOLVEMENT

Recently in Japan unusual complications with myeloma or mono- or poly-clonial gammopathies have been reported. All the cases have tetrads such as skin pigmentation, generalized edema, polyneuropathy, and dysglobuline-mia. Here I (YK) will call this syndrome "Dysglobulinemic cutaneo-visceral polyneuropathy" (Dysglobulinemic CVN). Including our cases, 23 cases (Japanese) are summarized (Table 6).

TABLE 6.   Dysglobulinemic C-V-N syndrome—23 Japanese Cases

1.	Sex: M:F = 3.6:1	
2.	Age of onset (mean)	46 yrs
2.	Mixed type polyneuropathy	100%
3.	Skin pigmentation	100
	Sclerodermoid	
	White nail	
	Hypertrichosis	61
4.	Edema, generalized	74
	Papilledema	52
	Hepatomegaly	65
5.	Gynecomastia (male)	67
	Diabetes	39

(H. Iwashita, Y. Kuroiwa)

There are a male preponderance with an average age of onset of 46 yrs, a clinically mixed type of polyneuropathy of the globe and stocking type, dark skin pigmentation with thickening of the skin (scleroderma-like) and edema, white nails, thick hypertrichosis in legs and chest, endocrine changes (gynecomastia and diabetes), liver and spleen enlargement, and dysglobulinemia. X-ray studies showed that in about half of these cases dysglobulinemia was caused by soli-tary myeloma. However, this type of myeloma has many features of solitary osteosclerotic myeloma (Fig. 2).

Needle biopsy of our case showed typical plasmocytoma of such solitary or localized osteosclerotic myeloma in the spine, and after irradiation, the skin changes gradually improved.

The pathogenesis of cutaneo-visceral and neural involvement has its roots in the dysimmune state due to plasmocytoma or other dysglobulinemic states (poly- or monoclonal), although some other metabolic pathogenesis might be also possible. Also some racial factors could be suspected due to the rarity of such conditions among Caucasian myeloma, although exact comparative studies remain to be done.

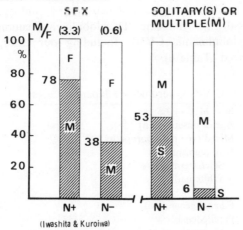

FEATURES OF MYELOMA (OSTEOSCLEROTIC) WITH NEUROPATHY

(Iwashita & Kuroiwa)

FIG. 2.   Features of (osteosclerotic) myeloma with neuropathy
        Note: N+ denotes myeloma with neuropathy.
        N−, myeloma without neuropathy.

TABLE 7.   DGL-C-V-N syndrome, laboratory

CBC: Normal	
SERUM PROTEIN	
Gammaglobulin increase	83
Monoclonal gammopathy	65
(lambda chain)	
CSF:	
gammaglobulin increase	100
(albulinocytologic diss.)	
EMG and Conduction Velocity:	
marked denervation	
Nerve Pathology: large fiber loss	
MYELOMA	
Solitary myeloma	75
Osteosclerotic	58

(Figures in percentages)

6. CONCLUSION

The role of immunodeficiency in neurological problems should be an important clue in the pathogenesis of various disorders, primary or secondary ones. In a condition where etiological agents are universally distributed in the world, selected affection of some individuals should be studied in terms of immunodeficiency. Dysimmune states due to other conditions, especially plasmocytoma, were also mentioned here. Genetic predisposition should be also studied through international comparisons.

REFERENCES

1. Gajdusek, D. C. and Gibbs, C. J. Jr.: NINDB Monograph, No. 2. Slow Latent and Temperate Virus Infections. U.S. Pub. Health Serv., Wash., DC. IX-X, 1965.
2. Ogawa, M., Okubo, H., Tsuji, Y., Yashu, Y., and Sonoda, K.: Chronic progressive encephalitis occurring 13 years after Russian spring-summer encephalitis. *J. Neurol. Sci.* 19:363, 1973.
3. Townsend, J., Baringer, J. R., Wolinsky, J. S., Malamud, N., Mednick, J. P., Panitch, H. S., Scott, R. A. T., Oshiro, L. S., and Cremer, N. E.: Progressive subella panencephalitis, late onset after congenital rubella. *New Engl. J. Med.* May, 8:990, 1975.
4. Aström, K. E., Mancall, E. L., and Richardson, E. P. Jr.: Progressive multifocal leucoencephalopathy. *Brain* 81:93, 1958.
5. Padgett, B. L., Walker, D. L., ZuRein, G. M., *et al.*: Cultivation of papova like virus from human brain with progressive multifocal leukoencephalopathy. *Lancet* 1:1257, 1971.
6. Weiner, L. P. and Narayan, O.: Virologic studies of progressive multifocal leukoencephalopathy. *Progr. Med. Virol.* 18:229, 1974.
7. Amako, K. and Mori, R.: Serological and morphological studies on progressive multifocal leukoencephalopathy. *Jap. J. Microbiol.* 16:155, 1972.
8. Kuroiwa, Y. and Shibasaki, H.: Epidemiologic and clinical studies of multiple sclerosis in Japan. *Neurology* 26 (6, Part 2): 8, 1976.
9. Saito, S., Naito S., Kawanami, S., and Kuroiwa, Y.: HLA studies on multiple sclerosis in Japan. *Neurol.* 26 (6, part 2):49, 1976.
10. Mori, R., Nagasawa, K., Umene, K., Miyazono, J., Shibasaki, H., and Kuroiwa, Y.: Cytotoxic activity of peripheral blood lymphocytes against HeLa cells persistently infected with measles virus: Depressed capacity in multiple sclerosis. *Neurol.* 26 (6, part 2): 77, 1976.
11. Utermohlen, V. and Zabriski, J. B.: A suppression of cellular immunity in patients with multiple sclerosis. *J. Exp. Med.* 138:1591, 1973.
12. Iwashita, H., Inoue, N., and Nagamatsu, K.: Polyneuropathy, pigmentation, diabetes mellitus and monoclonal gammopathy. *Clinc. Neurol.* (Tokyo) 11: 492, 1971.

182 Y. Kuroiwa and R. Mori

13. Imawari, M., Akatsuka, N., Ishibashi, M., et al.: Syndrome of plasma cell dyscrasia, polyneuropathy and endocrine disturbances: Report of a case. Ann. Intern. Med. 81:490, 1974.
14. Iwashita, H., Ohnishi, A., Asada, M., Kanazawa, Y., and Kuroiwa, Y.: Polyneuropathy, skin pigmentation, edema and hypertrichosis in localized osteosclerotic myeloma. Neurology 27:675, 1977.

DISCUSSION

Dr. SELIGMANN: I think that one of the very interesting features in this disease is that your monoclonal immunoglobulin chain almost always is an IgG. And this this reminds me of another quite different condition which is mucinoses papuleuses a skin disease in which you find always a slow migrating monoclonal IgG with the same type of light chains. This fact points to the possibility that this monoclonal protein in this peculiar disease could have the same antigen-binding activity with a known antigen. Since we are unable to screen for the antigen because we do not know what it is, I think that one of the ways of exploring the possible identity of the variable regions of the chains of the monocolonal immunoglobulin in all these patients is to look for shared ideotypic determinants in the monoclonal immunoglobulin in all these patients.

Dr. GOOD: What troubles me is why you think of this as multiple sclerosis. Why not think of it as another demyelinating disease? I think that the association of MS with B-7 and DW-2 is not nearly as tight, and the latest evidence from Kunkel's laboratory is that the association with a determinant on the B-lymphocyte is virtually 100 per cent. So you may find a further association of the majoristic compatibility region if you go further. We have done extensive studies of the leucocyte migration inhibition and the generation of MIF in multiple sclerosis and they are equivalent with the measles virus. That does not mean that we do not think that there might be an association with measles virus, but we cannot any longer take seriously the migration with the measles virus by itself.

Dr. HAYASHI: Coproski showed that parainfluenza infection in the nude mice did not cause any lesions. However, when injected intracerebrally it produced severe white matter lesion. So one thing I want to mention is that in regard to central nervous system infection, you have to study T-cell/B-cell interaction to produce antibodies locally. And one more thing is viral infection. When you think about viral infection, a very well known fact is that virus can be mutate, or mutant, can arise in or during, in vivo infections and one very classical example of that is the influenza virus. And so, when you have the influenza virus infect patients or animals, then produce antibody, then some selective mutant can arise during that period, and SSPE patients may very well be caused by that kind of thing. Measles-related virus agent found in SSPE patients may mean that it is a mutant from measles virus caused by antibody reaction.

Associated Diseases in Selective IgA Deficiency

Tadashi Kanoh

ABSTRACT

First, we give a pathogenetic concept of disorders of the IgA system and propose a rational definition and classification of selective IgA deficiency. Secondly, we discuss the clinical aspects of selective IgA deficiency on the basis of a study of 27 patients and present an extremely interesting case of acquired selective IgA deficiency. Thirdly, the results of family studies of selected patients and their significance are discussed. Fourthly, a summary of the immunological abnormalities seen in our cases is presented. Finally, we present a brief preliminary report of a unique familial pulmonary fibrosis coexistent with secretory component deficiency.

We may reasonably conclude that selective IgA deficiency has a variety of clinical and immunological aspects. Various clinical features in selective IgA deficiency seem mostly to arise from or to have relation to a defect of the IgA system. Thus, there is no doubt that immunodeficiency of this type is one of the most fascinating subjects for investigation of the immunologic system of defense.

INTRODUCTION

Since the first description by West et al.[1] of an isolated lack of serum IgA being associated with a variety of diseases, many reports have appeared in the literature about selective IgA deficiency in apparently healthy subjects[2-5] and in association with significant diseases.[3,6,7] The biological role of IgA antibodies is not clearly defined. Secretory IgA (S-IgA) has viral neutralizing activity[8] in the absence of complement fixation and may protect the mucous surfaces by preventing mucosal adherence and subsequent proliferation of bacteria.[9] Nasal washings from normal and allergic individuals have been found to contain IgA

First Division, Department of Internal Medicine, Kyoto University School of Medicine, Kyoto, Japan blocking antibodies.[10] Another possible biological function of S-IgA may be to limit absorption of nonviable antigens through the gastrointestinal and respiratory epithelia.[11] Thus, IgA deficiency seems to predispose a variety of clinical problems. There is no question, however, that some people with selective IgA deficiency get along well.[2-5] This provides a challenge in understanding S-IgA as an immune protective system of the mucous surfaces.

The purpose of this report is to give a pathogenetic concept of disorders of the IgA system, to propose a rational definition and classification of selective IgA deficiency, to describe the clinical spectrum of selective IgA deficiency on the basis of study of 27 patients and to discuss the results of family studies on selected patients, and to present a summary of the results of immunological studies. In addition, a brief preliminary report of a unique familial pulmonary fibrosis coexistent with secretory component deficiency will be presented.

DISORDERS OF THE IgA SYSTEM

In order to maintain an adequate function of the IgA system, each of the following four critical functions should be intact: (1) production of serum IgA, (2) local synthesis of dimeric IgA, (3) synthesis and accumulation of secretory component by the epithelium, and (4) appearance of S-IgA in the secretions, binding of secretory component to dimeric IgA, and subsequent external transport of S-IgA. From the level of defect in these functions, disorders of the IgA system can be divided into three major categories: (1) selective IgA deficiency which lacks serum IgA, (2) secretory IgA deficiency which lacks S-IgA in the presence of serum IgA, and (3) others[12,13] which have neoplastic or abnormal IgA-producing cells incapable of producing complete molecules of IgA. In addition, deficiency of serum IgA and S-IgA can be subdivided into five or four theoretical types, respectively (Table 1).

SELECTIVE IgA DEFICIENCY

Definition

Based on a review of the literature and our experience with 27 patients, we have given a definition of selective IgA deficiency as follows: (1) a serum IgA level less than 5 mg/100ml, and (2) no deficiency of other major immunoglobulins (IgG and IgM). We differ with Ammann and Hong[7] on the diagnostic criteria of this abnormality. Namely, normal humoral and cellular immunity are not included by us in this type. Associated diseases of selective IgA defi-

TABLE 1.   Disorders of the IgA system

		serum IgA	secretory IgA	local synthesis	S-component	our cases
Normal		+	+	+	+	
Selective IgA deficiency	*1	−	−	−	+	26
	2	−	−	+	+	
	3	−	−	−	−	
	4	−	−	+	−	
	*5	−	+	+	+	1
Secretory IgA deficiency	1	+	−	−	+	
	2	+	−	+	+	
	*3	+	−	−	− ⎫	
	*4	+	−	+	− ⎭	3
Others	*1	α-chain disease (Seligmann, 1968)				
	*2	absence of light-heavy chain assembly (Moroz, 1971)				

*Already-known types

ciency, for example autoimmune diseases, sometimes show a subtle deficiency of cellular immunity. It is needless to mention that other types of primary immunodeficiency diseases listed in the WHO classification,[14] such as ataxia telangiectasia, should be excluded. Moreover, the cases under 3 years of age

TABLE 2.   Primary immunodeficiency diseases examined in our laboratory (1968–1976)

Infantile X-linked agammaglobulinemia	5
Selective immunoglobulin deficiency (IgA)	27
Transient hypogammaglobulinemia of infancy	2
X-linked immunodeficiency with hyper-IgM	2
Thymic hypoplasia (DiGeorge syndrome)	
Episodic lymphopenia with lymphocytotoxin	
Immunodeficiency with normal or without hyperimmunoglobulinemia	
Immunodeficiency with ataxia telangiectasia	9
Immunodeficiency with thrombocytopenia and eczema (Wiskott-Aldrich syndrome)	
Immunodeficiency with thymoma	
Immunodeficiency with short-limbed dwarfism	
Immunodeficiency with generalized hematopoietic hypoplasia	
Severe combined immunodeficiency	
(a) autoxomal recessive	3
(b) X-linked	5
(c) sporadic	
Variable immunodeficiency (common, largely unclassified)	14
	67

were excluded from this study, for it is impossible to differentiate them from
the so-called "slow starter" type.[1]

Sixty-seven patients with primary immunodeficiency diseases were studied in
our laboratory during the past 8 years. Twenty-seven patients with selective
IgA deficiency ranging from ages 4 to 59 years were included among them.
The ratio of male to female was 13 to 14 (Table 2).

Classification

Comparing our data with those from the literature we will attempt to propose a rational classification of selective IgA deficiency from two aspects:
pathogenetic and clinical (Table 3). Viewed from the pathogenetic aspect,
there are two categories which may be termed (1) primary and (2) secondary.
All cases of selective IgA deficiency are not of primary and/or of congenital
nature. Selective deficiency of IgA rarely develops during the course of illness

TABLE 3.   Classification of selective IgA deficiency

Pathogenetic aspect:	
I. Primary	
Sporadic/Familial/Hereditary	
Congenital/Primary acquired	
II. Secondary	
Acquired	
Clinical aspect:	
I. Asymptomatic	
1. Apparently healthy persons	3 cases*
2. Apparently healthy relatives of patients with hypogam-maglobulinemia or other immune disorders	
II. Symptomatic	
1. Respiratory diseases	14 cases*
2. Gastrointestinal diseases	9
3. Chronic or recurrent infections	9
4. Allergic disorders	7
5. Autoimmune diseases	6
6. Cirrhosis or hepatitis	3
7. Viral infections	2
8. Malignancy	2
9. Thymic abnormalities	1
10. Chromosomal abnormalities	3
11. Epilepsy or seizures	13
12. Mental retardation	3
13. Other psychoneuropathies	3
14. Endocrinopathies	2
15. Miscellaneous	2

*The actual numbers of affected patients are shown in the right column.

by the known mechanism (secondary acquired).[15,16] Viewed from the clinical aspect, selective IgA deficiency can be divided into the two categories which can be termed (1) asymptomatic and (2) symptomatic. Although immunodeficiency of this type has been often said to be not uncommon in apparently healthy individuals, in our Japanese series about 10 percent of the cases were asymptomatic. Admittedly, the other 24 patients had certain significant associated diseases. The patients had 3 or more associated diseases on the average.

Clinical spectrum

Infectious diseases. Table 4 presents the chronic or recurrent infections seen among the patients so affected. As previously observed,[3,7,17,18] the predominance of respiratory infections was comfirmed. However, in contrast to those having additional immunological defects, they were generally mild. Not only bacterial, but also viral and fungal[19] infections were seen. Here we would like to pay attention to the association of selective IgA deficiency with viral hepatitis. Three of our patients had been in excellent health before they had viral hepatitis. Following the hepatitis, symptoms related to immunodeficiency appeared. IgA deficiency may follow infection with viruses capable of producing hepatitis. Moreover, high fever of unknown origin seems to occur more frequently than expected.

TABLE 4. Types of chronic or recurrent infection seen among 27 patients with selective IgA deficiency

*Bacterial;	otitis media	3 cases
	upper respiratory infection	10
	pneumonia	5
	urinary tract infection	3
	lymphadenitis	1
	skin	1
	diarrhea	2
*Viral;	hepatitis	3
	herpes zoster	1
	aseptic meningitis	1
*Fungal;	skin	2
	respiratory tract	1
*High fever of unknown origin		6

Gastrointestinal manifestations.   The gastrointestinal manifestations in patients with a lack of IgA are protean.[7,20-25] Special attention should be given to the fact that atrophic gastritis, in which the serum gastrin level is usually high, was associated with a low level of serum gastrin in some cases of selective IgA deficiency (Fig. 1). Atrophic gastritis of this type may have a causal relation to the occurrence of gastric carcinoma. In contrast to the results from Occidentals,[21,24] no case of celiac disease or pernicious anemia was seen in our Japanese series.

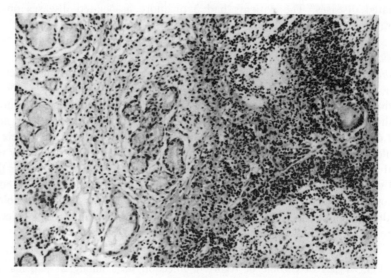

FIG. 1. Histologic picture of atrophic gastritis with low level of serum gastrin (25 pg/ml) in a 25-year-old woman (Case 10). H.E. stain, × 100

Autoimmune diseases.   A variety of autoimmune diseases have been reported in association with selective IgA deficiency (Table 5). The most common disease observed seems to be rheumatoid arthritis. In our series, however, systemic lupus erythematosus was most frequently seen. In our experience, most of the patients with autoimmune disease complicated with selective IgA deficiency had significant symptoms reflecting a defective defense mechanism (Fig. 2). The several mechanisms by which IgA deficiency could lead to autoimmune disease have been discussed. It is believed that the combined occurrence of selective IgA deficiency and autoimmune diseases can be explained by a deficiency of local immunity or associated thymic abnormalities. However, we have confirmed that autoimmune disease preceded the occurrence of IgA deficiency (acquired selective IgA deficiency).[16] Therefore, IgA deficiency may be induced by autoimmune mechanisms. As stated later, we found a high

To. Hi.   F.   Born in 1932

Isolated IgA deficiency
  Subacute hepatitis
  SLE
  Recurrent pneumonia

Nov. 1961	Raynaud syndrome	Aug.	Positive LE cell
May 1968	General malaise / Jaundice	Sept.	Isolated IgA deficiency
	Hypergammaglobulinemia (4.7 g%)		IgG 3760 mg%, IgA 0 mg%, IgM 368 mg%, IgD 7 mg%,
Sept.	Pharyngitis		K / L ratio 1.2, ANF (+++), LET (+++)
		Oct.	Renal insufficiency
Mar. 1969	Pneumonia		
May	High fever of unknown origin	Mar. 1970	Pneumonia
July	Exanthema / Stomatitis aphthosa	Apr.	Expired

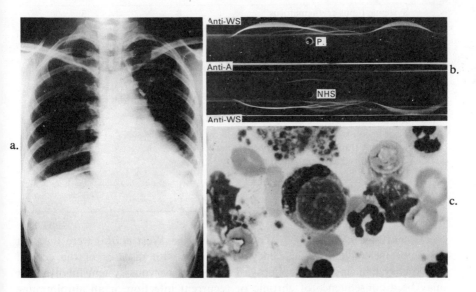

FIG. 2.   Marked susceptibility to infection occurring in a patient with SLE and selective IgA deficiency (Case 14).
a.   Chest X-ray film showing pneumonia in the left lower field.
b.   Immunoelectrophoretic pattern showing lack of IgA.
c.   Typical LE cell.

percentage of various autoimmune phenomena and immunologic abnormalities.

Malignancy.   Malignancy has been seen in selective IgA deficiency. Carcinoma of the esophagus, stomach, colon, and lung and malignant lymphomas have been reported.[20,26] To the list uterine carcinoma has now been added. Special attention should be paid to the fact that all of these carcinomas are in areas where secretory antibody is normally present. IgA deficiency may be associated with malignancy in a number of ways. The possible association of a defect of the IgA system with deficient thymic immunity in these patients might be related to an increased incidence of malignancy.

TABLE 5.   Autoimmune diseases associated with selective IgA deficiency

	Literature	Hong	Kanoh
Systemic lupus erythematosus	8	2	3
Rheumatoid arthritis	26		
Dermatomyositis	2	1	1
Pernicious anemia	6		
Thyroiditis	4	4	(1)
Cerebral vasculitis		1	1(PN)
Idiopathic Addison disease	2		
Sjögren syndrome	2		
Lupoid hepatitis	2	3	(1)
Transfusion reaction	7		
Idiopathic thrombocytopenic purpura	1		
Coombs positive hemolytic anemia	2		
Pulmonary hemosiderosis	3	2	
Regional enteritis	1		
Ulcerative colitis	1		1

Nervous system diseases.   To our knowledge, West *et al.*[1] were the first to report selective IgA deficiency in patients with diseases of the central nervous system, including epilepsy. The central nervous system involvement may be a consequence of chronic or recurrent infection or an autoimmune process, or both, since a high incidence of infection and autoimmune disease in selective IgA deficiency is well known. However, a satisfactory explanation should be given for the fact that about half the cases had epilepsy treated with anticonvulsants (Table 6). Since we reported selective IgA deficiency in a patient with postencephalitic epilepsy in 1968,[27] we have paid special attention to the effect of anticonvulsants, especially phenytoin, on the IgA system.[82] In addition, we found variable common immunodeficiency (2 cases) in epilepsy

TABLE 6. Drugs used in epileptics with selective IgA deficiency

Epilepsy/Seizures	13 cases
Anticonvulsant treatment	12 cases
phenytoin alone	6 cases
phenytoin + phenobarbital	2
carbamazepine alone	1
trimetadione + phenobarbital	1
phenobarbital alone	1

patients receiving phenytoin; these patients lacked both serum and secretory IgA. In one patient an abnormal serum IgA (5 mg/100ml) rose to 20 mg/100 ml when phenytoin was withdrawn, in parallel with a rise in the numbers of IgA-containing plasma cells in the jejunal mucosa. Immunohematological abnormalities are common in patients with selective IgA deficiency and in patients on anticonvulsants. One patient with selective IgA deficiency and epilepsy had systemic lupus erythematosus. As discussed later, antinuclear antibodies and anti-IgA antibodies were in some patients with immunodeficiency diseases and epilepsy, and of 35 epileptics treated with phenytoin, three had antinuclear antibodies and seven had anti-IgA antibodies. From these results, we conclude that:

(1) Phenytoin can mainly affect the IgA system, but sometimes other immunoglobulins also.

(2) Selective IgA deficiency may be induced by the drug through the development of autoimmunity.[16,29] Besides the defective secretion and increased catabolism of IgA, the suppression of lymphoid tissue by anti-IgA antibodies may be implicated in the pathogenesis of selective IgA deficiency, as shown in animal experiments.[30,31]

(3) Phenytoin may directly affect IgA-producing cells in the gut-associated lymphoid tissues.

(4) Autoimmunity induced by the drug could occur in conjunction with immunodeficiency diseases. Anticonvulsants, mainly phenytoin, have been linked with a broader spectrum of immunopathies, including lymphoma. These findings would be pertinent to the pathogenesis of malignant lymphomas, which also can be induced by the drug.[32]

Thymic abnormalities. IgA-antibody production seems to be highly thymus-dependent; intact T-cell function is required for normal IgA-antibody production.[33] IgA deficiency has been observed in homozygous nude mice. In humans, various diseases having defective T-cell immunity are associated with IgA deficiency.[19] For example, investigation of ataxia-telangiectasia revealed a high percentage of IgA deficiency.[34] Several cases of thymic abnormalities, including thymoma,[35] associated with lack of IgA have been reported (Fig. 3).[29] It has been suggested that some of the patients who lack IgA are deficient in a subpopulation of helper T-cells.[36]

Acquired selective IgA deficiency

According to our experience, a gradual reduction in serum IgA is seen in ataxia-telangiectasia. Several cases of acquired selective IgA deficiency have been reported.[16,37] In our series, there were 5 cases of acquired selective IgA deficiency (2 with autoimmune disease and 3 with epilepsy), in which serum IgA became selectively less than 5 mg/100ml during the course of illness (Table 7). Of these patients four had anti-IgA antibodies. An extremely interesting case was that of a 58-year-old man with periarteritis nodosa-like disease. He de-

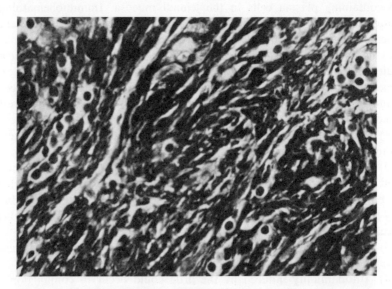

FIG. 3. The thymus from a 24-year-old woman with selective IgA deficiency (Case 1).[19] The prominent feature is a relatively increased epithelial element arranged in whirls. Lymphocytes are scanty and scattered among the epithelial cells. H.E. stain, × 400

TABLE 7. Five cases of acquired selective IgA deficiency

Case 4	57M	Cerebral vasculitis or PN	Anti-IgA(−)
Case 6	21F	SLE, chronic thyroiditis	Anti-IgA(+)
Case 16	21M	Epilepsy, Recklinghausen's dis.	Anti-IgA(+)
Case 24	4M	Epilepsy	Anti-IgA(+)
Case 25	4M	Epilepsy	Anti-IgA(+)

veloped a rapid deficiency of serum IgA within several months. Subsequent to this disappearance of IgA, he had repeated attacks of asthma, probably based on respiratory infection. He showed persistent deficiency of serum IgA during two years' observation (Fig. 4).

It is clear that selective IgA deficiency is not always primary and/or congenital. It has been inferred from studies of these acquired cases that the following mechanisms might be operative in the pathogenesis of acquired selective IgA deficiency in a complicated manner under genetic factors:

(1) Suppression of IgA production and/or increased catabolism of IgA by autoantibodies to IgA (secondary acquired).

(2) Direct suppression of IgA production by certain drugs or viral infections or indirect suppression or hypercatabolism of IgA through the production of anti-IgA antibodies (secondary acquired).

Of course, the possibility that IgA deficiency which occurs in the course of illness is not related to the disease and is coincidental cannot be ruled out (primary acquired).

Family studies

Familial occurrences of selective IgA deficiency have been reported on several occasions,[38-42] but the mode of inheritance is not entirely clear. In Japan no examples of familial selective IgA deficiency have been recognized. We have examined 6 families of 27 patients with selective IgA deficiency. Familial aggregation of IgA deficiency was not detected. However, some relatives, particularly in 2 families, had a marked elevation of IgA, an abnormality also detected by Huntley and Stephenson[38] in relatives of IgA-deficient patients, and other immunoglobulin abnormalities. The presence of acquired selective IgA deficiency and the finding of selective IgA deficiency in only one of identical twins[43] suggest the possibility that some environmental factors may be implicated in the development or expression of IgA deficiency.

Immunological studies

A variety of immunologic tests were performed on selected patients. Almost all of the symptomatic cases showed at least one or more immunologic reactivities. These are summarized in. Table 8. These findings support the concept that a lack of IgA is not the only manifestation selective IgA deficiency has shown in the immunological aspect. Immunodeficiency of this type seems to be much more complicated in the clinical as well as in the immunological sense than expected.[7,16,19,21,25,26,29] There are, as yet, many unsolved problems concerning the nature of selective IgA deficiency.

Ge. Oka.   58 M

Isolated IgA deficiency

— —— —— Corticosteroids / ACTH ————————

============ Anabolic steroids ============

+ Erythema

+ Increased brain pressure +   +   +   +   + + +   +   +   + +

      + Bronchitis   +   +   + +

             + Pleuritis   + Pneumonia

                        + Asthmatic attack + + + +++ +++

a.   + Candidiasis

Dec. '69	May '70			Dec. '70	May '71	Dec. '71
T. P. 7.5 g%	7.6			7.4	6.0	7.2
γ-glob. 1.4 g%	0.6			0.7	0.5	0.6
IgA 322 mg%	192	0	0	0		0
IgG 984	741	843	1010	640	741	831
IgM 60	50	42	42	42	42	57
IgD 0.1			2	4		
IgE 320 ng/ml		175				
K/L 1.9		3.9				
R F (+2 ME) x 40 (0)		x 80 (x 40)				
ANF +		−				
LET +		−				
β_1A 111 mg%		82				

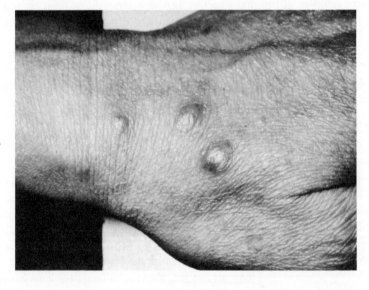

b.

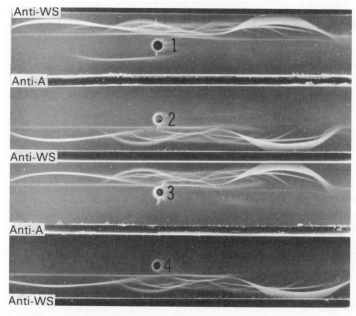

Fig. 4.   Acquired selective IgA deficiency occurring in a 58-year-old
man with periarteritis nodosa-like syndrome (Case 4).
a. A scheme of clinical course.
b. Skin lesions due to vasculitis.
c. Serum immunoelectrophoresis: (1) Jan. 1970, (2) May 1970, (3)
   Mar. 1971, and (4) Mar. 1972.

SECRETORY IgA DEFICIENCY

Secretory IgA deficiency which lacks S-IgA in the presence of serum IgA
is a very rare immunodeficiency disease. Strober et al.[44] described a 15-year-
old boy with chronic intestinal candidiasis who had a normal serum IgA level
without S-IgA and free secretory component in his secretions. A preliminary
report of a unique familial pulmonary fibrosis associated with secretory component deficiency has been presented (Fig. 5). It remains to be elucidated
whether the secretory component deficiency of these cases belongs to type 3

TABLE 8.   A summary of immunologic abnormalities in 27 patients

1. Immunodeficiency
    Selective IgA deficiency, usually associated with S-IgA deficiency
    Impaired humoral immunity
    Low titer of isohemagglutinins
    Inability to develop IgA-secreting cells from IgA-producing cells
    Impaired cellular immunity
    Thymic dysplasia
    Decreased IgA-bearing lymphocytes in about 10% of the cases
2. Autoimmunity
    Association with autoimmune diseases
    LE cell/LE test
    Anti-thyroglobulin antibody
    ANF/Fluorescent autoantibody
    RF/Inverse RF
    Anti-immunoglobulin A, M, and D
3. Malignancy
    Uterine carcinoma
    Hodgkin's disease
4. Miscellaneous
    Increased IgG and/or IgM
    Abnormal K/L ratio
    Cryoglobulinemia
    7S-IgM
    Monoclonal IgG
    Anti-milk antibody
    Anti-bovidae antibody
    Hypocomplementemia
    Decreased PHA responsiveness
    Increased PHA responsiveness

or type 4 of the classification of secretory IgA deficiency proposed by us. In contrast to normal persons and to patients with ordinary selective IgA deficiency, three members of this family had deficiency of free secretory component and S-IgA in their secretions with high levels of serum IgA. In two of the three, chest X-rays and histological pictures of the lung showed typical pulmonary fibrosis. The remainder is, as yet, asymptomatic without evidence of chest disease. Moreover, it is of note that two members of the family had lung cancer with or without pulmonary fibrosis. The supposition that secretory component deficiency may be causally linked with pulmonary fibrosis or lung cancer is very attractive. Further analyses of this family are now in progress.

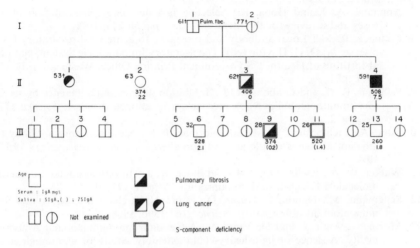

FIG. 5. A family with secretory component deficiency and pulmonary fibrosis.

Acknowledgments

I wish to express my heartfelt thanks to Professor Haruto Uchino, Kyoto University, and Professor Tomofusa Usui, Hiroshima University, for their interest and encouragement, and Dr. Shigeo Nomura, Hyogo Prefectural Amagasaki Hospital, for his cooperation. Grateful acknowledgment is made to many physicians who kindly gave us the opportunity to investigate patients with selective IgA deficiency.

REFERENCES

1. West, C. D., Hong, R., and Holland, N. H.: Immunoglobulin levels from the newborn period to adulthood and in immunoglobulin deficiency states. *J. Clin. Invest.* **41**:2054, 1962.
2. Rockey, J. H., Hanson, L. A., Heremans, J. F., *et al*: Beta-2A aglobulinemia in two healthy men. *J. Lab. Clin. Med.* **63**:205, 1964.
3. Kanoh, T.: Selective IgA deficiency. *Clin. Immunol.* **4**:149, 1972.
4. Vyas, G. N., Perkins, H. A., Yang, Y. M., *et al*: Healthy blood donors with selective absence of immunoglobulin A: prevention of anaphylactic transfusion reactions caused by antibodies to IgA. *J. Lab. Clin. Med.* **85**:838, 1975.
5. Kanoh, T.: Selective IgA deficiency in Japan. *Jap. J. Allergol.* **25**:241, 1976.
6. Claman, H. N., Merrill, D. A., Peakman, D., *et al*: Isolated severe gamma A

deficiency: Immunoglobulin levels, clinical disorders, and chromosome studies. *J. Lab. Clin. Med.* **75**:307, 1970.

7. Ammann, A. J. and Hong, R.: Selective IgA deficiency: Presentation of 30 cases and a review of the literature. *Medicine* **50**:223, 1971.
8. Chanock, R. M.: Local antibody and resistance to acute viral respiratory tract disease. *In*: D. H. Dayton (ed): The Secretory Immunologic System, National Institute of Health, US Government Printing Office, Washington, D. C., 1971, p83.
9. Williams, R. C. and Gibbons, R. J.: Inhibition of bacterial adherence by secretory immunoglobulin A: A mechanism of antigen disposal. *Science* **177**: 697, 1972.
10. Turk, A., Lichtenstein, L. M., and Norman, P. S.: Nasal secretory antibody to inhalant allergens in allergic and non-allergic patients. *Immunology* **19**:85, 1970.
11. Walker, W. A., Isselbacher, K. J., and Bloch, K. J.: Intestinal uptake of macromolecules: Effect of oral immunization. *Science* **177**:608, 1972.
12. Seligmann, M., Danon, F. Hurez, D., *et al*: Alpha-chain disease. A new immunoglobulin abnormality. *Science* **162**:1396, 1968.
13. Moroz, C., Amir, J., and De Vries, A.: A hereditary immunoglobulin A abnormality. Absence of light-heavy-chain assembly. Study of immunoglobulin synthesis in tonsillar cells. *J. Clin. Invest.* **50**:2726, 1971.
14. Fudenberg, H. H., Good, R. A., Goodman, H. C., *et al*: Primary immunodeficiencies. *Bull. Wld. Hlth. Org.* **45**:125, 1971.
15. Hancock, M. P., Huntley, C. C., and Sever, J. L.: Congenital rubella syndrome with immunoglobulin disorder. *J. Pediatr.* **72**:636, 1968.
16. Kanoh, T., Niwa, Y. and Yamaguchi, N.: A study of the pathogenesis of isolated IgA deficiency: Demonstration of three cases of acquired isolated IgA deficiency. *J. Jap. Soc. Intern. Med.* **64**:1353, 1975.
17. Buser, F., Butler, R., and Du Pan, R. M.: Susceptibility to infection and IgA deficiency in the infant. *J. Pediatr.* **72**:29, 1968.
18. Vassallo, C. L., Zawadzki, Z. A., and Simons, J. R.: Recurrent respiratory infections in a family with immunoglobulin A deficiency. *Am. Rev. Resp. Dis.* **101**:245, 1970.
19. Schlegel, R. J., Bernier, G. M., Bellanti, J. A., *et al*: Severe candidiasis associated with thymic dysplasia, IgA deficiency, and plasma antilymphocyte effects. *Pediatrics* **45**:926, 1970.
20. Fraser, K. J. and Rankin, J. G.: Selective deficiency of IgA immunoglobulins associated with carcinoma of the stomach. *Aust. Ann. Med.* **2**:165, 1970.
21. Ginsberg, A. and Mullinax, F.: Pernicious anemia and monoclonal gammopathy in a patient with IgA deficiency. *Am. J. Med.* **48**:787, 1970.
22. Bjernulf, A., Johansson, S. G. O., and Parrow, A.: Immunoglobulin studies in gastrointestinal dysfunction with special reference to IgA. *Acta Med. Scand.* **190**:71, 1971.
23. Mawhinney, H. and Tomkin, G. H.: Gluten enteropathy associated with selective IgA deficiency. *Lancet* **2**:121, 1971.
24. Falchuk, K. R. and Falchuk, Z. M.: Selective immunoglobulin A deficiency, ulcerative colitis, and gluten-sensitive enteropathy A unique association. *Gastroenterology* **69**:503, 1975.

25. Kanoh, T. and Uchino, H.: Primary immunodeficiency diseases in the adult. *J. Adult Dis.* **6**:1636, 1971.
26. Kersey, J. H., Spector, B. D., and Good, R. A.: Primary immunodeficiency diseases and cancer: The immunodeficiency-cancer registry. *Int. J. Cancer* **12**: 333, 1973.
27. Kanoh, T. and Wakisaka, G.: Clinical significance of hypoimmunoglobulinemia. *Acta. Haemat. Jap.* **31**:481, 1968.
28. Kanoh T. and Uchino, H.: Immunodeficiency and epilepsy. *Lancet* **1**:860, 1976.
29. Kanoh, T.: Thymic lesions associated with systemic immune disorders in man. *Acta. Haemat. Jap.* **34**:452, 1971.
30. Manning, D. D.: Induction of temporary IgA deficiency in mice injected with heterologous anti-immunoglobulin heavy chain antisera. *J. Immunol.* **109**: 1152, 1972.
31. Murgita, R. A., Mattioli, C. A., and Tomasi, T. B., Jr.: Production of a runting syndrome and selective γA deficiency in mice by the administration of anti-heavy chain antisera. *J. Exp. Med.* **138**:209, 1973.
32. Sorrell, T. C., Forbes, I. J., Burness, F. R., *et al*: Depression of immunological function in patients treated with phenytoin sodium (sodium diphenylhydantoin). *Lancet* **2**:1233, 1971.
33. Clough, J. D., Mims, L. H., and Strober, W.: Deficient IgA antibody responses to arsanilic acid bovine serum albumin (BSA) in neonatally thymectomized rabbits. *J. Immunol.* **106**:1624, 1971.
34. McFarlin, D. E., Strober, W., and Waldmann, T. A.: Ataxia-telangiectasia. *Medicine* **51**:281, 1972.
35. Case Records of the Massachusetts General Hsopital. *N. Engl. J. Med.* **284**:39, 1971.
36. Lawton, A. R., Royal, S. A., Self, K. S., *et al*: IgA determinants on B-lymphocytes in patients with deficiency of circulating IgA. *J. Lab. Clin. Med.* **80**:26, 1972.
37. Haddow, J. E., Shapiro, S. R., and Gall, D. G.: Congenital sensory neuropathy in siblings. *Pediatrics* **45**:651, 1970.
38. Huntley, C. C. and Stephenson, R. L.: IgA deficiency: Family studies. *North C. Med. J.* **29**:325, 1968.
39. Hilman, B. C., Mandel, I. D., Martinez Tello, F. J., *et al*: Familial hypogammaglobulinemia-A. *Ann. Allergy* **27**:394, 1969.
40. Tomkin, G. H., Mawhinney, H., and Nevin, N. C.: Isolated absence of IgA with autosomal dominant inheritance. *Lancet* **2**:124, 1971.
41. Douglas, S. D., Goldberg, L. S., and Fudenberg, H. H.: Familial selective deficiency of IgA. *J. Pediatr.* **78**:873, 1971.
42. Beermann, B. and Holm, G.: Familial IgA defects. *Scand. J. Haemat.* **12**:307, 1974.
43. Lewkonia, R. M., Gairdner, D., and Doe, W. F.: IgA deficiency in one of identical twins. *Br. Med. J.* **1**:311, 1976.
44. Strober, W , Krakauer, R., Klaeveman, H. L., *et al:* Secretory component deficiency: A disorder of the IgA immune system. *N. Engl. J. Med.* **294**:351, 1976.

DISCUSSION

Dr. SOOTHILL: I would like to comment on the epilepsy findings. I personally
found the concept of a drug producing deficiency of a single immunoglobulin
class quite incredible when Grobb reported it, and you quoted our prospective
study that confirmed this. We have done some more work on this quite extraordinary drug phenytoin. If you give it to mice, it not only suppresses IgA, it also
suppresses IgM and one of the IgG subclasses but not the other, so that the class
specificity of the effect of phenytoin varies from species to species. Next quite
incredible fact: In as far as the human effect is concerned Lorna Graham has
shown that if you add the drug in vitro to normal B-lymphocytes stimulated by
pokeweed mitogen phenytoin stops the production of IgA but not the production
of the other immunoglobulin classes. I find these phenomena incredible, but it
is truth because we and others have done prospective studies to confirm that the
deficiency is secondary, the deficiency of IgA in epilepsy is partly secondary, to
the drugs.
Dr. KANOH: I don't think that phenytoin exclusively suppresses the production of
IgA. Viewed from the clinical point, however, it is true that we can observe a
selective deficiency of IgA in some epileptics treated with the drug. Since IgA-
producing cells show the latest development in ontogeny and phylogeny, they
may be most labile and sensitive to the drug.
Dr. GOOD: I think it is very important to also recognize that epilepsy with extremely
high frequency of IgA deficiency occurs without hydantoin, and I think that the
words 'partially secondary' in the Grobb study are of the greatest importance.
When Miller and Van Felpmann and Grobb presented all of their details it
looked quite convincing that the IgA deficiency came first and that the hydantoin
accentuated this. I think that is even more incredible than having a selective
agent that selectively depresses the IgA.

I was very much intrigued by the association of the malignancy of the gastrointestinal tract with IgA deficiency. In our study with John Kershey and Bespech-
ter where we used a registry method to get the information, the associations, the
malignant associations with immunodeficiency in general have been largely lymphoreticular malignancies, especially what is called by most pathologists lympho-
cytoma, and gastric cancer. Gastric cancer just stands out like a sore thumb
among all of the cancers occurring in immunodeficiency, and its frequency is
relatively high, even for the United States, with a much greater increase than the
former. The real question from the studies that Tummi and I did a number of
years ago is whether the intestinal abnormality revealed by gastric malfunction
comes first. Whether there is something really abnormal about the gastrointestinal tract as a reflection of, perhaps, an epithelial abnormality, which then
ultimately plays out in a deficiency of development of the B-lymphoid system.
I think the possibility has to be entertained that the gastric cancer is related to
that abnormality which then has as its consequence immunodeficiency.

Dr. SELIGMANN: I was quite interested by the last family you presented, and I would like to ask the group what is the present status of patients with an absence of secretory component. Do you know any analysis, or something new since the report in the *London Journal of Medicine*? If other people found it, what is the status of infants with sudden death, and also in these patients with a deficiency of secretory components? It seems, as you nicely showed in your slide, that this abnormality has some IgA production in the secretory system in some, and maybe absent IgA production in some others.

Dr. KANOH: Like selective IgA deficiency, it seems probable that some cases of secretory component deficiency can be clinically asymptomatic. I think, however, one should keep in mind the possibility that such patients develop malignancies of gastrointestinal or respiratory tract as a reflection of an epithelial abnormality in a certain period later.

Dr. GOOD: I have really been very anxiously awaiting these patients with secretory component deficiency and now they are beginning to appear. Of course, we proposed when we began analyzing this issue, that there ought to be such patients, but among the patients with increased susceptibility to gastrointestinal infections and pulmonary infections, there are certainly very few. We have gone through many, many hundreds of patients finding a lot that have isolated IgA deficiency, but the secretory component seems to be a rare one. I still take exception to talking about this as secretory component. This has nothing to do with the secretory process; it is a transport component as South and I originally described, having to do with the transport of the secreted IgA, which is a dimeric molecule, across the intestinal tract and the component is produced by the epithelial cells. And now we are beginning to talk about a secretory deficiency of the transport component.

Selective IgA Deficiency and Hodgkin's Disease Associated with Hyperimmunoglobulinemia E

Yohnosuke KOBAYASHI,* Yuji KAGOSAKI*, Tadashi KANOH,**
and Tomofusa USUI*

ABSTRACT

An 8-year-old Japanese boy showed selective IgA deficiency and Hodgkin's disease associated with hyperimmunoglobulinemia E. Selective IgA deficiency was found at the age of five years and four months. Lymph node biopsies showed simple lymphadenitis at three years and five months, reticulosis at six years and five months, and eventually Hodgkin's disease at seven years and four months of age. Although it is impossible to determine the causal relationship between these two conditions, we have speculated that selective IgA deficiency was the primary disorder responsible for recurrent infections and that it permitted the activation and proliferation of latent oncogenic viruses, leading to lymphoid hyperplasia culminating in Hodgkin's disease.

Selective immunoglobulin A(IgA) deficiency is most commonly encountered in cases of primary immunodeficiencies and is also known to be frequently accompanied by various disorders, including respiratory infections, central nervous system disease, malignancies, allergic or autoimmune diseases.[1] However, its pathogenesis as well as the mechanism of association with the above conditions still remain to be elucidated. On the other hand, it is generally acknowledged that the frequency of malignancy, particularly of lymphoreticular origin, is significantly higher in patients with primary immunodeficiencies.[2] Especially Hodgkin's disease is often associated with immunological disturbances,[3] but its coexistence with selective IgA deficiency is extremely rare.

The purpose of this article is to present a case of selective IgA deficiency and

---
*Department of Pediatrics, Hiroshima University School of Medicine, Hiroshima, Japan
**The 1st Department of Internal Medicine, Kyoto University School of Medicine, Kyoto, Japan

Hodgkin's disease associated with hyperimmunoglobulinemia E and to discuss a possible causal relationship between these two disorders. An immunological survey of the family members in this case showed that the father also had hyperimmunoglobulinemia E.

CASE REPORT

The patient was an 8-year-old Japanese boy who had had frequent common colds during infancy. At two years and five months of age, he was found to have EEG findings of hypsarhythmia and was treated for infantile spasm with ACTH for about six months. Since then he has been placed on phenobarbital. Hydantoin, however, has never been given. Convulsions have not recurred. Following measles at the age of three years he had repeated otitis media and tonsillitis. At three years and five months of age, he was noted to have hepatomegaly and left cervical and bilateral inguinal lymphadenopathy. The diagnosis of "simple lymphadenitis" was then made by lymph node biopsy (Figs. 1 and 2). When he was five years and four months old, he was diagnosed as having selective IgA deficiency (IgG 970mg/100ml, IgA 0 mg/100ml, and IgM 128mg/

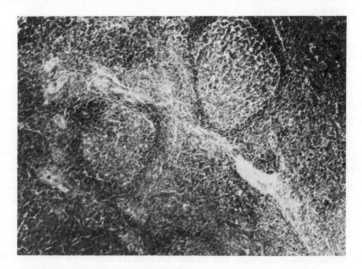

FIG. 1.   Section from left cervical lymph node showing follicular hyperplasia and proliferation of lymphocytes (3 years and 5 months old, H & E, ×48).

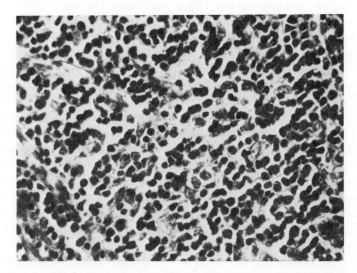

FIG. 2.   High-power magnification of Fig. 1 (3 years and 5 months old, H & E, ×480).

100ml by a single radial immunodiffusion test). In spite of antibiotic therapy, the right cervical lymph nodes increased progressively in size. At six years and three months of age, he was referred to Hiroshima University Hospital for further evaluation and treatment of a prolonged fever and lymphadenopathy of the right cervical region.

On admission the patient was well-developed and well-nourished. He was alert and intelligence was estimated to be almost normal. Physical findings were essentially negative except for slight hepatosplenomegaly and generalized lymphadenopathy. The tonsils were not visible. The lymph nodes were discrete, nontender, elastic soft and freely movable from the skin as well as the underlying structures. The largest one was the size of a hen's egg in the right cervical region.

The following laboratory findings were normal or negative: complete blood count, leukocyte differential, platelet count, urinalysis, serological tests for syphilis, liver function tests, blood urea nitrogen, serum creatinine, Paul-Bunnell test, thyroid test, Coombs test, rheumatoid factors, LE test, antinuclear antibody and anti-DNA antibody. Chromosome studies showed a normal male karyotype. The chest roentgenogram was normal. Bone marrow aspiration disclosed mild eosinophilia and absence of plasma cells. An EEG showed spike, spike and wave, high voltage fast waves. The total serum protein was 7.6g/

100ml with 4.7g of albumin and 1.0g of γ-globulin. The single radial immuno-diffusion test of serum showed an IgG of 1,152mg/100ml, IgA of 2.5mg, IgM of 245mg and IgE of 2,600IU/ml. IgA in serum was not detectable by immunoelec-trophoresis and showed only a trace in the Ouchterlony test; secretory IgA in the saliva was not detectable by the Ouchterlony method. No anti-IgA antibody could be detected in the serum at six years and five months of age, but a year later it was 2^4. Intermediate strength PPD and Candida skin tests showed false positive reactions. The number of immunoglobulin-bearing peripheral lym-phocytes were within the normal range, and 40% of peripheral lymphocytes showed E-rosette formation. Lymphocyte transformation in response to phy-tohemagglutinin was normal. The cutaneous application of 2% 2,4-dinitro-chlorbenzene (DNCB) followed by a challenge two weeks later failed to sensitize the patient. The phagocytic activities of leukocytes, chemotaxis, NBT reduction test and bactericidal activities were normal. Histologically, the lymph node removed from the right cervical region showed reticulosis (Figs. 3 and 4).

At seven years and one month of age, *i.e.*, nine months after the second lymph node biopsy, he was again admitted with an intermittent fever, night sweats and lymphadenopathy of the right cervical region, the largest node being the size of a small hen's egg.

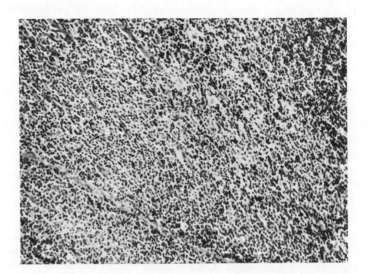

FIG. 3.   Section from right cervical lymph node showing lymph folli-cular hypoplasia and proliferation of reticular cells (6 years and 5 months old, H & E, ×120).

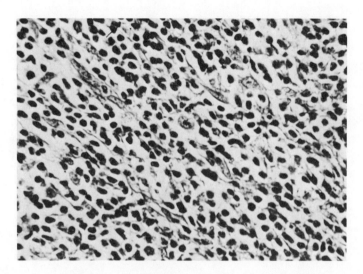

FIG. 4. Highpower magnification showing proliferation of lymphocytes and reticular cells and relatively few plasma cells (6 years and
5 months old, H & E, ×480).

A complete blood count showed a hemoglobin value of 9.8g/100ml, an erythrocyte count of 397 × 10⁴/cmm, a leukocyte count of 4,500/cmm with an
absolute lymphocyte count of 1,200/cmm, and a platelet count of 29.1 × 10⁴/
cmm. The total serum protein was 6.8g/100ml; an immunoelectrophoresis of
the serum showed a significant hypoalbuminemia (2.1g/100ml) and elevated
globulin fractions ($\alpha_1,\alpha_2,\beta,\gamma$). A chest roentgenogram showed enlarged lymph
nodes in the left hilus. Skeleton roentgenograms, lymphangiography, intravenous pyelogram and liver scanning were normal. Intermediate strength PPD
and Candida skin tests were negative. Lymphocyte transformation in response
to PHA was slightly depressed. The patient could be sensitized to 0.1% DNCB.
The lymph node biopsy of the right cerivcal region showed the morphological
features of Hodgkin's disease of the mixed cellularity type with hypoplastic
lymph follicles, relatively few lymphocytes, proliferation of reticular cells, numerous Hodgkin's cells and characteristic Sternberg-Reed cells (Figs. 5 and 6).
The clinical stage was estimated to be Hodgkin's disease stage II B. Following
combined chemotherapy with MOPP (nitrogen mustard 6mg/m², vincristine
sulfate 1.4mg/m², procarbazine 100mg/m² and prednisolone 40mg/m²) for 24
weeks (6 cycles), the size of the lymph nodes in the right cervical region gradually decreased. No febrile episodes, otitis media or tonsillitis had recurred. After

208   Y. Kobayashi *et al.*

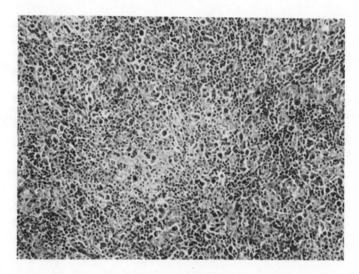

Fig. 5. Section from right cervical lymph node showing lymph
follicular hypoplasia, relatively few lymphocytes, marked proliferation
of reticular cells and diffuse fibrosis (7 years and 4 months old, H
& E, ×120).

chemotherapy, intermediate strength PPD and Candida skin tests were negative.
Lymphocyte transformation in response to PHA was markedly depressed, and
the patient could be sensitized to 0.1%-DNCB.

FAMILY STUDIES

The patient's parents and 6-year-old sister were healthy and none of his relatives had autoimmune diseases, malignancies or immunodeficiencies. An
immunoelectrophoresis and a single radial immunodiffusion test of the sera
of the family members showed the results in Table 1. The father was also noted
to have an elevated level of IgE.

COMMENTS

The patient reported here had a past history of recurrent viral as well as
bacterial infections since early childhood and marked lymphadenopathy, which

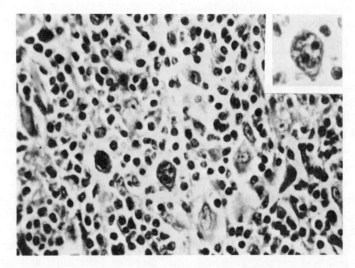

FIG. 6. Highpower magnification showing proliferation of reticular cells, numerous Hodgkin's cells and characteristic Sternberg-Reed cells (7 years and 4 months old, H & E, ×480).

TABLE 1. Immunological studies of family members

	Patient	Mother	Father	Sister
Total protein	7.6g/100ml	7.1	7.4	6.8
Albumin	62.2%	60.6	57.8	65.0
α_1-globulin	4.1	4.5	4.8	3.3
α_2-globulin	12.6	8.2	8.8	10.7
β-globulin	8.5	10.6	10.2	9.0
γ-globulin	12.6	16.1	18.4	11.7
IgG	1,152mg/100ml	1,264	1,440	1,020
IgA	2.5	292	194	89
IgM	245	94	181	102
IgE	2,600IU/ml	870	2,130	

gradually evolved from simple lymphadenitis into Hodgkin's disease during a 4-year period of observation. During this period, he had successively been found to have selective IgA deficiency, hyperimmunoglobulinemia E and partial impairment of cell-mediated immunity. Although neither Hodgkin's disease nor selective IgA deficiency are uncommon entities in themselves, and the former is recognized as being often accompanied by immunological disturbances, the association of these two disorders has been extremely rare, so this case provided us with a good opportunity for evaluating the possible causal relationships among the successive occurrences of the above-mentioned conditions in this patient.

In animal experiments, there is evidence that an immunosuppressive state is associated with an increased incidence of malignancies.[4] It is also true in humans, and there is a report that the incidence of malignancy in this group is roughly 10,000 times greater than in the general age-matched population, especially in Wiskott-Aldrich syndrome and ataxia telangiectasia, in which there is a 10% incidence of malignancy.[2] The malignant neoplasmas in these patients are mostly of lymphoreticular origin, such as leukemia or lymphoma. The malignant disorders reported to be associated with selective IgA deficiency are various and include lymphoma, leukemia, and carcinomas in areas where secretory IgA is normally present.[5-10] The association with Hodgkin's disease, however, has to our knowledge been reported only in one individual.[11] Although IgA was not specifically investigated, one of the cases reported by Hoffbrand bears some resemblance to our present patient.[12] In the beginning his patient had chronic lymphadenitis, repeated infections, and was later shown to have hypogammaglobulinemia and eventually developed Hodgkin's disease 30 years after the initial episode of cervical lymphadenopathy. Hoffbrand attributed lymphadenopathy and recurrent infections to a long-standing immunological deficiency, which preceded the onset of Hodgkin's disease.[12] Fraser and Rankin reported a case of selective IgA deficiency associated with carcinoma of the stomach and also mentioned the possibility that IgA deficiency may result in a defect in homeostatic regulation of potentially neoplastic cells.[13]

The terminal stage of Hodgkin's disease has frequently been stated to be responsible for hypogammaglobulinemia, which, however, is not likely to be the case in this patient, as the temporal sequence indicates that IgA deficiency developed prior to the onset of Hodgkin's disease.

Viral etiology has been firmly established in a number of animal malignancies,[14] and a certain virus has been intimately implicated in the causation of some kinds of human neoplasms, such as Burkitt lymphoma. No direct evidence has yet proved the infectious origin of Hodgkin's disease, but it is an attractive hypothesis that Hodgkin's disease may be due to a virus of low virulence, when we take into consideration clusters or even "epidemics" of the disease in certain districts or in consecutive patients who have had close contact with each other.[15]

Certain medications, especially hydantoin,[16] are known to induce IgA deficiency. In this patient, phenobarbital had been given for about three years before IgA deficiency was first found and has been continued to be given up to the present time. It cannot yet be determined whether or not phenobarbital might have played any role in the development of IgA deficiency in this patient. A significant elevation of IgE is unknown. Although hypoimmunoglobulinemia E is frequently observed in patients with malignancies or primary immunodeficiencies, except in the Wiskott-Aldrich syndrome, it has not always been described in patients with IgA deficiency.[17,18] One of the interesting features of hyperimmunoglobulinemia E in this patient is that IgE remained persistently elevated throughout the course of clinical observation, including the period of intensive immunosuppressive therapy with MOPP. The hyperimmunoglobulinemia E of the father is entirely unexplained. It may be a fortuitous finding or foretell a certain pending condition, necessitating further observations.

Although it is impossible at the moment to determine a causal relationship between the two disorders, we have been inclined to consider that a defect in the immunological surveillance system caused by IgA deficiency and a partial impairment of cell-mediated immunity have permitted the activation and proliferation of latent oncogenic viruses, leading eventually to Hodgkin's disease. Another explanation for the combination of these two disorders is that they are different expressions of a common defect, whether of genetic origin or of infectious etiology, which remains in the area of speculation.

Acknowledgements

This work has been supported in part by a grant for the research of immunologic disorders from the Ministry of Health and Welfare and by Scientific Research Grants (Project Nos. 144052 and 157253) from the Ministry of Education, Science and Culture of Japan.

REFERENCES

1. Ammann, A. J. and Hong, R.: Selective IgA deficiency. *in* "Immunologic disorders in infants and children", edited by E. R. Stiehm and V. A. Fulginiti 1973, pp 199–214.
2. Gatti, R. A. and Good, R. A.: Occurrence of malignancy in immunodeficiency disease, A literature review. *Cancer* **28**:89, 1971.
3. Aisenberg, A. C.: Manifestations of immunologic unresponsiveness in Hodgkin's disease. *Cancer Res.* **26**:1152, 1966.
4. Häyry, P., Rago, D., and Defendi, V.: Inhibition of phytohemagglutinin and alloantigen-induced lymphocyte stimulation in Ransher leukemia virus. *J. Nat. Cancer Inst.* **44**:1311, 1970.
5. Miller, W. V., Holland, P. V., Sugarbacker, E., Strober, W., and Waldmann, T. A.: Anaphylactic reactions to IgA: A difficult transfusion problem. *Am. J. Clin. Pathol.* **54**:618, 1970.

212 Y. Kobayashi *et al.*

6. Recant, L. and Hartroft, W. S.: Clinicopathologic conference, Rademacher's disease. *Am. J. Med.* **32**:80, 1962.
7. Binder, H. J. and Reynold, R. D.: Control of diarrhea in secondary hypogammaglobulinemia by fresh plasma infusion. *New Engl. J. Med.* **277**:802, 1967.
8. Ammann, A. J. and Hong, R. H.: Selective IgA deficiency: Presentation of 30 cases and a review of the literature. *Medicine* **50**: 223, 1971.
9. Kanoh, T.: Dysgammaglobulinemia. *Naika* **32**:111, 1973 (in Japanese)
10. Hamondi, A. B., Ertel, I., Newton, W. A., Jr., Reiner, C. B., and Clatworth, H. W., Jr.: Multiple neoplasms in an adolescent child associated with IgA deficiency. *Cancer* **33**:1134, 1974.
11. Nadrop, J. H. S., Voss, M., Buys, W. C., van Munster, P. J. J., van Tongeren, J. H. M., Aalberse, R. C. and van Loghem, E.: The significance of the presence of anti-IgA antibodies in individual with an IgA deficiency. *Eur. J. Clin. Invest.* **3**:317, 1973.
12. Hoffbrand, B. I.: Hodgkin's disease and hypogammaglobulinemia: A rare association. *Brit. Med. J.* **1**:1156, 1964.
13. Fraser, K. J. and Rankin, J. G.: Selective deficiency of IgA immunoglobulins associated with carcinoma of the stomach. *Aust. Ann. Med.* **2**:165, 1970.
14. Dmochowski, L. and Grey, C. E.: Studies on submicroscopic structure of leukemias of known or suspected viral origin: a rview, *Blood* **13**:1017, 1958.
15. Vianna, N. J., Greenwald, P., Brady, J., Polan, A. K. Dwork, A., Mauro, J., and Davies, J. N. P.: Hodgkin's disease: Case with features of a community outbreak. *Ann. Int. Med.* **77**:169, 1972.
16. Hyman, G. A. and Sommers, S. C.: The development of Hodgkin's disease and lymphoma during anticonvulsant therapy. *Blood* **28**:416, 1966.
17. Spitz, E., Gelfand, E. W., Sheffer, A. L., and Austen, K. F.: Serum IgE in clinical immunology and allergy. *J. Allergy Clin, Immunol.* **49**:337, 1972.
18. Buckley, R. H. and Fiscus, S. A.: Serum IgD and IgE concentrations in immunodeficiency disease. *J. Clin. Invest.* **55**:157, 1975.

DISCUSSION

Dr. GOOD: Of course, the other way of looking at it is that there is a basic abnormality of the T-cell system. You revealed a very profound deficit of T-cell function in the failure to sensitize the 2-4-dinitrochlorobenzene. And one thing that is eminently clear now is that the T-cell system is essential for the differentiation and development of the IgA producing cells. Witness, of course, the nude mouse, the defects in ataxia-telangiectasia. So is the crucial issue not whether or not you are able to reconstruct the T-cell deficit by effective treatment of the Hodgkin's disease? Although we have demonstrated. The very, very long persistence of abnormalities of the T-cell function in patients with Hodgkin's disease, they come back very properly toward normal and the question then is, what has been your experience? Was your treatment effective, and what has happened to the capacity to sensitize to 2-4-dinitrochlorobenzene? After MOPP treatment?

Dr. KOBAYASHI: Almost improved.

Dr. GOOD: Does he remain IgA deficient? You mean he remains IgA deficient, although there has been a return of the T-cell function toward normal. Why did you choose to treat this patient with MOPP rather than with radiation? Did he have a more disseminated disease?

Dr. KOBAYASHI: No. His legion is rather localized on the neck. Of course his main treatment included MOPP, and also he was irradiated.

Heterogeneity of Lymphocytes in Primary Immunodeficiency Disease

Masakatsu Kubo,* Michisato Murata,** Takeshi Okabe,* Nobuyuki Kitani,* Yusuke Tomita,* Makoto Hori,* and Yoshiyuki Kokubun*

ABSTRACT

Peripheral blood lymphocytes from ten patients with primary immunodeficiency disease were evaluated for T and B cell surface markers. Marked reduction in T cells was observed in one case each of SCID, thymic hypoplasia and common variable immunodeficiency. Surface immunoglobulin-bearing lymphocytes were reduced in two cases of congenital agammaglobulinemia, one case each of common variable immunodeficiency and immunodeficiency with normal or hypergammaglobulinemia. Complement receptor lymphocytes were diminished in one case each of congenital agammaglobulinemia and common variable immunodeficiency.

These results suggest that the primary immunodeficiency diseases associated with abnormality of serum immunoglobulin may have considerable heterogeneity in this entity when examined at the cellular level.

INTRODUCTION

Primary immunodeficiency disease is known to arise from a defect in the lymphocyte and lymphoid tissues, which is responsible for humoral and cellular immunity. Up to date, this syndrome has been classified chiefly on the basis of clinical characteristics, inheritability, immunoglobulin level and autopsy findings. However, reclassification has been recently tried from the viewpoint of the cellular level of lymphocytes, according to the findings on what combinations of T cells, B cells and lymphoid stem cells are responsible for the occurence of primary immunodeficiency and to what extent these cells are damaged.[1] We attempt to do a more detailed classification of primary

*Department of Pediatrics, The Jikei University School of Medicine, Tokyo, Japan
**Department of Immunology, Institute of Medical Science, University of Tokyo, Tokyo, Japan

216   M. Kubo *et al.*

immunodeficiency disease at the cellular level of lymphocytes, using ten cases of this syndrome.

THE SUBJECTS

The diagnosis of primary immunodeficiency disease was made on the basis of the criteria set forth by the Japanese Welfare Ministry, with reference to that of the World Health Organization.[1,2] The subjects were a boy (aged 6 months) with severe combined immunodeficiency (X-linked type), a boy (aged 7) and a girl (aged 4) with congenital agammaglobulinemia (sporadic type), a female infant (aged 6 months) suffering from immunodeficiency with normal or hypergammaglobulinemia, a boy (aged 7) with dysgammaglobulinemia type II by Hobb's classification, three males (aged 3, 7 and 27) with common variable immunodeficiency, a female newborn (aged one month) complicated with 18-trisomy and thymic hypoplasia, and a female infant (aged 11 months) who ran a particular clinical course of T cell deficiency.

METHODS

1. Lymphocyte preparation, identification of monocyte and lymphocyte subpopulations
From heparinized peripheral blood, mononuclear cells were isolated by the Ficoll-Hypaque gradients methods.[3] Subpopulations of peripheral blood lymphocytes were quantitated using the methods described by Yata and Jondal *et al.*[4,5] T cells were identified by the formation of spontaneous rosettes with sheep erythrocytes (E rosette). Cells with complement receptor were identified by formation of EAC rosettes. Surface immunoglobulin-bearing lymphocytes were identified by direct immunofluorescence using antiheavy chain immunoglobulin. Antiserum was ultracentrifuged at 10,000 × g for 15 minutes prior to each test to remove aggregated immunoglobulin.[6] For identification of monocytes, 0.1 ml of human serum and 0.1 ml of sterilized yeast solution (2.5 × 10^9/ml) were added to 0.2 ml of mononuclear cell suspension (5 × 10^6/ml), and the mixture was incubated at 37°C for 30 minutes. The percentage of the phagocytic cells was calculated after fuchsin staining.[7] Percentage value of cells with complement receptor obtained from lymphocyte subpopulations was corrected for monocyte content of cell suspension.

2. Phytohemagglutinin (PHA) response to lymphocytes
PHA response to lymphocytes was determined by the whole blood culture

technique of Pauly *et al.*,[8] measured by calculating the logarithm ratio of counts from ³H-thymidine incorporation of stimulated to unstimulated culture.

3. Serum immunoglobulin concentration

Serum immunoglobulin concentration was estimated by the method of the single radial immunodiffusion technique.[9]

RESULTS AND DISCUSSION

The normal individual's lymphocyte subpopulations of peripheral blood were 61.6 ± 6.0 % for T cells, and 27.3 ± 4.9 % for complement receptor lymphocytes. As for the surface immunoglobulin-bearing lymphocytes, the mean value was 1.97 % for IgM-bearing lymphocytes, 10.58 % for IgG-bearing lymphocytes, 1.45 % for IgA-bearing lymphocytes and 4.75 % for IgD-bearing lymphocytes. Lymphocyte blastogenesis on the stimulation of PHA (SI) was 2.0 ± 0.3.

Case 1 was severe combined immunodeficiency (SCI). Lymphocyte subpopulations in this case disclosed that T cells were markedly decreased to 14 %, while complement receptor lymphocytes were prominently increased to 79 %. SI declined to 1.0. Each of the immunoglobulin levels was low (Table 1). Since immunity in SCID is usually restored by bone marrow grafting, SCID might be caused by defective differentiation of lymphoid stem cells. Studies with the cellular level of lymphocytes in SCID provide more complicated

TABLE 1. Lymphocyte subpopulations in severe combined immunodeficiency and thymic hypoplasia

Case	1 Y. K.	2 K..K.
Diagnosis	SCID	Thymic hypoplasia
Sex	M	F
Age	6 M	1 M
Lymphocyte (/mm³)	2800	2924
E rosette (%)*	14	18
EAC rosette (%)**	79	63
PHA blast. (SI)	1.0	0.8
Serum immunoglublin (mg.dl)		
IgM	15	52
IgG	60	410
IgA	0	0

SI: Stimulation index. Logarithm ratio of counts per minute of stimulated to unstimulated culture. Normal individuals, 2.0 ± 0.3
* Normal individuals, 61.6 ± 6.0 % (mean ± SD)
** Normal individuals, 27.3 ± 4.9 % (mean ± SD)

aspects than previously believed in the nature of the disease, since there are
numbers of immunological variations in the subpopulations of lymphocytes in
patients with SCID, cases with deficiencies of both T and B cells,[10,11] cases
without deficiencies of T and B cells[22] and cases with a deficiency of T cells
(shown in this study). [12,13] Consequently, it can be assumed that SCID may
be a heterogeneous disease caused by defects occurring at various steps in the
maturation of T and B cells, manifesting either their quantitative or qualitative
deterioration.

Case 2 was thymic hypoplasia, complicated with 18 trisomy. Lymphocyte
subpopulations were 18 % for T cells and 63 % for B cells. PHA response to
lymphocytes was markedly reduced to 0.8. In a level of immunoglobulin,
serum IgA level was low, but the others remained normal (Table 1).

As seen in these two cases, a decreased proportion of lymphocytes forming
rosettes with sheep erythrocytes is considered to be a useful index in making
an early diagnosis of thymic hypoplasia.

Cases 3 and 4 were diagnosed as congenital agammaglobulinemia (sporadic
type) with an absence of any evident family history of immunodeficiency (Table
2). Case 4 was almost completely deficient in complement receptor and
surface immunoglobulin-bearing lymphocytes. It was noteworthy that null

TABLE 2. Lymphocyte subpopulations in congenital agammaglobulinemia (sporadic
type)

Case	3 K.U.	4 T.F.	Control
Sex	M	F	
Age	9 Y	4 Y	
Age at onset	6 M	4 M	
Lymphocyte (/mm³)	3800	4300	
E rosette (%)*	69	79	61.6 ± 6.0
EAC rosette (%)*	18	0	27.3 ± 4.9
PHA blast. (SI)	2.2	2.0	2.0 ± 0.3
Surface immunoglobulin(%)*			
IgM	1.7	0.5	1.97 ± 0.21
IgG	0.7	1.7	10.58 ± 0.97
IgA	0	0	1.45 ± 0.68
IgD	2.0	0	4.75 ± 0.43
Serum immunoglobulin (mg/dl)			
IgM	8	10	
IgG	24	64	
IgA	0	0	

SI: Stimulation index. Logarithm ratio of counts per minute of stimulated to unstimulated
culture.
* Mean ± SD

cells, devoid of the character of either T or B cells, were found to be 30 % of all the peripheral blood lymphocytes. In this case lymphocytes may be derived from either lymphoid stem cells or plasma cell-like mature ones, because they are lacking in complement receptor. But immunoglobulin containing cells were not detected in this case. It is therefore assumed that the lymphocytes in this case may not be plasma cell-like ones, but those of lymphoid stem cells at the cellular level. Case 3 showed a normal level of complement receptor, but exhibited a marked decrease in surface immunoglobulin-bearing lymphocytes. Yata et al. recently described several cases with X-linked agammaglobulinemia in which complement receptor lymphocytes were found to be at a normal level, while surface immunoglobulin-bearing lymphocytes were deficient. Their data indicated that the complement receptor of lymphocytes might also be present in immature B cells.[14] It is consequently assumed that case 4 in the present study might have developed due to the defect of B cells alone; while in case 3, the maturation of B cells might be impaired at the state in which complement receptor had appeared.

In cases 5, 6 and 7, immunodeficiency developed at the ages of 2 years or later and the diagnosis of common variable immunodeficiency was made (Table 3). Case 5 showed approximately normal T and B cells, being 61 and 19%, respectively. Serum IgG level, however, was remarkably reduced. Lymphocyte blastogenesis on PHA stimulation was slightly decreased. At 4 months after admission, both T and B cells diminished greatly and at the same time the immunoglobulin level was reduced. Such a shift in lymphocyte subpopulations is sometimes observed in the last stage of leukemia and after the administration of immunosuppressive drugs. In our case, however, atypical lymphocytes were not found in peripheral blood, nor any infiltration into lymphoid tissue by tumor cells was observed and no immunosuppressive drug was given. It is known in experimental animals that rinderpest virus in the paramyxovirus group destroyed lymphocytes of peripheral blood or T and B areas of the peripheral lymphoid tissue.[15] Also in humans, there may be a possibility that the cells responsible for immunity would be widely destroyed by virus. From the viewpoint of the cellular level of lymphocytes, the present case is considered to have developed by acquisition the pathological status equivalent to SCID. In cases 6 and 7, both T and B cells were normal. This finding suggests that there might be a defect either in the development of the B cells into the antibody-producing cells or in the secretory mechanism. As for the pathogenic mechanism of this disease, Waldmann et al.[16] indicated that T cells might inhibit the development of B cells into antibody-producing cells. Furthermore, Wernet et al.[17] suggested that the T cell factor might be necessary for the maturation of B cells.

TABLE 3.   Lymphocyte subpopulations in common variable immunodeficiency

Case	5 T.K.		6 T.W.	7 Y.T.	Control
Sex	M		M	M	
Age	2.6Y	3Y	25Y	14Y	
Lymphocyte (/mm³)	1800	900	2400	3200	
E rosette (%)**	61	62	72	73	61 6 ⊥ 60
EAC rosette (%)*	19	4	26	19	27.3 ± 4.9
PHA blast. (SI)	1.5	0		1.8	2.0 ± 0.3
Surface					
immunoglobulin (%)*					
IgM		0	9	5.5	1.97 ± 0.21
IgG		0	11	5.2	10.58 ± 0.97
IgA		0.2	5	2	1.45 ± 0.68
IgD		0		1.3	4.75 ± 0.43
Serum					
immunoglobulin					
IgM mg/dl	177	18	18	800	
IgG	140	16	220	20	
IgA	64	8	55	0	

SI: Stimulation index. Logarithm ratio of counts per minute of stimulated to unstimulated
      culture
 *   Mean ± SD
**   Mean and range

Case 8 showed a remarkable decrease in serum IgG and IgA. Lymphocyte
subpopulations were 76% for T cells and the normal percent for B cells identified by a cell marker of complement receptor. This case was diagnosed as
dysgammaglobulinemia type II according to Hobbs' classification (Table 4).

Case 9 showed a normal level of serum immunoglobulin, but with a remarkable decrease in the surface immunoglobulin bearing lymphocytes (Table 4).
Isohemagglutinin titer was lower than 8-fold. Specific antibody production
was not observed on stimulation with polymerized flagellin (POL). Some
insight into these observations is provided by studies on bursectomized
chickens shortly after hatching. Cooper et al.[18] reported that in a family of
SCID that the electrophoretic pattern of immunoglobulin was fairly abnormal
as compared with that of normal individuals, though its concentration was
normal. They suggest that immunoglobulin obtained from these patients might
have undergone a qualitatively abnormal change. The immunoglobulin
from our case was also mobilized with a considerable restriction in electrophoretic pattern, as compared with our control (Fig. 1). Normal level of
serum immunoglobulin plus an abnormal pattern of immunoglobulin on immunoelectrophoresis associated with a deficiency of B cell immunity as shown

TABLE 4. Lymphocyte subpopulations in dysagammaglobulinemia type 1 and immunodeficiency with normal gammaglobulinemia

Case	8 Y.H.	9 U.O.	Control
Sex	M	F	
Age	7 Y	6 M	
Age at onset	6 M	1 M	
Lymphocyte (/mm³)	2900	4000	
E rosette (%)	76	68	61.6 ± 6.0*
EAC rosette (%)	17	32	27.3 ± 4.9*
Surface immunoglobulin (%)			
IgM		0	1.97 ± 0.21*
IgG		1.1	10.58 ± 0.97
IgA		0.5	1.45 ± 0.68
IgD		0	4.75 ± 0.43
Serum immunodlobulin (mg/dl)			
IgM	79	120	
IgG	60	448	
IgA	8	63	

* Mean ± SD

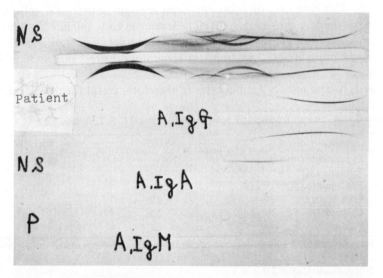

Fig. 1.   Immunoelectrophoresis of a sera from a patient of immunodeficiency with normal gammaglobulinemia (P) and a normal control (NS). The patients' IgG has restricted mobility.

in our case may provide us with the following hypothesis to explain the pathogenesis of this disorder. These phenomena may be primarily produced by the qualitative modification of surface immunoglobulin in a patient's lymphocytes. The surface changes of lymphocytes have failed to demonstrate the B cell function, since the surface immunoglobulin-bearing lymphocytes and isohemagglutin titer were simultaneously decreased. The failure to produce the specific antibody against POL is also one piece of strong evidence which supports the above possibility. The abnormal pattern of electrophoretic mobility in the patient's serum immunoglobulin is probably due to the production of a specific antibody against a certain antigen, accompanied with a lack of normal response against various antigens caused by the impairment of surface immunoglobulin receptors. The qualitative modified surface of the patient's lymphocytes may be brought about either by a disturbance of developmental process of B cells or constitutional chemical abnormality of surface immunoglobulin molecules due to a genetic mutation or the existence of a competitive blocking compound to immunoglobulin receptors. Case 9 can be interpreted as the so-called molecular disease of immunoglobulin.

Case 10 showed quantitative diminution of T cells in the early stage, and both quantitative and qualitative improvement of T cells was accomplished by administration of the transfer factor and clinical features were much improved (Fig. 2). This case may therefore represent the slow starter of T cells, which resembles the IgA slow starter. T cell deficiency in early infancy was observed in the cases of ectopic thymus. There is also another case, shown in Table 5. The stress brought about by transient respiratory distress may induce T cell deficiency.

The E rosette test for lymphocytes is, therefore, useful for the diagnosis of

TABLE 5.   A case of transient T lymphopenia (case 11. S.T. 4 day. M.)

Day	50/12/7	50/12/17
Lymphocyte (/mm³)	3200	2400
E rosette (%)*	11	72
EAC rosette (%)**	65	21
PHA blast.	0.9	
Ca (meq/1)	2.5	4.6
P (meq/1)	7.5	6.3

SI: Stimulation index. Logarithm ratio of counts per minute of stimulated to unstimulated culture
      Normal individuals: 2.0 ± 0.3
 *   Normal individuals: 61.6 ± 6.0 % (Mean ± SD)
**   Normal individuals: 27.3 ± 4.9 % (Mean ± SD)

Day	74/Dec.	75/Jan.	75/Feb.	75/June.	76/June.
Tranfer factor		↓↓↓		↓↓	
Abscess					
Moniliasis					
Diarrhea					
WBC /mm^3	12800	14400	7900	11500	8700
Ly(%)	47	40	49	81	43
Eo(%)	27	15	28	3	4
IgG mg/dl	1400		1400	1600	1500
IgM	260		180	52	190
IgA	56		240	142	82
IgE unit/ml	4000				4000
*E rosette(%)	28	20	67	73	69
**EAC rosette (%)	63	68	18	25	27
PHA blast.(S.I.)	1.1				
Skin test(Candida)	−	−	+	+	+

Fig. 2. Clinical course and immunological studies in a case of un-
classified immunodeficiency (case 10, R.K. 11 M.F.)
* Normal individuals: 61.6 ± 6.0 (Mean ± SD)%
** Normal individuals: 27.3 ± 4.9 (Mean ± SD)%
SI: Stimulation Index. Normal individuals: 2.0 ± 0.3 (Mean ± SD)

thymic hypoplasia in the newborn and in early infancy. On some occasions,
however, the T lymphocyte population is associated with transient T cell deficiency and prudence is necessary in the diagnosis of this disease.

Primary immunodeficiency disease displays considerable heterogeneity when
examined at the cellular level, even if the concentration of serum immunoglobulin is identical. Both quantitative and qualitative reduction in several types
of primary immunodeficiency disease may be produced by genetic abnormality,
as seen in DiGeorge syndrome, SCID or congenital enzyme deficiency.[19,20]
Furthermore, recent reports have indicated the possibility that T cells may
regulate the differentiation and the maturation of B cells.[16,17,21] It seems,
therefore, necessary to reclassify immunodeficiency diseases according to their
etiology.

Acknowledgements
We wish to thank Dr Y. Eto, for helpful discussion, and express our thanks
to Dr K. Yoshino for permission to study the polymerized flagellin antibody.

224   M. Kubo *et al.*

REFERENCES

1. Fudenberg, H. J., Good, R. A., Hitzing, W., Kunkel, H. G., Roitt, I. M., Rosen, F. S., Rowe, D. S., Seligmann, M., and Soothhill, J. R.: Primary immunodeficiency: Report of WHO committee. *Pediat.* **42**:927, 1971.
2. Kobayashi, N.: Diagnostic criteria of primary immunodeficiency, Japanese Welfare Ministry, 1974.
3. Böyum, A.: Isolation of mononuclear cells and granulocytes from human blood, *Scand. J. Clin. Invest.* **21**:77, 1968.
4. Yata, J., Tsukimoto, I., and Tachibana, T.: Human lymphocytes subpopulations: Human thymus lymphoid tissue antigen-positive lymphocytes forming rosettes with sheep erythrocytes and HTL antigen negative lymphocytes interacting with antigen-antibody complement complexes. *Clin. Exp. Immuno.* **14**:317, 1973.
5. Jondal, M., Holm, G., and Wigzel, H.: Surface markers of human T and B lymphocytes. I. A large population of lymphocytes forming nonimmune rosette with sheep red cells. *J. Exp. Med.* **136**:207, 1972.
6. Kawamura, A. and Murata, M.: Detection of immunoglobulin determinants on the cell surface of lymphocytes. *Clin. Immunol.* **8**:689, 1976. (in Japanese)
7. Miller, E. M.: Phagocytosis in the newborn infant: Humoral and cellular factors. *J. Pediat.* **74**:255, 1969.
8. Pauly, J. L., Sokel, J. E., and Han, T.: Whole blood culture technique for functional studies of lymphocyte reactivity to mitogen, antigen, and homologous lymphocytes. *J. Lab. Clin. Med.* **82**:500, 1973.
9. Mancini, G., Carbonara, A. O., and Heremans, T. F.: Immunochemical quantitation of antigens by single radial immunodiffusion. *Immunochemistry.* **2**:235, 1965.
10. Keightley, R. G., Lawton, A. R., and Cooper, M. D.: Successful fetal liver transplantation in a child with severe combined immunodeficiency. *Lancet* **i.** 850, 1975.
11. Yata, J., Tsukimoto, I., Arimoto, T., Goyak N., and Tachibana, T.: Human thymus lymphoid tissue antigen, complement receptor and rosette formation with sheep erythrocytes of their lymphocytes of primary immunodeficiency. *Clin. Exp. Immuno.* **14**:309, 1973.
12. Buckley, R. H., Gilbertsen, R. B., Shiff, R. I., Ferreira, E., Sonal, S. O., and Waldmann, T. A.: Heterogeneity of lymphocyte subpopulations in severe combined immunodeficiency. *J. Clin. Invest.* **58**:130, 1976.
13. Cooper, M. D. and Lawton A. R.: Circulating B cells in patients with immunodeficiency. *Amer. J. Path.* **69**:513, 1972.
14. Yata, J. and Tsukimoto, I.: Maturation of cell surface structure of human B lymphocytes. *Lancet* **1425**, 1972.
15. Yamamouchi, K., Chino, F., Kobune, F., Fukuda, A., and Yoshikawa, Y.: Pathogenesis of Rinderpest virus interaction in rabbits. *Infection and Immunity* **9**:199, 1974.
16. Waldmann, T. A., Durm, M., Broder, S., Blackman, M., Blease, B. M., and Strober, W.: Role of suppressor T cells in pathogenesis of common variable hypogammaglobulinemia. *Lancet* **609**, 1974.

17. Wernet, P., Siegal, F. R., Dicker, H., Fu, S., and Kunkel, H. G.: Immunoglobulin synthesis *in vitro* by lymphocytes from patients with immunodeficiency: Requirement for a special serum factor. *Proc. Nat. Acad. Sci.* 71:531, 1974.
18. Lawton, A. R., Frank, L. Y., and Cooper, M. D.: A spectrum of B-cell differentiation defects, immunodeficiency in man and animals. Birth Defects (Bergsma, ed.), Vol. XI. National Foundation, Sinauer, Associates. Sunderland, Mass. 1975, p. 28.
19. Yount, T., Nichols, P., Ochs, H. D., Hammer, S. D., Scott, R. C., Chen, S. H., and Wodgewood, R. J.: Absence of erythrocytes adenosine deaminase associated with severe combined immunodeficiency. *J. Pediat.* 84:173, 1974.
20. Giblett, E. R., Amman, A. J., Sandman, R., Wara, D. W., and Diamond, L. K.: Nucleoside-phosphorylase deficiency in a child with severely defective T cell immunity and B cell immunity. *Lancet* i:1010, 1975.
21. Seeger, R. C., Robins, R. A., Stevens, R. H., Klein, R. B., Waldman, D. T., Zeltzer, P. M., and Kessler, S. W.: Severe combined immunodeficiency with lymphocytes, *in vitro* correction of defective immunoglobulin production by addition of normal T lymphocytes. *Clin. Exp. Immuno.* 26:1, 1976.
22. Yata, J., Tsukimoto, I., and Nakagawa, T.: Specificity of lymphocytes in primary immunodeficiency. *Diagnosis and Treatment.* 61:17, 1973. (in Japanese)

Functional Abnormalities of the Lymphocytes from Patients with Lesch-Nyhan Syndrome

Toshiro NAKAGAWA, Tsugutoshi AOKI, and Junichi YATA

INTRODUCTION

There are two different metabolic pathways of purine synthesis: *de novo* and salvage pathways. Purine ribonucleotides are synthesized from low molecular weight precursors by the *de novo* pathway or by direct reactions of purine bases with 5-phosphoribosyl-1-pyrophosphate (PRPP) catalysed by purine phosphoribosyl-transferase enzymes, including hypoxanthine guanine phosphoribosyltransferase(HGPRT), in salvage pathways.

The relative contributions of these two pathways differs from one tissue to another. The Lesch-Nyhan syndrome is a disease in which HGPRT is deficient in all body tissues and therefore the salvage pathway is blocked.[1]

In this study, we estimated DNA and RNA synthesis of the lymphocytes from this syndrome after stimulation with various mitogens and studied the dependency on the salvage pathway of the metabolic activation of the lymphocytes by each mitogen.

MATERIALS AND METHODS

The lymphocytes were isolated by Ficoll-sodium metrizoate gradient centrifugation[2] from the peripheral blood of two patients with Lesch-Nyhan syndrome and normal individuals, and were suspended in RPMI-1640 (Gibco) supplemented with 15% fetal calf serum (Microbiol. Assoc. Inc.) in a concentration of 5×10^5 mononuclear cells per millilitre.

Each of the mitogens was added to one millilitre of cell suspension and incubated at 37°C for 70 hr in a CO_2 incubator. Concentration of the mitogens used in this study was 10 μl/ml for phytohemagglutinin-P (PHA, Difco), 10 μg/ml for concanavalin A (ConA, Sigma), 10 μg/ml for pokeweed mitogen

Department of Pediatrics, School of Medicine, Toho University, Tokyo, Japan

228   T. Nakagawa *et al.*

(PWM, Gibco) and 100 μg/ml for lipopolysaccharide (LPS, E. coli 0111:B4, Difco). Two μCi of ³H-thymidine (³H-TdR) or ¹⁴C-uridine (¹⁴C-UdR) were added to each tube after 70 hr. Cultures were further incubated for 2 hr. Trichloroacetic acid-precipitable ³H-TdR or ¹⁴C-UdR of the harvested cultures on filter paper disks were assayed for radioactivity and thus DNA or RNA synthesis of the cells was evaluated.

RESULTS

The enzyme HGPRT is virtually absent in erythrocytes (Table 1). Lymphocytes stimulated with PHA did not show incorporation of ¹⁴C-hypoxanthine and ¹⁴C-guanine, while they incorporated ¹⁴C-adenine (Table 2). These results indicate the lack of the salvage pathway catalysed by HGPRT in the Lesch-Nyhan syndrome.[1] The spontaneous incorporation of ³H-TdR and ¹⁴C-UdR was low in lymphocytes from patients as compared with those from controls.

The lymphocytes from the patients responded well to PHA both in DNA

TABLE 1. Biochemistry

| | Phosphoribosyltransferase activity in erythrocyte hemolysates (mu M/mg protein/hr) | | Serum | |
	HGPRT	APRT	Uric acid (mg/100ml)	BUN (mg/100ml)
Normal ranges in our laboratory	89–115	23–38	3.5–6.0	8–15
Patient 1	0.6* 0.09**	52* 49**	11.2	23
Patient 2	0.1 0.2	45 53	9.3	18
Father of Pt. 2	N.T. 102	N.T. 28	5.1	11
Mother of Pt. 2	N.T. 103	N.T. 28	4.3	14

* Evaluated by the method of Seegmiller *et al.*
** Evaluated by the method of Rubin *et al.*

TABLE 2. Metabolic defect in patients with Lesch-Nyhan syndrome

| | Incorporation of purines into PHA-stimulated lymphocytes (cpm) | | |
	¹⁴C-adenine	¹⁴C-hypoxanthine	¹⁴C-guanine
Healthy controls	24,593 +4,630	17,700 +8,950	14,861 +1,055
Patient 1	29,675	116	59
Patient 2	38,650	240	145

and in RNA synthesis, while their responses to ConA were extremely decreased (Figs. 1 and 2). The ratio of the count from patients' lymphocytes to those of normal lymphocytes was mean 0.82 for RNA stimulation, whereas it was mean 0.08 for ConA stimulation. When the ratios of the counts for PHA to those for ConA were compared, it was approximately 1 in normal individuals by both ^{3}H-TdR and ^{14}C-UdR uptake, while it was about 6 by ^{3}H-TdR and 12, 13 by ^{14}C-UdR in patients.

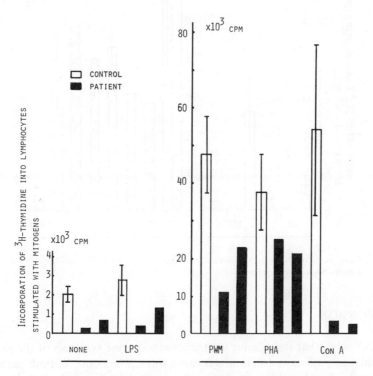

FIG. 1.   Responses to mitogens of lymphocytes from patients with Lesch-Nyhan syndrome.

The lymphocytes from the patients responded less to PWM by DNA and RNA synthesis than normal. They also did not incorporate ^{14}C-UdR by the stimulation of LPS, which had been shown to induce RNA synthesis in normal lymphocytes.

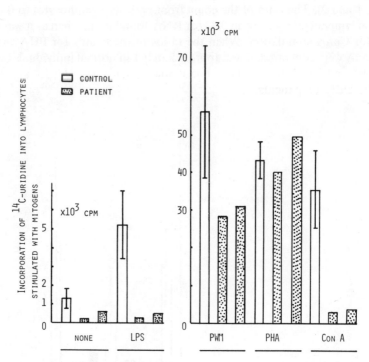

FIG .2.   Responses to mitogens of lymphocytes from patients with
Lesch-Nyhan syndrome.

DISCUSSION

It is known that the relative contribution to purine synthesis of the *de novo*
and salvage pathways differs in various tissues. For example, both pathways
are operating in fibroblasts[3] whereas there is little or no *de novo* purine biosynthesis taking place in brain tissue.[4] Some lymphoma cells do not show
salvage pathway metabolism.[5]

There is accumulating evidence which indicates that the cells responding
to PHA and those to ConA are distinct populations of T-lymphocytes.[6-8]
We observed in our study that the HGPRT deficient lymphocytes responded
well to PHA but not to ConA. This may indicate that PHA-induced purine
synthesis does not necessarily require the salvage pathway, while it is essential
for ConA-induced purine synthesis, or alternatively that the ConA-responsive

T lymphocyte population is reduced because of a defect of HGPRT which might be engaged in the development of this T lymphocyte population.

Recently, Ballet and colleagues observed that coformycin, a potent inhibitor of adenosine deaminase (ADA), inhibits proliferative response to PHA, but not those to ConA or PWM.[9] Moreover, their previous reports have demonstrated that maturation of precursor cells into T lymphocytes is very sensitive to coformycin, while that of immunoglobulin-secreting cells is not impaired. In comparison of their results with our present data, PHA-induced purine synthesis seems to be more dependent on ADA while HGPRT seems essential for ConA, PWM and LPS responses.

Further studies of the purine metabolism in patients with various enzyme defects would provide a better understanding of the functions of human lymphocytes.

REFERENCES

1. Seegmiller, J. E., Rosenbloom, F. M., and Kelley, W. N.: *Science* **155**:1682, 1967.
2. Böyum, A.: Scand. *J. Clin. Lab. Invest., suppl.* **97**:77, 1968.
3. Rosenbloom, F. M., Henderson, J. F., Caldweu, I. C., Kelley, W. N., and Seegmiller, J. E.: *J. Biol. Chem.* **234**:1166, 1968.
4. Howard, W. J., Kerson, L. A., and Appel, S. H.: *J. Neurochemist* **17**:121, 1970.
5. Brockmen, R. W.: *Cancer Res.* **25**:1596, 1965.
6. Jubert, A. U., Hersh, E. M., and McBride, C. M.: *Surg. Gynec. Obstet.*, **136**:567, 1973.
7. Lindahl-Kiessling, K.: *Exp. Cell Res.*, 70:17, 1972.
8. Wisloff, F. and Froland, S. S.: *Int. Archs. Allergy appl. Immunol.* **45**:456, 1973.
9. Ballet, J.-J., Insel, R., Merler, E., and Rosen, F. S.: *J. Exp. Med.* **143**:1271, 1976.

COMMENT

Dr. GOOD: Well, I am really delighted to see this because everyone who has studied Lesch-Nyhan up until now has talked about the lymphocyte functions being normal, but Lesch-Nyhan's ought to have an immunological abnormality and it is very entertaining that you have to find one that probably involves a subpopulation of the T-lymphocytes.

Immunodeficiency and Common
and Disabling Disease

J. F. SOOTHILL

Patients with recognised severe immunodeficiency, which is largely inherited by single gene systems,[1] experience frequent infection, a wide range of allergic disease, and, perhaps, frequent cancer. Management of these diseases has been improved as a result of the diagnosis of the fundamental cause—the intrinsic deficiency of the patient. Such allergic diseases occur frequently in the population generally, causing chronic disability—especially asthma, eczema, arthritis and nephritis. Since genetic variation may be polygenic as well as Mendelian, is there evidence that minor relative immunodeficiency, especially in the neonatal period, may underly some of this disease, and can such an understanding contribute to prevention or treatment of the disease?

Immunodeficiency and common infection

All children have respiratory infection, some more than others. There is often lymphoid hyperplasia in the upper respiratory tract, and in Britain one in ten children have their tonsils removed for these infections, though there is no clear evidence that it helps. Such infections occur frequently in some children with isolated IgA deficiency when there may be considerable lymphoid hyperplasia. We therefore investigated patients with recurrent sore throats immunologically and found that the serum IgA tended to be rather low (though only a few were below the lower limit of normal—the 2.5 percentile—since the syndrome is more frequent than this). The ones with higher IgA had streptococci in their tonsils, and no more trouble after tonsillectomy (but penicillin might have done as well), but the ones with lower IgA had *Haemophilus influenzae*, and had as much trouble after tonsillectomy as before.[2,3] Here, understanding of the immunodeficiency element clearly influences treatment of a common disease. But since lymphoid hypertrophy has some of the features of allergy, and the common allergies are influenced by neonatal antigen ex-

Department of Immunology, Institute of Child Health, University of London, England

233

perience, similar protective measures (see below) might prevent much of the trouble.

Bone and joint infection in the first year of life is rare, but commonly chronically disabling. In prospective and retrospective studies of such children we found that at least half have defects of the antibody (including isolated IgM deficiency) complement or phagocytes.[4] Of relevance to management was the high incidence of wound infection in late reconstructive surgery in these children. Protection of the vulnerable minority from infection (*e.g.* breast-feeding) may reduce such troubles. Host factor variation as well as infection experience should influence planning of a suitable environment for children; even within the conventional "normal range", relevant variation occurs.

Immunodeficiency and atopic allergy

Allergy is an even commoner cause of chronic disability. In children eczema and asthma predominate. It is customary to assume that allergy results from damage due to spontaneous overaction of one of the mechanisms outlined by Coombs and Gell[5] on an antigen specific basis, perhaps linked to postulated IR genes and so to tissue type. But the commonest type of allergy—the state of atopy—is clearly antigen-nonspecific and allergy often occurs in immuno-deficient children (especially of IgA) and there is an increased proportion of relatively IgA deficient subjects in atopics.[6] We therefore considered that perhaps the damaging mechanism may be intrinsically normal, but chronically overstimulated by excessive contact with antigen, because another mechanism, which would normally exclude, eliminate, or otherwise inactivate the antigen, was defective.

Since IgE antibody, the characteristic response of an atopic, is largely pro-duced in the submucosa, the most likely defect would be of secretory IgA, the principle immunoglobulin of mucous secretions, and, since IgA is the immunoglobulin most involved in transient immunodeficiency, it was possible that a higher proportion of childhood allergy had an IgA deficiency basis than the data of Kaufmann and Hobbs would suggest. We took advantage of the strong familial tendency of atopy, and watched the development of immune responses and of atopy in newborn offspring of allergic parents. Serum IgA was significantly lower at 3 months in those who subsequently developed atopy (eczema, or positive skin prick tests to common allergies) than in those who did not (Fig. 1).[7] Again, only some lay below the conventional "normal range", as would be expected in atopy, which represents perhaps 20% of the population. We identified the immunodeficiency by serum IgA concentra-tion, but this does not necessarily mean that secretory IgA was the causative deficiency. It could be associated with another transient deficiency, such as that

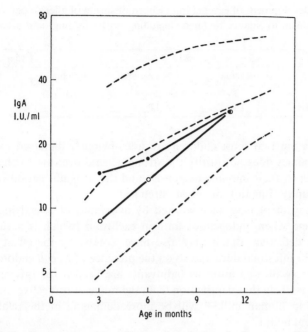

FIG. 1.   Log mean values of serum IgA during the first year of life in infants of reaginic parents.
○ = those with evidence of atopy. ● = those without. Means ±2 S.D. for healthy British children are approximately indicated.

of suppressor T cells, which influence IgE antibody production in experimental animals.[8]

However it works, we regarded this as important, because of the possibility that avoidance of sensitization during this deficient phase might result in stable freedom from disease. This is likely since, though so strongly familial, in pairs of identical twins, one may be allergic and the other not, and, whereas children born in Britain of immigrant parents have as much allergy as British children, those immigrating as infants have far less.[9] We therefore followed the development of eczema and atopy in offspring of atopic parents, some of whom attempted six months of antigen avoidance (including exclusive breast feeding) and others who did not. Eczema was much less frequent in those who did, and it was prevented, not delayed, since there was virtually no more in the second six months, when management was conventional (Table 1).[10] This establishes that variation in the child's immunity function influences the planning of appropriate management, even when within the normal range.

TABLE 1. Development of eczema in newborn offspring of allergic parents brought up on an antigen avoidance regimen (including breast feeding) and a conventional regimen

	6/12		1 year	
	Eczema	No eczema	Eczema	No eczema
Regimen	2	24	3	23
Conventional	10	17		

The observation that most children are not obviously damaged by artificial feeding as babies does not justify the strong general decision to change to it. Infants differ in their immune responses, and the neonatal period is the time when immunity function is most stretched.

This management may have worked by avoidance of sensitizing antigens during a time when endogenous antigen exclusion (which is a function of IgA,[11]) was defective. But it may also have worked by the effect of breast feeding on the intestinal flora and so on the presence of E. coli endotoxin as an adjuvant for swallowed antigens (adjuvants are needed for IgE response in animals). It is likely that deprivation from the range of protective mechanisms which exist in human milk[12] will be more damaging in the relatively immunodeficient infant.

But this is only one of the immunodeficiencies within the normal range (above the 2.5 percentile) which contributes to allergy (Table 2). Miller[13] described two families with infants in whom opsonization for phagocytosis of killed bakers' yeast by normal polymorphonuclear leucocytes was defective, in association with fatal bacterial infection, diarrhea and eczema. This function is defective in 1 in 20 of the population and is responsible for 1 in 4 of unexplained frequent infections in children[14]; 1 in 4 of children with eczema and adults with hay fever have this defect (Soothill & Harvey—unpublished

TABLE 2. Immunodeficiency within the normal range (>5%) which contributes to vulnerability to immunopathological disease

Antigen specificity	Mechanism	Deficiency	Environmental influence
specific?	IR genes?	HLA-related	—
non-specific	antigen exclusion	IgA (transient)	infant feeding, birth season
		complement (alternative pathway)	infant feeding? birth season?
	antigen elimination	low affinity antibody	nutrition, infection
		macrophage clearance (PVP)	nutrition, infection
		cystic fibrosis gene	

data). The defect is one of the alternative pathways of complement, since insulin or bacterial endotoxin fails to activate their complement.[15] There is reason to suspect that the effect of this dominant gene is influenced by neonatal environmental factors; perhaps the main function of the alternative pathway of complement is the inactivation of bacterial endotoxin in the neonatal period before an IgG response to it has been developed. It is likely that allergy was prevented in such children too in our "antigen avoidance" program.

These findings led to the proposition that neonatal contact with seasonal antigens might influence the incidence of allergy in children in allergic families. It does,[16] so that, in Britain, avoidance of being born in September or October would reduce the chances of allergy in a vulnerable infant. There are less grounds for optimism for prevention in those vulnerable because of another common, genetically determined defect of a surface immunity function. Both homozygotes (1 in 2000 in Britain) and heterozygotes (1 in 20) for cystic fibrosis have a factor which depresses cilial function; they also have an excess of atopy.[17]

Atopy and tissue type

Though atopy is highly familial (50% of the children of atopic parents are atopic), its many syndromes vary not only between but within families—some have eczema and asthma, and others just hayfever. These differences are linked to certain common HLA haplotypes (antigen combinations)—for instance complicated eczema is associated with HLA Al B8, and hay fever with HLA A3 B7,[18] Fig. 2. These associations are maintained in the different immunodeficiency groups (see above), when they are analysed separately, and both are influenced by neonatal antigen experience. Such complicated interactions of multiple gene systems, and of environment, are likely in the etiology of common disease.

Immunodeficiency and other allergy

Allergic damage, other than that elicited by IgE in atopics, requires persistence of antigen in the presence of an immune response to it. We have shown that such differences exist in different inbred strains of mice[19] in relation to production of low affinity antibody response to unadjuvantised antigen,[20] and poor clearance function of macrophages.[21] These differences are antigen-nonspecific and breeding experiments show them to be of polygenic inheritance,[22] but such environmental factors as diet can influence them strongly.[23] The immunopathological significance of this heterogeneity is still to be fully established. It is different from the mouse strains selected for high or low agglutinating antibody responses by Biozzi et al.,[24] where some

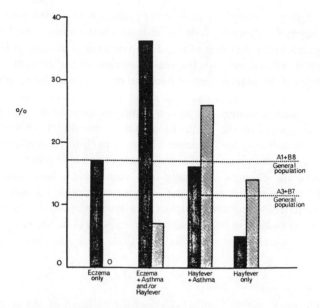

FIG. 2.   Frequencies of the antigen combinations A1 + B8 (solid columns) and A3 + B7 (hatched columns) in atopic patients classified by clinical manifestations.

The general population frequencies for these antigens are indicated by the horizontal lines.

infections are worse in "high responders". Such common disabling diseases as arthritis or nephritis may well depend on such variation.

Immunodeficiency and other common disabling diseases

Patients with severe immunodeficiency are vulnerable to a number of other chronic disabling diseases, for which the damaging mechanism is less clear, besides frequent infection and atopic allergy. These include epilepsy, auto-allergic disease and perhaps cancer. Idiopathic epilepsy in childhood (especially febrile convulsions, and temporal lobe epilepsy) is often associated with primary IgA deficiency, as well as with secondary IgA deficiency resulting from phenytoin treatment.[25,26] This, and the association of epilepsy with a defect of the alternative pathway of complement,[14] raises the possibility that optimal neonatal antigen experience may be helpful here too. The role of relative immunodeficiency in other forms of immunopathology, including autoallergy, and in cancer, still needs systematic study.

These studies have established that variation of immune response can underlie special vulnerability to common diseases. The immunodeficiency element can interact with other genetic characteristics, and the manifestations of both can be modified by appropriate management. Because of the special vulnerability of the newborn, neonatal management appropriate for the child is especially important in preventing chronic disease.

REFERENCES

1. Cooper, M. D. *et al.*: Meeting report of the 2nd international workshop on primary immunodeficiency diseases in man. *Clin. Immunol. and Immunopathol.* **2**:416, 1974.
2. Donovan, R. and Soothill, J. F.: Immunological studies in children undergoing tonsillectomy. *Clin. Exp. Immunol.* **14**:347, 1973.
3. Donovan, R.: Clinical and immunological studies on children undergoing tonsillectomy for repeated sore throats. *Proc. Roy. Soc. Med.* **66**:413, 1973.
4. Kuo, K. N., Lloyd-Roberts, G. C., Orme, I. M., and Soothill, J. F..: Immunodeficiency and infantile bone and joint infection. *Arch. Dis. Childh.* **50**:51, 1975.
5. Coombs, R. R. A. and Gell, P. G. H.: Classification of allergic reactions responsible for clinical hypersensitivity and disease. Chapter 25 *In*: Clinical Aspects of Immunology, (P. G. H. Gell, R. R. A. Coombs, and P. J. Lachmann, eds.), Blackwell Scientific Publications, Oxford, 1975.
6. Kaufman, H. S. and Hobbs, J. R.: Immunoglobulin deficiencies in an atopic population. *Lancet* **ii**:1061, 1970.
7. Taylor, B., Norman, A. P., Orgel, H. A., Stokes, C. R., Turner, M. W., and Soothill, J. F.: Transient IgA deficiency and the pathogenesis of infantile atopy. *Lancet* **ii**:111, 1973.
8. Tada, T., Okumura, K., and Taniguchi, M. J.: Regulation of homocytotropic antibody formation in the rat. *J. Immunol.* **108**:1535, 1972.
9. Smith, J. M.: The prevalence of asthma and wheezing in children. *Br. J. Dis. Chest.* **70**:73, 1976.
10. Matthew, D. J., Taylor, B., Norman, A. P., Turner, M. W., and Soothill, J. F.: Prevention of eczema. *Lancet* **i**:321, 1977.
11. Stokes, C. R., Soothill, J. F., and Turner, M. W.: Immune exclusion is a function of IgA. *Nature* **255**:745, 1975.
12. Bullen, C. L.: *In*: Symposia of the Swedish Nutrition Foundation XIV. Almqvist and Wiksell International, Stockholm, 1977.
13. Miller, M. E. and Nilsson, U. R.: A familial deficiency of the phagocytosis-enhancing activity of serum related to a dysfunction of the fifth component of complement. *New Eng. J. Med.* **282**:354, 1970.
14. Soothill, J. F. and Harvey, B. A. M.: Defective opsonization, a common immunity deficiency. *Arch. Dis. Childh.* **51**:91, 1976.
15. Soothill, J. F. and Harvey, B. A. M.: A defect of the alternative pathway of complement. *Clin. Exp. Immunol.* **27**:30, 1977.
16. Soothill, J. F., Stokes, C. R., Turner, M. W., Norman, A. P., and Taylor, B.:

Predisposing factors and the development of reaginic allergy in infancy. *Clin. Allergy*. **6**:305.

17. Warner, J. O., Norman, A. P., and Soothill, J. F.: Cystic fibrosis heterozygosity in the pathogenesis of allergy. *Lancet* i:990, 1976.

18. Turner, M. W., Brostoff, J., Wells, R. S., Stokes, C. R., and Soothill, J. F.: HLA in eczema and hay fever. *Clin. Exp. Immunol.* **27**:43, 1977.

19. Alpers, T H , Steward, M. W., and Soothill, J. F.: Differences in immune elimination in inbred mice. The role of low affinity antibody. *Clin. Exp. Immunol.* **12**:121, 1972.

20. Soothill, J. F., and Steward, M. W.: The immunopathological significance of the heterogeneity of antibody affinity. *Clin. Exp. Immunol.* **9**:193, 1971.

21. Morgan, A. G. and Soothill, J. F.: The relationship between macrophage clearance of PVP and affinity of anti-protein antibody response in inbred mouse strains. *Nature* **254**:711, 1975.

22. Katz, F. E. and Steward, M. W.: The genetic control of antibody affinity in mice. *Immunology* **29**:543, 1975.

23. Coovadia, H. M. and Soothill, J. F.: The effect of protein restricted diets on the clearance of 125 I-labelled polyvinyl pyrrolidone in mice. *Clin. Exp. Immunol.* **23**:373, 1976.

24. Biozzi, G., Asofsky, R., Lieberman, R., Stiffel, C., Mouton, D., and Benacerraf, B.: Serum concentrations and allotypes of immunoglobulins in two lines of mice genetically selected for "high" or "low" antibody synthesis. *J. Exp. Med.* **132**:752, 1971.

25. Seager, J., Jamieson, D. L., Wilson, J., Hayward, A. R., and Soothill, J. F.: IgA deficiency, epilepsy and phenytoin treatment. *Lancet* ii:632.

26. Fontana, A., Grob, P. J., Sauter, R., and Joller, H.: IgA deficiency, epilepsy and hydantoin medication. *Lancet* ii:228, 1976.

The Patterns of Infections with Bacteria or Fungi in Immunodeficient Mice

Kikuo NOMOTO, Shoichi SHIMOTORI, Tsunenori MIYAKE, Shizuko MURAOKA, Kenichi MATSUO, and Kenji TAKEYA

ABSTRACT

Protection against various pathogenic microorganisms is known to depend upon humoral and cellular elements, both of which are composed of specific and nonspecific mechanisms. In this study, mutual contributions of T cell-mediated cellular immunity as a specific mechanism and non-immune phagocytosis as a nonspecific mechanism were analyzed with regard to protection against some kinds of so-called "intracellular parasites." Athymic nude mice were used as T cell-deprived hosts. Macrophage functions were suppressed by lethal irradiation or injection with dextran sulfate 500 (DS-500), carbon particles and silica. Normal littermates of nude mice were used as the hosts equipped with T cell functions. BCG, *Listeria monocytogenes* or *Candida albicans* was injected intravenously into various hosts and the numbers of viable organisms per organ were estimated by the method of quantitative viable count at various times after the injection.

(1) BCG did not grow in normal hosts regardless of the strains of BCG. However, the French strain of BCG grew progressively in nude mice and raised lesions in various organs. The Japanese strain did not grow in nude mice.

(2) *Listeria* grew transiently in normal mice after infection and was eliminated from the liver and spleen by day 9 or 14. In nude mice, viable cells of *Listeria* were detected consistently in these organs beyond 21 days. A persistent form of infection was observed in nude mice. However, *Listeria* grew progressively and extensively within a period as short as 3 days, when mice were deprived of macrophage functions before infection.

(3) After infection with *Candida*, the numbers of viable organisms in the liver decreased gradually in normal and nude mice from the initial stage of infection. The numbers in the kidney decreased in normal, but increased in nude mice at a late stage. When the hosts were exposed to lethal irradiation

Department of Microbiology, School of Medicine, Kyushu University, Fukuoka, Japan

242   K. Nomoto *et al.*

3 days before infection, *Candida* grew progressively in the liver and kidney from the initial stage.

In general, protection appears to depend principally upon non-immune phagocytosis and cellular immunity at the early and late stages of infection, respectively. The requirement for T cell-mediated immunity appears to be different according to the species or strains of microorganisms, stages of infection and target organs of infection.

INTRODUCTION

Protection against various microorganisms is known to depend upon humoral and cellular elements, both of which are composed of specific and nonspecific mechanisms. However, the contribution of individual mechanisms to protection against each of the organisms has not yet been analyzed in quantitative terms, since all or most such protective mechanisms occur concurrently in the same individuals in most of the experimental systems used up to the present time. Alteration of the patterns of infection has to be studied in hosts deprived of each of the elements participating in resistance against infection, in order to ascertain the contribution of each element and to establish experimental models reflecting severe infections in immunodeficient patients.

Nude mice have been proposed as hosts deprived congenitally of the thymus. However, the presence of several per cent of θ-positive lymphocytes was reported by several investigators. The present authors examined the presence of T cell functions in nude mice by the use of thymus-dependent antigens. When normal mice were subjected to thymectomy at birth, T cell-dependent immunological capacities were depressed profoundly but several per cent of θ-positive lymphocytes were detected in their peripheral blood. When neonatally thymectomized mice were immunized repeatedly with thymus-dependent antigen, for example sheep red blood cells, T cell functions specific for the antigen recovered gradually to the normal level.[1] The residual θ-positive cells in neonatally thymectomized mice proved to be T cells in terms of their functions in immune response. On the other hand, repeated stimulation with such kinds of antigens did not augment the functions of T cells in nude mice. Thus, nude mice can be used as T cell-deprived hosts at least in terms of functions in immune response, although antigenic stimulation occurs persistently in infected hosts. Macrophage functions were suppressed by lethal irradiation or injection with dextran sulfate 500 (DS–500), carbon particles or silica. Macrophage function proved to be depressed at least transiently by these treatments. When nude mice were subjected to these treatments, we could use the mice as T cell-and macrophage-deprived hosts. Tumor-bearing mice were used as hosts deficient in protection against infection, since North et al.[2] reported the depression of macrophage-dependent protective mechanism at an early stage of the tumor-bearing state and the present authors observed the depression of T cell-dependent protective mechanism at a late stage of the tumor-bearing state.

In the present study, we are concerned with cellular elements. Therefore, *Mycobacteria, Listeria* and *Candida* were chosen as standard parasites, since it was suggested that the contribution of humoral antibodies was not important in protection against these microorganisms.

MATERIALS AND METHODS

Animals.   Athymic nude mice (*nu/nu*) of BALB/c background and their normal littermates (*nu/+*) were purchased from Central Laboratory for Experimental Animals (Tokyo). They were raised in a specific-pathogen-free (SPF) condition. In our laboratory, they were maintained in a clean, but not germ-free room. Pellets, drinking water and equipment were sterilized. Their cages were covered with filter caps to minimize microbial contamination. ddN mice were maintained under conventional conditions.

Infection.   Viable organisms 2–3 $\times$ 10^3 of *Listeria monocytogenes*, 1–6 $\times$ 10^5 of *Candida albicans* (line-24), 2 $\times$ 10^6 of the Japanese strain of BCG or 3.5 $\times$ 10^5 of the French strain of BCG were suspended in saline and injected intravenously.

Determination of organisms in organs.   At various times after infection, mice were bled by cutting the femoral artery, and then the lung, liver, kidney and spleen were removed. Individual organs were homogenized separately in 10 ml of solutions suitable for individual microorganisms with Teflon homogenizers. The homogenized suspensions were diluted serially 10–fold with solutions and 0.1 ml of each dilution was spread on agar media. Trypticase soy agar medium, Candida GS agar medium and Ogawa's medium were used, respectively, for *Listeria, Candida* and BCG.

X-irradiation.   Mice were exposed to 900 R of whole body irradiation and used as the hosts for infection 3 days later. X-rays were delivered from a Shimazu 250 kVp machine operating at 200 kVp with 1 mm Cu and 1mm Al filtration at 100 cm of focus-target distance.

Blockade of reticuloendothelial system.   Carbon particles (Pelikan ink) were suspended in saline containing 1 % gelatin at a concentration of 25 mg/ml and 0.2 ml of the suspension was injected intravenously on days −1 and 0, and intraperitoneally on day 1. DS-500 (molecular weight 500,000) was dissolved in 0.15 M NaCl at a concentration of 5 mg/ml. A dose of 50 mg/kg was injected intraperitoneally on day −1 or days −1 and 0 according to the method of Hahn.[3] Silica of 2μ of an average diameter was suspended in saline at a concentration of 50 mg/ml according to Zisman.[4] One ml of the suspension was injected intraperitoneally three times on days −1, 0 and 1. These mice were infected with microorganisms on day 0.

Tumor-grafting.   A homotransplantable tumor, sarcoma-180, was transferred through outbred ddN mice in an ascites form. Viable tumor cells of 1 × 10^6 were inoculated subcutaneously into ddN mice. Tumors grew progressively to reach diameters of 10 to 15 mm 3 weeks later. The tumor-bearing mice were injected intravenously with *Listeria* cells 5 hr or 3 weeks after the tumor-grafting.

RESULTS

Growth of Listeria *in nude mice*
     Viable cells of 2.6 × 10^3 of *L. monocytogenes* were inoculated into *nu/nu* and *nu/+* mice on day 0. Live bacteria in the liver and spleen were counted 3, 6, 9, 12, 15 and 21 days later. Three animals were taken out from each group at each time point. Numbers of viable bacteria in both organs were almost the same in *nu/nu* and *nu/+* mice on day 3 (Fig. 1). Live bacteria began to disappear on day 6 and day 9, respectively, from the spleen and liver of *nu/+* mice and were eliminated completely by day 12. On the other hand, approximately 10^5 viable bacteria were detected in both organs of *nu/nu* mice during the observation period of 21 days.

Growth of Listeria *at an early stage of infection in irradiated mice*
     Viable cells 2.0 × 10^3 of *L. monocytogenes* were inoculated into *nu/nu, nu/+* and irradiated *nu/+* mice on day 0. Live bacteria were counted 1, 24, 48 and 72 hr later. In the spleens of the three groups, live bacteria were hardly detectable 1 hr after infection (Fig. 2). The numbers of bacteria increased rapidly to reach over 10^4 per spleen by 24 hr in all the groups. The numbers of live bacteria increased slightly in *nu/nu* and *nu/+* mice thereafter, while bacteria increased progressively and extensively to reach over 10^7 by 72 hr in the

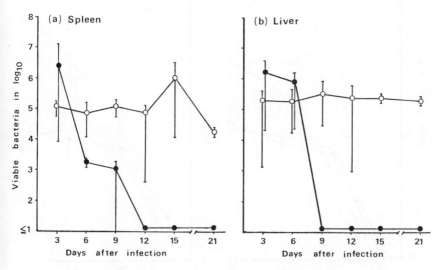

FIG. 1.   Growth of *L. monocytogenes* after an intravenous inoculation of 2.6×10^3 live bacterial cells into nude mice (○) and normal
littermates(●).
Each point represents an average per organ and bars represent ranges.

irradiated *nu/+* mice. Similar patterns of bacterial growth were observed
in the liver of these groups, although total numbers of bacteria per organ were
larger in the liver than in the spleen of the corresponding groups (Fig. 2).

Effect of reticuloendothelial blockade on the growth of Listeria

Viable cells 3.0×10^3 of *L. monocytogenes* were inoculated into *nu/nu* and
nu/+ mice treated with DS-500, carbon or silica, as mentioned above. Viable
bacteria in the spleen and liver were counted 3 days after infection and averages
of five animals are presented in Fig. 3. Bacterial growth was remarkably enhanced by treatment with DS-500 or carbon in *nu/nu* and *nu/+* mice. The
numbers of bacteria in the mice treated with such agents reached 10^8 to 10^9
in the spleen and 10^9 to 10^{10} in the liver, while bacteria in both organs were
less than 10^5 in the non-treated *nu/nu* and *nu/+* mice. Bacterial growth was
enhanced also by treatment with silica, although the degree of enhancement
was rather low as compared with that of the other two agents. No difference
in the enhancement of bacterial growth was detectable between *nu/nu* and *nu/+*
mice with respect to the three agents.

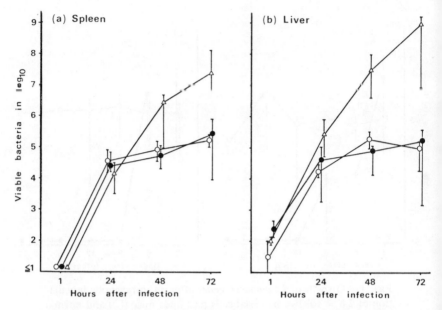

Fɪɢ. 2.   Growth of *L. monocytogenes* after an intravenous inoculation of 2.0 × 10³ live bacterial cells into nude mice(○), normal
littermates (●) and irradiated littermates(△).
Each point represents an average per organ and bars represent ranges.

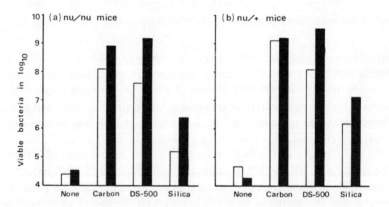

Fɪɢ. 3.   Growth of *L. monocytogenes* at 3 days after an intravenous
inoculation of 3.0 × 10³ live bacterial cells into nude mice and littermates which were treated with carbon, DS-500 or silica.
Open and closed columns represent the number of bacteria in the spleen and
liver, respectively. Each column represents an average of five animals.

Growth of Listeria *in tumor-bearing mice*

Viable cells 2.1 × 10³ *L. monocytogenes* were inoculated into ddN mice 5 hr after tumor-grafting. Viable bacteria in the liver and spleen were counted 24, 48 and 72 hr after the infection. Bacterial growth in the liver was enhanced substantially in tumor-bearing mice and approximately 1000 times as many bacteria in tumor-bearing mice as compared to the controls, were detected at 72 hr after infection (Fig. 4). The growth of bacteria in the spleen was not affected by the tumor-bearing state.

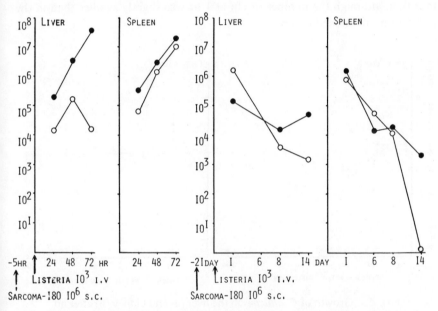

FIG. 4. Growth of *L. monocytogenes* after an intravenous inoculation of 2.1 × 10³ and 2.6 × 10³ of live bacterial cells, respectively, at 5 hr and 21 days after tumor-grafting.
○: normal controls, ●: tumor-bearing mice. Each point represents an average of 16 mice.

Viable cells 2.6 × 10³ of *L. monocytogenes* were inoculated into ddN mice 3 weeks after tumor-grafting. Viable bacteria in the liver and spleen were counted 1, 6, 8 and 14 days later. Elimination of bacteria from the spleen was suppressed markedly in tumor-bearing mice, while bacteria were eliminated completely from control mice by 14 days after infection. The elimination of bacteria at a late stage of infection from the liver was also suppressed in tumor-bearing mice (Fig. 4).

Growth of Candida *in nude mice and irradiated nude mice*

Live organisms 1.5 × 10⁵ of *C. albicans* were inoculated into nude mice, normal littermates and 900 R-irradiated nude mice. The numbers of colony-forming units (cfu) per liver and kidney were estimated at 1 hr and at 1, 2, 5 and 20 days after infection. Most of the irradiated nude mice died within 3 to 4 days after infection. The numbers of cfu were approximately 1 × 10⁵ in the livers of nude mice and normal littermates at 1 hr after infection and declined in the same fashion in both the groups thereafter (Fig. 5). In irradiated nude mice, on the other hand, the numbers of cfu increased slightly 2 days after infection, although the number of cfu at 1 hr was slightly smaller than in the two groups mentioned above.

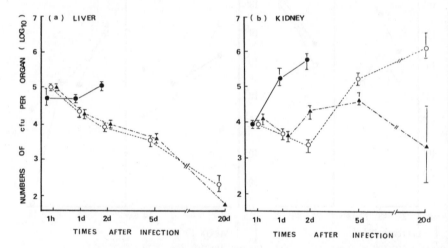

FIG. 5.   Growth of *C. albicans* in the liver (a) and kidney (b) after an intravenous injection of 1.5 × 10⁵ cfu into nude mice, normal littermates and irradiated nude mice.
Live organisms per organ were counted at various times after the injection. ▲: normal littermates, ○: nude mice, ●: irradiated nude mice. Each point represents an average of three animals and bars represent the ranges. The units of "h" and "d" represent hour and day, respectively.

In the kidneys of the three groups, approximately 1 × 10⁴ cfu were detected at 1 hr after the inoculation of *C. albicans*. The numbers of cfu were maintained within almost the same range from 1 hr to 20 days in normal littermates, although a slight reduction was detected at the initial and late stages (Fig. 5). In nude mice, the number of cfu increased progressively after a slight reduction in the initial stage. In irradiated nude mice, the number of cfu increased progressively in the 2 days after the inoculation without such a reduction in the initial stage observed in the other two groups.

In irradiated nude mice, the capacity to eliminate candida cells from the peripheral blood after intravenous inoculation was depressed to a remarkable extent at 3 days after the exposure to 900 R. When candida cells were added to the macrophage monolayers obtained from such irradiated nude mice, the ability to digest the engulfed candida cells was suppressed profoundly as compared with those obtained from non-irradiated nude mice.

The effects of other treatments on the growth of C. albicans were very weak as compared with those on the growth of L.monocytogenes.

Growth of the Japanese and French strains of BCG in nude mice

Viable organisms 2.0 × 10⁶ of the Japanese strain of BCG were inoculated into nude mice and normal littermates. Viable bacteria in the lung, liver, kidney and spleen were counted at 2, 4, 7 and 10 weeks after the inoculation. The Japanese strain of BCG scarcely increased in any organ of *nu/nu* and *nu/+* mice during the observation period.

Two weeks after injection with the French strain of BCG, no difference was detectable between *nu/nu* and *nu/+* mice (Fig. 6). At 4 weeks after injection, greater numbers of viable bacteria were detected in the liver and kidney of *nu/ nu* than in those of *nu/+* mice. The number in each organ decreased in *nu/+* mice thereafter, but increased progressively in *nu/nu* mice.

DISCUSSION

Protection against a variety of microorganisms has been considered to depend upon T cell-mediated immunity, although the degrees of contribution of such a type of resistance may be different among individual organisms. Increased susceptibilities of nude mice to experimental infections have been reported with respect to *L. monocytogenes*,[5] BCG,[6] *Babesia microti* and *Plasmodium berghei yoelii*.[7] According to Emmerling *et al.*,[5] viable organisms of *Listeria* were eliminated from the spleen of normal littermates in the typical course of an experimental infection, but were retained persistently in nude mice from an initial to a late stage of infection. Our results confirmed their results.

We expected the occurrence of a fulminating course of the infection with *L. monocytogenes* in nude mice, since resistance against such bacteria is generally considered to depend largely upon T cell-mediated immunity. Nonetheless, nude mice showed a persistent infection but not a fulminating course.

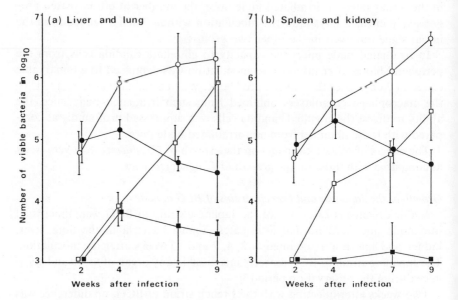

FIG. 6.   Numbers of viable bacteria per organ at various times after an intravenous inoculation with 3.5×10^5 viable cells of French strain.
(a) Open and closed circles indicate the numbers in the liver, respectively, of *nu/nu* and *nu/+* mice. Open and closed squares indicate the numbers in the lung of *nu/nu* and *nu/+* mice, respectively. (b) Open and closed circles indicate the numbers in the spleen of *nu/nu* and *nu/+* mice, respectively. Open and closed squares indicate the numbers in the kidney of *nu/nu* and *nu/+* mice, respectively: Bars represent ranges.

The contribution of other mechanisms must be taken into account in understanding resistance against *L. monocytogenes* as a whole. Possible candidates for such resistance may be the protection by phagocytes, including nonimmune macrophages and polymorphonuclear cells, and that by humoral immunity. In the present study, the contribution of phagocytes was studied by the use of mice in which phagocyte functions were suppressed by several agents. Bacterial growth came close to a plateau of approximately 10^5 per organ in 24 hr in non-irradiated *nu/nu* and *nu/+* mice. This plateau was maintained beyond 72 hr, while bacteria grew progressively and extensively in irradiated mice. The defense mechanism, by which extensive growth at an early stage of infection was inhibited in non-irradiated mice, appears to be independent of the presence of T lymphocytes. Lethal irradiation proved to gvie severe damage to various elements in hosts. Experiments with irradiation did not rule out the possibility that the damage to elements other than phagocytes enhanced the growth of *L. monocytogenes*. Then we carried out similar experiments with mice treated with DS-500, carbon particles and silica, all of which proved to suppress macrophage functions. Bacterial growth at 72 hr after infection was enhanced remarkably by these treatments. Such enhancing effects were detected in all of the nude mice, normal littermates, C3H/He, AKR and C57BL/6 mice. Therefore the mechanism suppressed by such treatment appears to be thymus-independent. Non-immune phagocytosis and T cell-mediated immunity appear to contribute to protection against *Listeria*, at an early and a late stage of infection, respectively.

Tumor-bearing state of hosts appears to induce the deficiencies of macrophage-dependent resistance and T cell-mediated protective immunity, respectively, at the initial and late stages of the tumor-bearing state. At an intial stage as early as 5 hr after tumor-grafting, resistance against *L. monocytogenes* was suppressed in the liver but not in the spleen. The depression was prevented by treatment with zymosan, which activated macrophages directly. When *L. monocytogenes* was inoculated into tumor-bearing mice at a stage as late as 21 days after tumor-grafting, complete elimination of bacteria at the late stage of infection was suppressed. The depressed protective immunity was restored by a polysaccharide which proved to restore T cell functions of tumor-bearing mice. The deficiencies of protection against infection in cancer patients will become an important research project in terms of secondary immunodeficiencies.

The pattern of infection with *C. albicans* was substantially different from that with *L. monocytogenes*. In the liver, the numbers of cfu of *Candida* declined progressively in both nude mice and normal littermates. This elimination may depend primarily upon phagocytosis and digestion by the fixed macrophages in the liver, and such functions may not require the contribution of T cell-mediated immunity for their expression.

In the kidney, the pattern of the growth of *Candida* was entirely different. At the late stage of infection, *C. albicans* grew progressively in nude mice, but not in their normal littermates. Normal littermates did not completely eliminate candida cells from their kidneys but inhibited their growth to a considerable extent. Since fixed macrophages are not so numerous in the kidney as in the liver, the accumulation of macrophages induced by T cell-mediated cellular immunity may be required for effective protection against *C. albicans*. Louria et al.[8] reported that infection progressed only in the kidney after an experimental infection in mice. Dobias[9] and Hasenclever and Mitchell[10] also reported that lesions in the kidney were less extensive in immunized than non-immunized mice. Thus, nonimmune phagocytosis appears to be the main protective mechanism in the liver regardless of the stage of infection. T cell-mediated immunity appears to be required for the elimination of candida cells from the kidney at the late stage of infection.

The Japanese strain of BCG appears to be eliminated by nonspecific defense mechanisms composed mainly of normal macrophages, since there was no difference in bacterial growth between T cell-deprived mice and controls. On the other hand, specific immunity mediated by T lymphocytes appears to be re-

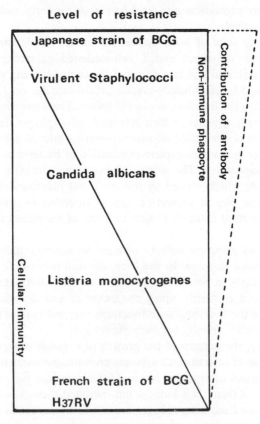

Level of resistance

FIG. 7. Tentative evaluation of the mutual contribution of non-immune phagocytosis and T cell-mediated immunity to protection against various microorganisms.

The results in the present paper and those in our preliminary experiments were included.

quired for resistance against the more virulent French strain. Phipps strain of BCG appears to be comparable to the French strain in virulence, since Phipps strain was found to grow in nude mice but not in normal littermates by Sher et al.[6]

We evaluated the mutual contribution of nonimmune phagocytosis and T cell-mediated immunity tentatively, as shown in Fig. 7. The figure includes the results in this paper and the results from our preliminary experiments. Mutual contribution appears to be different among individual microorganisms. Therefore, severe or chronic infection with individual organisms may be expected to occur in the cases in which the principal defense mechanism against the invading microorganisms is depressed congenitally or secondarily. Therapy or prevention of severe or chronic infection in immunodeficient patients may be promoted more efficiently, if the mutual relationships between nonimmune and immune mechanisms in the resistance against infection is understood more precisely. Contribution of humoral elements will be analyzed in studies along the line of the present paper.

REFERENCES

1. Takeya, K. and Nomoto, K.: Characteristics of antibody response in young or thymectomized mice. *J. Immunol.* **99**:831, 1967.
2. North, R. J., Kirstein, D. P., and Tuttle, R. L.: Subversion of host defense mechanisms by murine tumors. I. A circulating factor that suppresses macrophage-mediated resistance to infection. *J. Exp. Med.* **143**:559, 1976.
3. Hahn, H.: Effects of dextran sulfate 500 on cell-mediated resistance to infection with *Listeria monocytogenes* in mice. *Infect. Immunity* **10**:1105, 1974.
4. Zisman, B., Hirsh, M. S., and Allison, A. C.: Selective effects of antimacrophage serum, silica and anti-lymphocyte serum on phagocytosis of herpes virus infection of young adult mice. *J. Immunol.* **104**:1155, 1970.
5. Emmerling, P., Finger, H., and Bockemühl, J.: *Listeria monocytogenes* infection in nude mice. *Infect. Immunity* **12**:437, 1975.
6. Sher, N. A., Chaparas, S. D., Greenberg, L. E., Merchant, E. B., and Vickers, J. H.: Response of congenitally athymic (nude) mice to infection with *Mycobacterium bovis* (Strain BCG). *J. Nat. Cancer Inst.* **54**:1419, 1975.
7. Clark, I. A. and Allison, A. C.: *Babesia microti* and *Plasmodium berghei yoelii* infections in nude mice. *Nature* (London) **252**:328, 1974.
8. Louria, D. B., Brayton, R. G., and Finkel, G.: Studies on the pathogenesis of experimental *Candida albicans* infections in mice. *Sabouraudia* **2**:271, 1963.
9. Dobias, B.: Specific and non-specific immunity in *Candida* infections: Experimental studies of the role of *Candida* cell constituents and review of literature. *Acta. Med. Scand.* **176** (suppl. 421):1, 1964.
10. Hasenclever, H. F. and Mitchell, W. O.: Acquired immunity to candidiasis in mice. *J. Bacteriol.* **86**:401, 1963.

DISCUSSION

Dr. GOOD: Margaret Chide has shown that the nude mice that are infected with hepatitis virus do have quite a number of T-lymphocytes with T-lymphocyte function. And there could be differences between the influence of different organisms on the induction of the T-cell component. And it was very clear that a very small number of post-thymic T-cells could go a long way to produce this resistance to the *Candida* infection. Even small numbers of cells that might be induced differently by the different organisms might result in the differences in the French strain and the Japanese strain of the BCC.

Dr. AIUTI: We have several patients with chronic mucuscandidiasis in whom we found a very elevated antibody against *Candida*, and after treatment with the transfer factor, we could reconstitute cellular immunity and we observed a decrease of the titer of antibody. So we think that the role of antibodies is practically nil or, at least, not important.

III. COMPARATIVE AND ANALYTICAL
EPIDEMIOLOGY OF IMMUNODEFICIENCY

Inheritance, Incidence and Epidemiology of Severe Combined Immunodeficiency Syndromes

W. H. HITZIG and A. B. KENNY

ABSTRACT

Severe combined immunodeficiency (SCID) is distinguishable from agammaglobulinemia by its profound blood lymphopenia and dysplasia of lymphatic tissues, in particular the thymus. SCID was once considered a clearcut entity, but it is now accepted to belong to a heterogeneous group. This was first indicated by *genetic findings*, namely the two modes of auto-somal recessive *vs.* sexlinked inheritance. Since 1972 the autosomal recessive cases have been further subdivided, through testing the activity of the enzyme adenosine-deaminase (ADA), into equal groups of ADA deficient and ADA normal cases. Finally, reports of dysostosis, hair anomaly and reticular dysgenesis combined with SCID are not rare. In addition, rare sporadic non-heritable cases were observed, *e.g.* after intrauterine rubella infection.

The incidence of SCID has been estimated at 1:30,000 (Switzerland) to 1:100,000 (USA), or even at 1:16,000 in autopsy material. A detailed analysis of incidence is presented.

Epidemiology: SCID has been observed in every country, every population, and every ethnic group as soon as doctors became suspicious of the disease. Cases have been seen in Caucasians, Jews, Japanese, Arabs and Negroes, and in all continents. Since the systematic collection of ADA deficient patients, the apparent predominance of the sex-linked form in the USA *vs.* prevailing autosomal recessive transmission in Europe seems doubtful.

Within each genetic group characteristic clinical features have now been recognized. This is of a certain importance for therapeutic approaches.

INTRODUCTION

The term "combined immunodeficiency" was coined only a few years ago.

Department of Pediatrics, University of Zürich, Switzerland

It is appropriate to recall briefly its historical development. In 1958 a malignant form of agammaglobulinemia was distinguished from the well-known Bruton type by reason of its distinctive feature, namely a profound lymphopenia.[1,2] At that time, this disease was believed to be rare and exceptional.

By 1961, eleven well-studied and 20 suspected cases were described.[3] Some of them were of siblings or cousins of the patient whose illness was termed in 1950 by Glanzmann and Riniker "Lymphozytophthise".[4] This syndrome was characterized by a deficiency of both humoral and cellular immunity reactions. For about one decade it was known as the "Swiss type of agammaglobulinemia". In 1968, at the workshop on Sanibel Island, we reported on 71 well-documented cases differing only in patterns of inheritance.[5] We considered them representative of a single disease entity. To the present time many additional case reports have appeared in the literature and have provided two important modifications of the original disease description.

First, and of prime importance, was the detection in 1972 of deficiency in blood cells and serum of the enzyme adenosine deaminase (ADA).[6] Since then two other enzyme deficiencies have been described, of nucleotide phosphorylase and of inosine deaminase.

Secondly, the patterns of inheritance have been clarified.

In addition, many minor modifications have been pointed out. Certain authors have gone so far as to state that each case represented a different individual variety of "combined immunodeficiency". Such an interpretation of the observed cases so broadens the scope of this disease entity that the original concept of SCID is threatened with destruction.

To state clearly what I am talking about I repeat the earlier given definition: "severe combined immunodeficiency is a congenital and usually hereditary deficiency of both humoral and cellular immunity characterized clinically by the early onset of severe infections and a rapid progressive course with early demise. Pathologically it is characterized by lymphoid and plasma cell aplasia and thymic dysplasia."

PATTERN OF THE DISEASE

In 1968 we[5] reviewed 71 well-documented cases of SCID in an attempt to delineate a picture of this disease. We have now updated the list of clinical and pathological signs by evaluating 328 fully investigated cases of our own and from the literature (Table 1). In addition to the data from the unequivocal patients, there are data on 59 siblings and 47 other relatives who died with

TABLE 1. Severe combined immunodeficiency

Well-documented cases			328
Siblings			59
Other relatives			47
Total			434

Sex	♂	♀	Not stated	Total
	300	108	26	434

Familial cases: in 93 sibships		
Certain cases	179	
Siblings	59	285
Other relatives	47	

suggestive signs. This brings the total number of cases to 434. The following facts emerge from this compilation:

1) There is a clear predominance of males in a proportion of nearly 3:1.

2) Familiality is a frequent feature: 285 of the total 434 cases occurred in 93 sibships. The other cases were without recorded familial background.

3) Clinical signs and laboratory data are quite uniform (Table 2):

a) Severe infections in the majority of the cases started in the very first weeks of life and recurred frequently or never cleared. They were polytopic, *i.e.*, they affected the 3 main contact surfaces of the body (skin, respiratory and intestinal mucosa) and resulted occasionally in septic invasions. All untreated infants died within the first months of life.

TABLE 2. Severe combined immunodeficiency (evaluation of 171 cases)

		1968	1976
Number of cases		70	111
Clinical signs (%)			
Diarrhea		86	47
Respiratory infections		89	63
Moniliasis		79	63
Skin infection, rash		67	30
Septicemia		57	26
Laboratory findings (%)			
Lymphopenia (<1000)		90	51
Hypogammaglobulinemia		97	61
PHA(79 cases)	(—)		78
	(↓)		21
MLC (41 cases)	(—)		80
	↓		19
	+		1

b) Laboratory data established the frequent occurrence of severe lymphopenia. More important, the functions of lymphocytes were always deficient. Immunoglobulin values were usually very low, in the range of agammaglobulinemia. Antibody formation was never found. The thymus was very small or absent. Sometimes it could be visualized by chest X-ray. In a few cases, however, thymus biopsy made at an early stage of the disease was reported to reveal a normal amount of thymic tissue.

c) Post mortem histological findings (Table 3) were striking and specific in the lymphatic organs. The gut-associated lymphoid tissue was virtually absent. The normal architecture of lymph nodes and thymus was destroyed,

TABLE 3. Histologic findings in 244 cases of SCID

Lymph nodes and spleen		
hypoplastic, reticular or epitheloid	235	
not mentioned	9	
Thymus		
not found	10	
<1g	32	
<2g	21	
<5g	17	
5–12g	8	
normal	2	
small	110	
not mentioned	44	244
Hassall's corpuscles		
absent	154	
present	19	
not mentioned	61	
no thymus	10	244

and the number of lymphocytes in these organs was extremely reduced. One of the most striking features was the diminution of thymus tissue. In 10 cases no thymus at all was found. Albeit, it should be remarked that in 27 cases the weight of the thymus was near the normal range. This weight, however, included all the connective and adipose tissue which is usually greatly enlarged in SCID patients. In addition, the absence of Hassall's corpuscles, formerly considered a *sine qua non* in this disease by several authors, was not confirmed in 19 cases. In 1971 we[7] presented indirect evidence for a possible progressive destruction of thymus tissue and of Hassall's corpuscles. Such destruction has since then been confirmed by other investigators in a few biopsied cases.

ENZYME DEFICIENCY IN SCID

A new and revolutionary element has been introduced into our understanding of the pathogenesis of SCID by the detection of a deficiency of adenosine-deaminase (ADA) in blood cells and serum.[6] Absence or inactivity of this otherwise ubiquitous enzyme is now considered to be causally related to SCID. When this enzyme is inactive, adenosine-monophosphate and cyclic adenosine-monophosphate accumulate, and this accumulation exerts a toxic effect on the lymphoid system.[8] *In vitro* studies with lymphocyte cultures have shown that the toxicity is due to the inhibition of phosphoribosyl-pyrophosphate synthetase, an enzyme essential for the formation of precursors of purine and pyrimidine nucleotides. *De novo* synthesis of these nucleotides is essential for lymphocyte proliferation.

Lack of activity of ADA may be due to true absence or to inactivation by an inhibitor of the enzyme. Presence of such an inhibitor has recently been described by Trotta and coworkers.[9] Upon dilution or after aging of red cell lysates of two children with ADA deficiency, the enzyme activity rose to almost normal levels. We confirmed these findings in the blood of 3 heterozygous carriers.

This ADA enzyme deficiency serves as a unique genetic marker. Homozygotes are readily identifiable by virtually absent enzyme activity. They are SCID patients. The heterozygotes who show no signs of immunodeficiency can now be identified through exhibition of significantly redued ADA activity. Such genetic identification provides the first incidence of the use of an enzyme deficiency for the detection of the heterozygotic state in an immunological disease. It is a most valuable tool for genetic counselling in affected families.

Deficiency of adenosine-deaminase has been confirmed in a number of families. In our own material,[10] 8 sibships of previously deceased patients were reinvestigated, and in 3 pairs of parents the enzyme deficiency was present in a heterozygous form. As an example I present the previously published[7] pedigree of one family because of apparently incomplete manifestation of the SCID syndrome in 3 boys, that is, they exhibited almost normal immunoglobulins during a prolonged period of time. On reviewing the literature we could confirm that SCID patients with ADA deficiency tend to have nearly normal immunoglobulin concentrations but very low lymphocyte counts.

An additional feature of a small group of SCID patients is the presence of cartilagenous anomalies leading to short stature. It has been termed "short limbed dwarfism".[11] All the patients studied up to now were ADA deficient, whereas children with SCID and normal ADA never presented this type of dysostosis.

Deficiency of a second enzyme of the nucleotide pathway has recently been described.[12] Purine-nucleoside-phosphorylase was absent in a 4-year-old girl with hypoplastic anemia suggestive of Blackfan-Diamond anemia, with retarded somatic and mental development and suffering recurring infections. Up to the present time 3 other patients with the same enzyme deficiency have been detected. The difference in the clinical appearance is striking.

INHERITANCE IN SCID

In the small group of ADA deficient patients the autosomal recessive transmission is proven and the heterozygotes can be identified. In the much larger remaining group with normal or unknown ADA, the mode of inheritance in familial cases can be classified as autosomal recessive if girls are among the patients. Several families were first described as examples of sex-linked inheritance, but later the birth of an affected girl clarified the situation and necessitated classification in the autosomal group. Present data (Table 4) show that in the group with autosomal recessive transmission slightly less than 1/2 of the patients tested so far were ADA deficient. This proportion is not statistically significant because of the small number of patients.

TABLE 4.   Inheritance in severe combined immunodeficiency 1950–1976

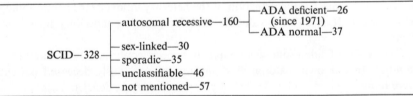

The small group of probably sex-linked cases, less than 10% of the total, is still subject to the criticism that no positive diagnostic criteria are available. In a great number of non-familial cases (138 SCID patients) the hereditary pattern is not clear. It is obvious that diagnostic criteria for the identification of the healthy gene carriers are highly desirable.

Sporadic, non-hereditary cases certainly exist, but estimates of their frequency are impossible. Intrauterine infection is a proven etiology of this condition; graft-versus-host disease with chimerism another possibility.[13] I want also to remind you that severe infantile malnutrition due to exogenous socioeconomic factors can produce a phenocopy of SCID with depletion of the lymphoid system and thymic dysplasia. The end-stage is indistinguishable from the hereditary and congenital disease, although SCID in kwashiorkor is probably acquired.

EPIDEMIOLOGIC INCIDENCE

Table 5 shows the distribution of the cases found in the literature up to June 1976. This table of course is subject to all the deficiencies of screening the world literature for a certain disease, and we have knowledge of a considerable number of unpublished observations. Even so, however, the very uneven geographic distribution is probably not real, but due to different diagnostic criteria.* The diagnosis is presumably often missed in countries with high infantile mortality. But also in developed countries with higher medical standards the diagnosis may be missed, and cases of SCID should be suspected in death certificates within the categories of infection, malnutrition, diarrhea, unexpected sudden death, etc. In our own hospital, we missed the diagnosis twice within the last year: One case was diagnosed as whooping cough—pertussis-like cough was described as a clinical sign of the rarely missing pneumopathy— and the other patient died of erythrodermia which later turned out to be due to graft-versus-host reaction caused by a previous blood transfusion. In both cases the diagnosis was made only by the pathologist at post mortem examination.

TABLE 5. Epidemiology of SCID (June 1976)

Europe	118
North America	204
South America	3
Japan	2
New Zealand	1
	328

In this connection, Berry's re-evaluation of about 1000 autopsies[14] of infants who died at the Hospital for Sick Children in London should be recalled. When he reviewed the histological material he found evidence for profound

* Material presented at this Symposium by Hayakawa for the new Japanese IDS registry proves this assumption: a retrospective investigation revealed 28 cases of SCID observed over a ten-year period in Japan.

lymphatic anomaly and/or thymus involvement in 16 cases. Even if this figure is an overestimation due to selection at Great Ormond Street and possibly also to incorporation of some doubtful cases, it shows anyway that SCID has never been recognized as an entity before the disease was known to the pathologist. The same is certainly true, and even more important, for clinicians who still quite often are not aware of this disease.

It has been questioned whether such diagnostic failures are of practical importance. Until recently SCID has been considered to be an extremely rare disease of purely academic interest, the study of which has admittedly contributed a good deal to the understanding of normal functions of the immune system. However, based on our new figures this view must be challenged. As a hereditary trait the disease might be more frequent than suspected. This had no importance as long as the infantile death rate due to infectious diseases was very high, but in the last two decades it has become a sizable figure.

Even more important is the possibility of genetic counselling. As mentioned, ADA deficiency can now be diagnosed in the heterozygous carriers. In addition prenatal diagnosis has been possible in a few cases using fibroblast cultures grown from amniotic fluid. The first such case was predicted by Dr. Rochelle Hirschhorn to be a homozygote for ADA deficiency, i.e., a SCID patient. Since the gestational age was already over 20 weeks, pregnancy was carried to term, and the diagnosis was confirmed in the healthy-looking newborn baby. In one of our families the firstborn ADA deficient twins both died of the disease. The second pregnancy was similarly monitored with the help of Dr. Rochelle Hirschhorn. She measured intermediate ADA activity in amniotic fluid fibroblasts and predicted heterozygosity. This diagnosis was confirmed in cord blood and again at the age of 3 months. The boy is now 5 months old, thriving and free of infections. He presents normal lymphocyte counts and functions, but slightly subnormal immunoglobulin concentration.

Thus, the possibilities of detection of heterozygote gene carriers and of prenatal diagnosis of ADA inactivity offer a sound base for genetic counselling in affected families. This example could stimulate increased endeavours towards clarification of the other, still obscure etiologic factors of the SCID syndrome.

REFERENCES

1. Hitzig, W. H., Biro, Z., Bosch, H., and Huser, H. J.: Agammaglobulinämie and alymphozytose mit schwund des lymphatischen gewebes. *Helv. Paed. Acta* 13:551, 1958.

2. Tobler, R. and Cottier, H.: Familiäre lymphopenie mit agammaglobulinämie und schwerer moniliasis. Die "essentielle lymphocytophthise'' als besondere form der frühkindlichen agammaglobulinämie. *Helv. Paed. Acta* **13**:313, 1958.
3. Hitzig, W. H. and Willi, H.: Hereditäre lympho-plasmocytäre dysgenesie ("alymphocytose mit agammaglobulinämie"). *Schweiz. Med. Wschr.* **91**:1625, 1961.
4. Glanzmann, E. and Riniker, P.: Essentielle lymphocytophthise. Ein neues krankheitsbild aus der säuglingspathologie. *Ann. Paediatr.* **175**:1, 1950.
5. Hitzig, W. H.: The Swiss type of agammaglobulinemia. *Birth defects* **4**:82, 1968.
6. Giblett, E. R., Anderson, J. E., Cohen, F., Pollara B., and Meuwissen, H. J.: Adenosine-Deaminase deficiency in two patients with severely impaired cellular immunity. *Lancet* **1972/II**:1067.
7. Hitzig, W. H., Landolt, R., Müller, G., and Bodmer, P.: Heterogeneity of phenotypic expression in a family with Swiss-type agammaglobulinemia: Observations on the acquisition of agammaglobulinemia. *J. Pediat.* **78**:968, 1971.
8. Ishii, K. and Green, H.: Lethality of adenosine for cultured mammalian cells by interference with pyrimidine biosynthesis. *J. Cell Sci.* **13**:1, 1973.
9. Trotta, P. P., Smithwick, E. M., and Balis, M. E.: A normal level of adenosine deaminase activity in red cell lysates of carriers and patients with severe combined immunodeficiency disease. *Proc. Nat. Acad. Sci. USA* **73**:104–108, 1976.
10. Ackeret, C., Plüss, H. J., and Hitzig, W. H.: Hereditary severe combined immunodeficiency and adenosine deaminase deficiency. *Pediat. Res.* **10**:67, 1975.
11. Gatti, R. A., Platt, N., Pomerance, H. H., Hong, R., Langer, L. O., Kay, H. E. M., and Good, R. A.: Hereditary lymphopenic agammaglobulinemia associated with a distinctive form of shortlimbed dwarfism and ectodermal dysplasia. *J. Pediat.* **75**:675, 1969.
12. Giblett, E. R., Ammann, A. J., Sandman, R., Wara, D. W., and Diamond, L. K.: Nucleoside-Phosphorylase deficiency in a child with severely defective T-cell immunity and normal B-cell immunity. *Lancet* *1*:1010, 1975.
13. Kadowaki, J., Thompsen, R. I., Zuelzer, W. W., Woolley, P. V., Jr., Brough, A. J., and Gruber, D.: XX/XY lymphoid chimaerism in congenital immunological deficiency syndrome with thymic alymphoplasia. *Lancet* **II**:1152, 1965.
14. Berry, C. L. and Thompson, E. N.: Clinico-pathological study of thymic dysplasia. *Arch. Dis. Child.* **43**:579, 1968.

DISCUSSION

Dr. GOOD: I would like to know any examples where the familial form of ADA deficiency, or some other, has been associated with a progressive disease.

Dr. HITZIG: For the care of public health, it is much more important to be able to avoid the disease, and if we have means for sound genetic counselling, we might be able to avoid the birth of new cases.

Dr. GATTI: If you do the immunologic studies at birth on a child that is ADA deficient in a family where you have already documented one case, what do the studies look like?

Dr. COOPER: It is my understanding that it is heterogenetic. That in some of these patients T- and B-cells will be there for a time and then some or all will be lost; some are missing right from birth as has been the case with our cases.

Dr. GOOD: I think the point that I am making is that there *is* heterogeneity, there is no question about the heterogeneity, of the ultimate phenotypic expression, but it is diagnosable by immunological analysis at birth. Although there is heterogeneity, the criteria of severe combined immunodeficiency, if you use these definitions that Hitzig first set out, which we have amplified through the years using the T- and B-cell analyses, you can make the diagnosis at birth, and I think confusion in the literature is due to cases of other origins that may be virus infection or something else, which look like this in the terminal stage.

Dr. GATTI: First I was interested in what you said about the possibility that the X-linked cases may not really be X-linked but undefined, or yet to be defined, or that there were some which were recessive; is that what you were implying?

Dr. HITZIG: Yes.

Dr. GATTI: That is an interesting observation because, as you probably are aware, the family that we first transplanted was a very well-documented X-linked family where there are now, I think, 14 males who have been affected over three generations. Since that case there have been others, and they have all been male. On the other hand, in the second generation there were two females that died of recurrent infections, and finally an overwhelming fatal infection. They were two sisters in the same family, and they were four years old and five years old, I believe. This family was also documented as X-linked in Boston, another branch of the family. I wonder if any of the other X-linked families have been looked at in retrospect with this thought in mind?

Dr. GOOD: I think that there is no question about the hereditary nature in that family. It is transmitted through the female to the male; it is either X-linked on the X-chromosome, or it is X-limited. You may have a more or less defective cellular function depending upon the influence of the inactivated, which X-chromosome is inactivated, so I really do not accept that there is not an X-linked form of combined immunodeficiency. It is the sporadic male cases where you do not know whether or not they are X-linked, or when you have multiple cases in a family with two males, you do not know whether they are X-linked or auto-somal.

Dr. COOPER: What would you think would be the most reliable feature for the diagnosis of G. V. H. disease?

Dr. HITZIG: Well, the skin manifestations are very variable, and therefore we put them all together under the term of rashes. Apart from skin infections where germs could be identified, rashes which first have been described as morbilliform are very frequent and very variable. In most cases the thought did not even arise that this might be graft rashes. We have been taught to consider this possibility by the pathologists only. Now the outspoken graft-versus-host reactions are easy to recognise if you know the diagnosis; it is a very severe disease, and I think for the clinician the most important thing is to avoid blood transfusions without absolute need. And several of the cases which we have seen just got a simple blood transfusion and some of them for not very strict reasons, just to correct a slight anemia. But the few lymphocytes which you transmit with a simple blood transfusion can be sufficient to cause graft-versus-host reaction. If you have a suspicion of this disease, I think as a clinician you should do a skin biopsy and send it to a pathologist who is familiar with this disease, and then he will confirm it for you. The second feature is diarrhea, which, as I showed, is one of the presenting symptoms of the disease, and is therefore very unreliable, but in the stools you can find desquamating epithelial cells. This is very simple to do, but I think this comes only in the second line.

Dr. GOOD: With Slade and Woodruff at our place we have made an exhaustive study now of the histopathology of graft-versus-host disease and it is unique. The characteristic is the epithelial invasion by lymphocytes in the production of *satellite* necrosis, and, in the epithelium of the skin, mummified cells with the adjacent lymphocyte. Exactly the same lesion is present in the colon.

Dr. HITZIG: We have forgotten one further feature. That is liver involvement. I have seen a patient in hospital after a fetal liver infusion who had severe hepatitis, or severe icterus for a long time and then recovered, and that is another feature of graft-versus-host reaction.

Dr. COOPER: My point is why we have persisted in using a younger fetal liver to try, as Dr. Hitzig has tried many times, to use this as a successful source for stem cells. The crucial issue number one will be stem cells that are growing up in the environment of a histologically incompatible recipient will become tolerant, and if not, will they attack the recipient? I agree with you that if you get a source of stem cells before any have been influenced by the thymus, then one will not likely get graft-versus-host disease. Many times when graft-versus-host disease has been diagnosed after this it has been a misdiagnosis because the diagnostic features are not unique, they are common to many other problems.

Dr. GOOD: The pathological features are unique but I think that the evidence about the post-thymic T-cells is excellent. It is not absolute that it is the post-thymic T-cells. It may be that you have to be free of the things that we call mature lymphocytes, you know, either B or T. With the best reagent for eliminating the cells which can initiate the graft-versus-host reaction you can cross major histocompatibility barriers in rats and mice, and now in dogs. If you take their marrow, and with *antiserum*, appropriate *antiserum*, properly *absorbed* and *properly specific,* you can avoid a graft-versus-host reaction even after fatal radiation which is a very sensitive test, just as we do with fetal liver, and with spleen and bone marrow if we got them under appropriate biological dissection.

Dr. COOPER: Will these stem cells be able to kill virus-infected cells of the recipient type? Will the Zinkernagel phenomenon be operative and will the donor cells, lacking the same histocompatibility determinants as skin cells, let us say, infected, will the infected cells be killed by these histo-incompatible cells?

Dr. GOOD: Unequivocally yes, and the data from the Notre Dame study, where they have been able to show that they not only are able to treat effectively, but to prevent the occurrence of RNA tumor virus-induced malignancy, going across major barriers and having a completely histo-incompatible system. So that although the Zinkernagel system is a fascinating one, it at least is not essential for the defense against certain viruses or there may be other ways of achieving the same thing.

Dr. COOPER: Then let us take your patient with the fetal liver transplant, where allogeneic stem cells, presumably raised up to become T-cells and B-cells, already existed in the recipient. Did they get together and make antibodies as they should?

Dr. GOOD: No, I think that what happened there was that we developed in this patient suppressor T-cells. We could demonstrate that. Then when we introduced or knocked out the existing lymphoid system and introduced a system that had both T and B from the donor we had full immunologic function. I am not absolutely certain that T and B cooperation can work with major histo-incompatibility between the T and the B. I think it is very likely that it will not work. I think for the experiments in animals that that is the case. But I think that we still need the critical studies on humans to prove that. I do not think humans are going to be different from the animals, however, and I would try under those circumstances to introduce an entirely new immunologic system, both B and T.

Dr. COOPER: Could I ask one last question and that is, has anyone tested patients who have been restored with allogeneic stem cells of whatever sources; has anyone been able to demonstrate delayed hypersensitivity which again may require histocompatibility for I-region, or comparable determinants?

Dr. GOOD: Well, the answer to your question do any of these patients who have been restored with stem cells from a foreign source have delayed hypersensitivity is unequivocally, yes. Every one of our patients we call fully reconstituted have a full spectrum of cell-mediated immunity; I mean, they do have delayed allergy in the classical sense: to antigens to which you sensitize them to, to 2–4 dinitrochlorobenzene, to antigens that they have a natural infection to, to all of these things. But that really is not the critical issue I think, because they are reconstituted with respect to both their B and T cell systems. The critical issue would arise if they were reconstituted with one and not with another. I think that is a very untenable situation; that is what we call an imcomplete reconstitution, and we keep going after them.

Dr. GOOD: We have a mismatch at the HLA locus in camp, although we had match at what we call the Four-locus. Originally, in the Copenhagen case we had a mismatch at both of the HLA, and a match at the D locus. And in the experimental animals, where this has been successful, we had mismatches across the strongest histocompatibility barriers, both with biologic dissection and with antigenic dissection. In other words, if you remove the fully differentiated cells, put in stem cells in rats across the AGB barrier, those animals are fully reconstituted and they are normal. The only difference in them is that the donor cells are tolerant of the recipient, but they can function immunologically very well.

Dr. TADA: I think there is a lot of controversy over the histocompatibility requirement for T/B cell cooperation and especially in the bone marrow transplantation, the cooperation between the macrophage and the T-cell. Recent experiments show that in order to induce adoptive DL-type hypersensitivity, K and D region identities are required to induce a good response. In that sense, I think the Zinkernagel system just fits this experiment, but in other cases, there are no definite histocompatibility requirements. I think that at the moment we can consider there are several different possibilities, like adoptive differentiation and negative and positive selection, and also radical exclusion, if you use F-1. But I do not think there is any clear-cut demonstration of the histocompatibility requirement in human cases, and I do not think we can give a good answer at the moment.

Analysis of Registered Cases of Immunodeficiency in Japan

Hiroshi HAYAKAWA, Nobuko IIZUKA, Junichi YATA, Kiyomi YAMADA, and Noboru KOBAYASHI

We would like to present data from an epidemiological survey on primary immunodeficiency diseases and some related diseases in Japan.

Although interest in these rare but important diseases has been growing among most physicians recently, a nationwide epidemiological survey has never been performed in our country.

This project on primary immunodeficiency diseases in Japanese people has been planned with a grant from the Ministry of Health and Welfare of Japan. Not only primary immunodeficiency diseases but also some diseases with neutrophil dysfunction and others were surveyed at the same time because very little data on these diseases are available on Japanese people.

The initial study was planned to include the total population of the recognized various immunodeficiency diseases throughout Japan during the previous ten years (from 1966 to 1975).

Approximately 1700 hospitals and institutes which had departments of pediatrics and/or internal medicine and had more than 200 beds for in-patients were listed as the subjects of this survey and were mailed the initial questionnaire.

Almost all outstanding hospitals and institutes in our country could be included according to criteria and almost all individuals with immunodeficiency diseases might be taken care of by these hospitals.

Finally among 641 collected replies, 183 (28.5 %) hospitals reported any cases of immunodeficiency while the other 458 hospitals reported no cases at all (Table 1).

In total so far 628 cases have been reported. Among them transient hypogammaglobulinemia of infancy was the most frequent disease (116 cases). Selective IgA deficiency, selective immunoglobulin deficiency other than IgA and infantile sex-linked agammaglobulinemia followed it (93, 77 and 70 cases,

The All-Japan Immunodeficiency Registration Center (Representative, N. Kobayashi), Department of Pediatrics, University of Tokyo, Tokyo, Japan

TABLE 1.   The total number of reported cases with primary immunodeficiency (Initial survey)

1. Infantile sex-linked agammaglobulinemia	70	(11.1%)
2. Thymic hypoplasia (DiGeorge)	23	(3.7%)
3. Severe combined immunodeficiency	26	(3.8%)
4. Immunodeficiency with generalized hematopoietic hypoplasia	1	(0.2%)
5. Selective immunodeficiency (IgA)	93	(14.8%)
6. Selective immunodeficiency other than IgA	77	(12.3%)
7. Immunodeficiency with ataxia telangiectasia	46	(7.5%)
8. Immunodeficiency with thrombocytopenia and eczema (Wiskott-Aldrich)	28	(4.5%)
9. Immunodeficiency with normal or hyper-immunoglobulinemia	11	(1.8%)
10. Transient hypogammaglobulinemia of infancy	116	(18.5%)
11. Variable immunodeficiency	29	(4.6%)
12. Immunodeficiency with thymoma	3	(0.5%)
13. Immunodeficiency with short-limbed dwarfism	1	(0.2%)
14. Chronic granulomatous disease	40	(6.5%)
15. Chediak-Higashi disease	11	(1.8%)
16. Other dysphagotosis of the neutrophils	6	(0.9%)
17. Chronic mucocutaneous candidiasis	12	(1.9%)
18. Complement deficiencies	2	(0.3%)
19. Other unclassified cases suspected of primary immunodeficiency	33	(5.3%)
Total	628	

hypoplasia, severe combined immunodeficiency and Wiskott-Aldrich syndrome (23, 26 and 28 cases, respectively) and about twice as many as these three were reported with ataxia telangiectasia (46 cases). As far as neutrophil dysfunction is concerned, 40 cases with chronic granulomatous disease and 11 cases with Chediak-Higashi disease were included.

However, this initial questionnaire could not identify each case, so duplication of the reported cases is inevitable. So the second questionnarie was designed to be capable of identifying each case and surveying the prognosis of it. It was also planned to check the complication of malignancies, collagen and autoimmune diseases, allergic diseases and some other related diseases in the patients themselves and their family members. The second questionnaire was mailed to every doctor who reported cases in the initial survey.

Until August 15, 1976, 352 cases (54.9 % of the initially reported numbers) have been again registered with full information.

Tentatively we classified the immunodeficiency diseases as: T cell deficiency group, B cell deficiency group, T and B cell deficiency group, neutrophil dysfunction group, and others.

Tables 2–6 show the total numbers of the cases in the second survey. Table respectively). Almost the same number of cases were reported with thymic 2 shows the T cell deficiency group. Eight boys and three girls were registered with thymic hypoplasia. Among them only three cases (27.3%) were reported alive at the time of registration.

TABLE 2. The total number of registered cases with primary immunodeficiencies
T Cell Deficiency

	Male	Female	Total
Thymic hypoplasia	8	3	11
Chronic mucocutaneous candidiasis	3	4	7
Total	11	7	18

The other disease of this group, chronic mucocutaneous candidaisis was rather few in number. However, most cases with this disease might be taken care of by some dermatologists, so actually many more cases might have been missed from this survey.

Table 3 shows the B cell deficiency group. 43 cases of infantile sex-linked agammaglobulinemia were collected. Although more than 90% of the patients reported that they had experienced some severe infections, most of them had been successfully controlled and 77.3% of the cases were alive at the time of registration. In the initial survey 116 individuals with transient hypogammaglobulinemia of infancy were reported, but most of them were missing from the second survey, and only 29 cases (25%) were registered. Prognosis at the time of the registration was more favorable (96.6% alive) in this disease than in the others.

As far as selective IgA deficiency was concerned 42 cases were registered here. As Dr. Kanoh has shown, this disease seems to be rather rare in Japanese

TABLE 3. The total number of registered cases with primary immunodeficiencies
B Cell Deficiency

	Male	Female	Total
X-linked agammaglobulinemia	43	0	43
Selective IgA deficiency	23	19	42
Selective Ig deficiency other than IgA	13	2	15
Immunodeficiency with normo- or hyper-gammaglobulinemia	1	1	2
Transient hypogammaglobulinemia of infancy	18	11	29
Total	98	33	131

people. But some more missing cases might not have been seen here. In Table 4 various diseases shown in this table were classified as both T and B cell deficiency group. Among them 28 individuals were registered with severe combined immunodeficiency. This disease was so severe that only two cases (7.1%) were reported surviving at the time of registration. All cases were complicated with severe infections and no adenosine deaminase deficiency was demonstrated among these 28 patients.

TABLE 4. The total number of registered cases with primary immunodeficiencies
T and B cell deficiency

	Male	Female	Total
Severe combined immunodeficiency	20	8	28
Ataxia telangiectasia	19	11	30
Wiskott-Aldrich syndrome	21	1	22
Immunodeficiency with thymoma	1	1	2
Gatti-Lux syndrome	0	1	1
Common variable immunodeficiency	32	18	50
Total	93	40	133

Other diseases of this group included 30 cases with ataxia-telangiectasia, 22 cases with Wiskott-Aldrich syndrome (mostly male but one female), 50 cases with common variable immunodeficiency, and others.

There were 34 cases with chronic granulomatous disease, mostly male, 4 cases with Chediak-Higashi disease and other unclassified neutrophil dysfunction syndrome in this registration, as shown in Table 5.

TABLE 5. The total number of registered cases with primary immunodeficiencies
Neutrophil dysfunction disease

	Male	Female	Total
Chronic granulomatous disease	27	7	34
Chediak-Higashi disease	3	1	4
Others	2	1	3
Total	32	9	41

Figure 1 shows the approximate geographical distribution of all the registered cases. More exactly this figure shows how many patients were registered from which part of our country. The numbers in the parentheses mean the approximate population of each part (shown in ten thousand surveyed in 1973. It seems that there are no significant deviations in the geographical distributions of immunodeficiency patients throughout Japan.

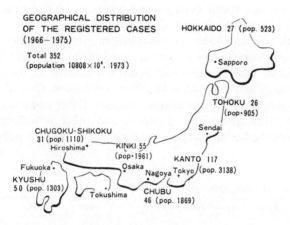

GEOGRAPHICAL DISTRIBUTION
OF THE REGISTERED CASES   HOKKAIDO 27 (pop. 523)
(1966—1975)

Total 352
(population 10808×10⁴. 1973)   •Sapporo

TOHOKU 26
(pop•905)

CHUGOKU-SHIKOKU   Sendai
31 (pop. 1110)
Hiroshima•   KINKI 55
(pop•1961)   KANTO 117
Fukuoka•.   Osaka
Nagoya Tokyo/(pop. 3138)
KYUSHU
50 (pop. 1303)
Tokushima   CHUBU
46 (pop. 1869)

FIG. 1   Geographical distribution of the registered cases (1966—1975)

Table 6 and the tables following show the complicated diseases observed in these immunodeficient patients. Table 6 shows an overview of the data obtained. Among all 352 cases 8 reported that they had developed some kind of malignancies by the time of registration. Kersey and coworkers reported that the overall incidence of malignancy in primary immunodeficiency syndromes was approximately 7 %, with a range from 2 % in severe combined immunodeficiency to 10 % in ataxia telangiectasia. Our incidence of 8 in 352 (2.3 %) seems somewhat lower than their results.

TABLE 6.   Complicated diseases observed in immunodeficiency patients

	Number of Cases	Malignancy	Collagen and auto-immune diseases	Allergic diseases	Other diseases
T-deficiency	18	0	0	2(11.1)	2(11.1)
B-deficiency	131	3(2.3)	16(12.2)	35(26.7)	19(14.5)
T & B deficiency	133	3(2.3)	12(9.0)	21(15.8)	13(9.8)
Neutrophil dysfunction	41	1(2.4)	1(2.4)	4(9.8)	2 (4.9)
Others	29	1(3.4)	3(10.3)	4(13.8)	4(13.8)
Total	352	8(2.3)	32(9.1)	66(18.8)	40(11.4)

It is uncertain whether this difference means there exists some racial difference or whether it is only due to the scale of the survey or a difference in survival period long enough to permit development of some malignancies.

The next column shows collagen and autoimmune diseases. 9.1 % of our overall cases reported some kind of this complication.

The fourth column shows complications of allergic diseases. Of interest is that B cell deficiencies seem to have a significantly high incidence of allergic diseases. Among them, 9 cases with bronchial asthma, 21 with eczema, three with drug allergy and one with milk allergy were listed. Overall 18.8 % of our cases were recognized to have allergic diseases. Other complications included cardiac anomalies, neurologic disorders and other miscellaneous diseases. Table 7 shows the list of malignancies observed in patients with immunodeficiency.

TABLE 7.   List of malignancy observed in patients with immunodeficiency

Code No	Type of immunodeficiency	Age	Sex	Type of malignancy
1. 208	Selective IgA deficiency	3Y	M	Hodgkin's disease
2. 156	Dysgammaglobulinemia Type 1	1Y	M	Brain tumor
3. 157	Dysgammaglobulinemia Type 1	7Y	M	Brain tumor
4. 240	Wiskott-Aldrich syndrome		M	Malignant lymphoma
5. 28	Wiskott-Aldrich syndrome	3M	M	Acute leukemia
6. 234	Common variable immunodeficiency	59Y	F	Gastric cancer
7. 23	Chediak-Higashi disease	1Y	M	Malignant lymphoma
8. 115	Congenital rubella syndrome	2M	F	Hepatoma

A patient with Wiskott-Aldrich syndrome, Chediak-Higashi disease and selective IgA deficiency developed malignant lymphoma and a couple of sibling cases with dysgammaglobulinemia suffered from brain tumor. Another case with Wiskott-Aldrich syndrome died of acute leukemia.

As far as collagen and autoimmune diseases are concerned, Table 8 shows the list of such diseases. Outstanding are 7 cases reported with rheumatoid arthritis in B cell deficiency, mostly in cases of X-linked agammaglobulinemia. Table 9 shows allergic diseases observed in patients with immunodeficiency.

Now we would like to turn to analyse the familial history of these immunodeficient patients. Table 10 reveals the pattern of the reported specific disease in the siblings of cases with immunodeficiency. The first column shows the number of the patients, the second column shows the reported number of siblings of the patients and the other columns show how many individuals among these siblings reported to be suffering from each specific disease.

TABLE 8. List of collagen disease and autoimmune disease observed in patients with immunodeficiency

T-deficiency: No case
B-deficiency: SLE 2. RA 7, Ulcerative colitis 2, Behcet 2, others 3
T & B-deficiency: Ulcerative colitis 1, RA 1,ITP 1, Hemolytic Anemia 1, pure red
                   cell anemia 2, aortitis 1, RF 1, nephrosis 1, others 3
Neutrophil dysfunction: Others 1
Others: Hashimoto's thyroiditis 1, glomerulonephritis 1, others 1

TABLE 9. List of Allergic diseases observed in patients with immunodeficiency

	Asthma bronchiale	Eczema	Drug allergy	Milk allergy	Others
T-deficiency	0	2	0	0	0
B-deficiency	9	21	3	1	2
T & B-deficiency	5	13	0	2	3
Neutrophil dysfunction	0	3	1	0	0
Others	2	2	0	0	0
Total	16	41	4	3	5

TABLE 10. Pattern of reported specific diseases in the siblings of cases with immunodeficiency

	Number of Cases	Number of Siblings	Immunodeficiency	Malignancy	Collagen and autoimmune diseases	Allergic diseases	Others
T-deficiency	18	18	0	0	0	0	0
B-deficiency	131	179	18(10.1%)	0	2(1.1%)	1(0.6%)	0
T & B deficiency	133	186	29(15.6%)	1(0.5%)	0	0	6(3.2%)
Neutrophil dysfunction	41	48	10(20.8%)	2(4.2%)	0	0	0
Others	29	37	4(10.8%)	0	0	0	5(13.5%)
Total	352	468	61(13.0%)	3(0.6%)	2(0.4%)	1(0.2%)	11(2.4%)

Overall, 61 individuals among 468 siblings (13.0 %) reported that they also had immunodeficiency diseases. Among them were included six pairs of X-linked agammaglobulinemia and ataxia telangiectasia, three pairs of Wiskott-Aldrich syndrome, common variable immunodeficiency and chronic granulomatous disease. Such diseases as malignancies, collagen and autoimmune diseases and allergic diseases did not seem significantly more frequent among these siblings of immunodeficiency patients. The following few tables show these specific diseases reported among family members other than siblings of the patients with immunodeficiencies. Table 11 shows reported immunodeficiency in the

TABLE 11.   Reported immunodeficiency in family (except siblings) of patients with immunodeficiency

	Number of registered cases	Total number of case	Total number of reported family members		Paternal side	Paternal family members		Maternal side	Maternal family members
T-deficiency	18	0	142		0	73		0	69
B-deficiency	131	9	1004	(0.9%)	2	501	(0.4%)	7	503(1.4%)
T & B-deficiency	133	15	875	(1.7%)	4	408	(1.0%)	11	467(2.4%)
Neutrophil dysfunction	41	8	409	(2.0%)	2	201	(1.0%)	6	208(2.9%)
Others	29	1	191	(0.5%)	1	90	(1.1%)	0	101
Total	352	33	2621	(1.3%)	9	1273(0.7%)		24	1348(1.8%)

family. The reported total number of family members was calculated and each case was listed up in two fashions according to whether he or she was a paternal or maternal relative. Overall 1.3 % of the family members reported some kind of immunodeficiency disease. Of interest is the fact that the maternal cases seem significantly more frequent than the paternal ones throughout all groups of immunodeficiency. A similar comparison was performed on malignancies seen in paternal and maternal relatives. Table 12 shows this data and a total of 2.2 % of these relatives were reported to have developed some malignancies. There were no significant differences in this incidence between paternal and maternal sides, and no difference was seen among some different immunodefi-

TABLE 12.   Reported malignancy in the family members (except siblings) of the patients with immunodeficiency

	Number of registered cases	Total number of cases	Total number of family members		Paternal side	Paternal family members		Maternal side	Maternal family members	
T-deficiency	18	1	142	(0.7%)	0	73		1	69	(1.4%)
B-deficiency	131	23	1004	(2.3%)	11	501	(2.2%)	12	503	(2.4%)
T & B-deficiency	133	26	875	(3.0%)	11	408	(2.7%)	15	467	(3.2%)
Neutrophil dysfunction	41	6	409	(1.5%)	4	201	(2.0%)	2	208	(1.0%)
Others	29	2	191	(1.0%)	1	90	(1.1%)	1	101	(1.0%)
Total	352	58	2621	(2.2%)	27	1273	(2.1%)	31	1348	(2.3%)

ciency diseases. Only 8 cases were seen to have collagen and autoimmune diseases among 2621 family members and this number was not enough for statistical analysis (Table 13). However Table 14 shows another interesting suggestion. This shows the reported allergic diseases such as bronchial asthma and eczema in the relatives of patients with immunodeficiency diseases. Among 2621 individuals, 33 (1.3 %) were reported as having some allergic diseases. Of outstanding interest is that in the families of patients with T deficiency a significantly high incidence of allergic diseases was revealed, especially in the maternal relatives.

Although no immunological evaluation on every individual had been

TABLE 13. Reported collagen diseases and autoimmune diseases in the family members (except siblings) of patients with immunodeficiency

	Number of registered cases	Total number of cases	Total number of reported family members		Paternal side	Paternal family members		Maternal side	Maternal family members	
T-deficiency	18	0	142		0	73		0	69	
B-deficiency	131	6	1004	(0.6%)	5	501	(1.0%)	1	503	(0.2%)
T & B-deficiency	133	1	895	(0.1%)	1	408	(0.2%)	0	467	
Neutrophil dysfunction	41	1	409	(0.5%)	0	201		1	208	(0.4%)
Others	29	0	191		0	90		0	101	
Total	352	8	2621	(0.3%)	6	1273	(0.5%)	2	1348	(0.1%)

TABLE 14. Reported allergic diseases in the family members (except siblings) of patients with immunodeficiency

	Number of registered cases	Total number of cases	Total number of reported family members		Paternal side	Paternal family members		Maternal side	Maternal family members	
T-deficiency	18	13	142	(9.2%)	1	73	(1.4%)	12	69	(17.4%)
B-deficiency	131	11	1004	(1.1%)	4	501	(0.8%)	7	503	(1.4%)
T & B-deficiency	133	5	875	(0.6%)	2	408	(0.5%)	3	467	(0.6%)
Neutrophil dysfunction	41	3	409	(0.7%)	1	201	(0.5%)	2	208	(1.0%)
Others	29	1	191	(0.5%)	0	90		1	101	(1.0%)
Total	352	33	2621	(1.3%)	8	1273	(0.6%)	25	1348	(1.9%)

280 H. Hayakawa *et al.*

performed, some kind of T cell deficiency, such as deficient suppressor T cell function, might be hypothesized in these cases and further evaluation should be performed on these people from this point of view.

Although our study has not been perfectly completed this kind of survey seems to give us many exciting suggestions for further studies on primary immunodeficiency and many other Nanbyo, or intractable chronic diseases including malignancies and collagen and autoimmune diseases. We would like to continue this registration to collect greater amounts and more exact information on this disease in our country. Racial difference in incidence of these diseases is another interesting subject, but to date too little knowledge has been obtained on a global scale.

DISCUSSION

Dr. SELIGMANN: I would have two questions because there were two things which were astonishing to me in your tables.

The first, of course, is the fact that you have a very small percentage of so-called variable immunodeficiency, which is what we could call the wastebasket, but which represents, obviously for us in Europe, and I would say probably also in the States, almost the majority of patients with true primary immunodeficiency. And I would have two specific questions about this. The first is, it is a possibility that although you try to have both the pediatrics cases and adult cases, you mainly had the pediatricians' answers to your questionnaire, because I saw there were many cases in children and infants, and if this is the case, that you had few adults coming into your register, it could explain the low incidence of variable which is shown much higher in adults than in children, so this would be a question.

Another question about this is, you found a high incidence of infantile X-linked, since it was 11 per cent and you include in your cases all complement deficiencies, neutrophil deficiencies and so on, so do all the cases which are labelled as infantile X-linked have a documented family history proving that there is really an X-linked transmission?

For my second question, that was my first question I extended, my second question is very short. I found extremely interesting the striking, high percentage of transient hypogammaglobulinemia which was 19 per cent and I would like to ask you the definition you have of transient hypogammaglobulinemia in infancy to put the cases into the register, and then perhaps John Soothill will come in to parse the difference between normal and abnormal.

Dr. HAYAKAWA: Yes. That is one of the biggest problem for us. As for your first question, your suggestion is a very important one and I think we should try to rearrange the cases into childhood cases and adult cases. This time we did not make such a classification and as I stated, this survey depends on the questionnaire method, so it is impossible to clarify the diagnosis so precisely, in other words, to confirm the definitive diagnosis. So it completely depends on how the reporting doctor diagnosed the patient. So we are going to the third project to clarify what you pointed out and this is the next problem for us, I think.

Dr. KOBAYASHI: I just would like to stress that this is a collaborated work all over Japan with pediatricians and some internists as well, whom we can trust their diagnosis. This is not our personal work, but our project team's work, involving more than a hundred doctors registering the cases at our registration center. This is not a population-based study, but a physician-based one. But we are very lucky because we get such good cooperation.

And the second point, a comparison with the incidence of leukemia and lymphoma, the all-Japan children's cancer registration, of which I am now also taking charge, has collected about 500 cases of leukemia and lymphoma for each year. This is only childhood cases up to 15 years old, so this makes one fourth of all the population. It is estimated that our children's cancer survey covers approximately 50 or 60 per cent of all cancer appearing in children. On the basis of this registration, it is calculated that the incidence of childhood leukemia is one out of 10,000 children. This incidence is similar to that of primary immunodeficiency in Japan. Coverage of immunodeficiency must be rather good, since immunodeficiency is a very complicated disease and so we expect these patients are being cared for in the hospitals which we send questionnaires to. I believe, at least for immunodeficiency, we collected more than 70 or 80 per cent of those cases.

But as you mentioned, diagnostic problems was present in earlier days, because of the general standard of diagnose was low and the knowledge was scanty. However at least for the last five years the diagnostic level has improved in Japan. When we started to organize this project team with a grant from the government, the diagnostic criteria were established and the booklets of criteria were distributed to the physicians all-over Japan. I believe this kind of study is very important and we would like to continue to do it in a more meaningful way, and for your comments we are very grateful and we will consider them in future study. Thank you.

Dr. HITZIG: I think it is only a beginning, because all retrospective studies are very unreliable. But the system which has been set up seems to me so wonderful and so promising that you must go on and continue this and then in one or two years you will come out with reliable figures which will certainly be important for the whole world.

IV. NATURE AND EFFECTIVENESS OF THE TREATMENTS FOR IMMUNODEFICIENCY

Therapy of Immunodeficiency Syndromes

Walter H. Hitzig

The therapeutic approaches to diseases are subject to changes and modifications, so much so that most of the treatments taught in medical school are obsolete if not forgotten within a few decades. This regrettable fact accounts for the reluctance of scientifically oriented doctors to risk their reputations with papers on therapy. On the other hand, for the patient, the therapeutic possibilities are of primary importance and usually the only interesting part of his illness. I shall restrict myself to a brief review of the therapeutic possibilities and approaches to immunodeficiency syndrome (IDS) tried in the last 25 years.[1]

A. CAUSAL THERAPY

Application of the rule "find the cause and eliminate it" has been possible in few instances of IDS, e.g. genetic counselling in hereditary cases and withdrawal of the drug in hydantoin-induced IgA deficiency. Genetic counselling in the hereditary forms of IDS, under favourable circumstances, can lead to suppression of the abnormal gene. The IgA deficiency due to the anti-epileptic drug hydantoin is reversible and expresses an innate predisposition to the disease. While this is the only known example of drug-induced IDS, it makes further investigations along similar lines worthwhile.

B. CONVENTIONAL (SUPPORTIVE) THERAPY

The introduction and widespread use of sulfonamides and antibiotics first prolonged the life of patients with the severe forms of IDS long enough to make investigation of the underlying defect possible. These agents are still indis-

Department of Pediatrics, University of Zürich, Switzerland

pensable in the management of IDS. In chronic granulomatous disease of childhood (CGD) it is claimed that the killing defect of the granulocytes of the patient can be favourably influenced by sulfonamides, Bactrim (Septrim) being widely used. If true, the sulfonamides in this instance would be a specific and not a conventional supportive antibacterial therapeutic agent.

Opportunistic infections are of great importance in all IDS with cell mediat ed immune deficiency (CMI-D), and can be due to bacterial, viral, fungal, and parasitic agents. Above all, I would like to mention pneumocystis carinii, a widely distributed and usually innocuous saprophyte which, however, in a high proportion of patients with CMI deficiency causes a fatal pneumonia. Pentamidine, the specific agent against pneumocystis carinii, is so dependable that several transplant teams use it prophylactically before bone marrow transplantation.

Antiviral agents for human use with few undesirable side effects are now available and have changed the usually resigned attitude toward the treatment of viral infections in IDS patients with CMI. These patients, on the other hand, are ideal subjects on which to test the efficacy of these new antiviral agents.

C. SPECIFIC THERAPY

Under this heading are included procedures used to repair the specific immune deficiency or its underlying cause and attempts to replace well-defined missing factors.

I. Replacement therapy
1. Replacement of antibodies
1.1. Gammaglobulin therapy,[1,2,3,4,5] first used in 1952 independently by Bruton, Janeway and Good, has withstood the test of time and together with supportive therapy has made active and pleasant lives possible for an increasing number of boys with congenital agammaglobulinemia. The drawbacks of gammaglobulin therapy are well known, notably the large volumes required (expensive and painful) and the shocklike reactions that sometimes occur, usually in patients who are completely agammaglobulinemic and therefore in greatest need of this therapy. The main cause of this reaction is the rapid intravenous activation of complement by immunoglobulin aggregates.[2] Tendency to aggregation is inherent in immunoglobulin molecules and is enhanced by concentration of the solution. Worldwide efforts to produce gammaglobulin preparations completely safe for intravenous administration (*i.e.*, with little or no aggregates) have not been entirely successful.[2,3,5,6,7,8]

Replacement of specific antibodies in "antibody deficiency syndromes" has been proposed and attempted but up to now the preparations used contain a spectrum of antibodies as prevails in the blood donor population.
1.2. Single class immunoglobulin replacement has been recommended, *e.g.* in IgA deficiency patients.[9] However, general considerations and clinical experiences show contraindications to its use. In many diseases due to the absence of a specific protein or enzyme, the injection of the missing protein ("cross-reacting material") provokes antibody production, presumably because the patient did not develop tolerance against it during his embryonal life. This jeopardizes the future management of the patient as subsequent injection of the protein may be dangerous because of possible anaphylactic shock, or be ineffective because the protein is rapidly inactivated by the previously formed antibodies. Because of this and because intravenous IgA is not excreted on the mucosal surfaces, IgA-free gammaglobulin preparations have even been requested by those treating IgA deficient patients. Preparation is possible by removal of IgA during the process or by using plasma from IgA deficient patients as starting material.
1.3. Whole untreated *plasma* instead of concentrated gammaglobulin has been recommended in order to avoid the previously mentioned shock-like reactions. The danger of transmission of hepatitis can be avoided by close supervision of donors or by using the "buddy" system, *i.e.*, by assigning each patient his own personal donor, preferably one of his relatives.
2. Replacement of cellular factors
   In IDS with cellular immunodeficiency it seemed logical to replace the missing immunocompetent cells. Cell infusions or simple blood transfusions were first tried, not surprisingly (in the light of present knowledge) with disastrous results: fatal graft versus host reactions (GvHR) following a single whole blood transfusion are well documented. Complete histocompatibility minimizes but does not remove the danger of GvHR. Nevertheless, this form of therapy is still used when a transient cellular replacement is desirable as in some lepra cases.
   During cellular immune reactions a number of mediator substances are produced. Purified and concentrated preparations of these mediators have been used therapeutically. A voluminous but controversial literature has accumulated for transfer factor.[10] Interferon seems to be useful in certain viral infections but is available only in a few centers. Thymic factors and extracts prepared by various methods have been used by many authors for T cell deficiencies.

II. "Cellular engineering"
   This term includes the various procedures used to influence permanently,

and hopefully with one single therapeutic action, the composition or function of a specific cell population or compartment. The first attempts with endocrine glands, almost a century ago, at first sight sensationally successful, turned out to be due to the hormone content of the transplanted organs. Modern approaches however intend true permanent organ grafting.

1 Transplantation of immunocompetent organs

This transplantation was tried as soon as their interdependence became known and a hypothesis of their functions was elucidated. Success of such treatments is usually considered to confirm the hypothesis, but one should also keep alternative explanations in mind. Historically, the grossly pathological thymus found in severe combined immunodeficiency (SCID) led to transplantation of thymus tissue, fetal thymus being preferred to circumvent possible GvHR. As these early attempts were not successful, fetal liver tissue, as a source of stem cells was transplanted together with fetal thymus.[11]

The questionable results of this combined therapy were overshadowed by the complete immunological reconstitution achieved with allogeneic bone marrow transplantation by the Minneapolis group. Since then, bone marrow has been transplanted in a large number of cases, and more than 35 children so treated are alive with normally functioning immune systems and normal development.

A strict requirement for the success of bone marrow transplantation is histocompatibility. Since the majority of SCID patients do not have HLA compatible donors, fetal liver and other sources of immunocompetent cells or their precursors are again being tried. Fetal liver transplantation has been successful lately in a few SCID patients.

2. *Correction of metabolic defects*

In rare cases of IDS a specific metabolic defect has been demonstrated. Up to now our case of transcobalamin II deficiency is unique, in which the lack of the vitamin B 12 transport protein led to hematological, gastrointestinal and immunological abnormalities. These were corrected by the simple administration of vitamin B 12 (1 mg/day, peroral or parenteral).

More frequent is adenosine deaminase (ADA) deficiency and SCID. In this condition stem cells are probably normal, but their function is progressively impaired by faulty metabolic pathways. Some of these patients were completely reconstituted by bone marrow transplants, 2 cases transiently by fetal liver transplantation and one child for a few weeks by blood transfusion.[13] As more similar metabolic defects in IDS are discovered, the therapeutic possibilities will increase.

III. Checking of inhibitors

An increasing number of cases of IDS have been shown to be due to circulating substances (autoantibodies or suppressor cells inhibiting a normal immune system). This discovery has opened up new therapeutic approaches. One patient with agammaglobulinemia due to an autoantibody was greatly improved by hydrocortisone. In those cases with suppressor cells, cytotoxic drug therapy might be used in the future.

TREATMENT OF IDS

A. Causal therapy
B. Conventional therapy:
   anti-infectious agents
   sulfonamides
   antibiotics
   antiviral, antifungal, antiparasitic agents
C. Specific therapy:
   I. Replacement of missing substance
      1. Antibodies in humoral immune deficiency (AMI)
         1.1. gammaglobulin
         1.2. IgA/M
         1.3. plasma
      2. Cellular factors in cellular deficiency (CMI)
         2.1. infusion of cells
         2.2. injection of mediator substances, transfer factor, Interferon, thymic factors, levamisol?
   II. "Cellular engineering"
      1. Transplantation of immunocompetent organs
         1.1. fetal thymus and liver
         1.2. adult bone marrow
         1.3. others
      2. Correction of metabolic defect
         2.1. transcobalamin II deficiency by vitamin B 12
         2.2. adenosine deaminase by blood transfusion
   III. Checking of inhibitors
      1. AMI: auto-antibodies
      2. CMI: immunosuppression?

REFERENCES

1. Hitzig, W. H.: Therapy of Immunological Deficieny Diseases, *In*: Immunologic Incompetence (B. M., Kagan and E. R. Stiehm, eds.), p. 203, Year Book Medical Publishers. Chicago, 1971.
2. Barandun, S., Skvaril, F., and Morell, A.: Prophylaxe und Therapie mit Gammaglobulin. I. Teil: Allgemeine Charakterisierung und klinische Anwendung

von Gamma-globulin-präparaten. II. Teil: klinische anwendung von gamma-globulin-präparaten. *Schweiz. Med. Wschr.* **106**:533–542 und 580–587, 1976.

3. Hitzig, W. H. and Müntener, U.: Conventional immunoglobulin therapy. *Birth Defects: Orig. Article Series* **11**:339–342, 1975.

4. Schwick, H. G., Fischer, J., and Geiger, H.: Human IgA- and IgM- globulins for clinical use. *Progr. Immunobiol. Standard* **4**:86–91, 1970

5. The Use of Human Immunoglobulin. Report of a WHO Expert Committee. *Wld. Hlth. Org. Techn. Rep. Ser.* **327**:1–29 1966.

6. Janeway, Ch. A., Merler, E., Rosen, F. S., Salmon, S., and Crain, J. D.: Intravenous gamma globulin. Metabolism of gamma globulin fragments in normal and agammaglobulinemic persons. *New Eng. J. Med.* **278**:919–923, 1968.

7. Steinbuch, M.: Notes on the production of plasma derivatives in France. *Vox Sang.* **23**:56–57 1972.

8. Stephan, W.: Hepatitis-free and stable human serum for intravenous therapy. *Vox Sang.* **20**:442–457, 1971.

9. Schwick, H. G.: A survey of the production of plasma derivatives for clinical use. *Vox Sang.* **23**:82–91 (1972.

10. Hitzig, W. H. and Grob, P.: Transfer factor. *Progr. Clin. Immunol.* **2**:69–100 1974.

11. Hitzig, W. H., Kay, H. E. M., and Cottier, H.: Familial lymphopenia with agammaglobulinaemia. An attempt at treatment by implantation of foetal thymus. *Lancet* **II**:151, 1965.

12. Hong R., Kay, H. E. M., Cooper, M. D., Meuwissen, H., Allan, M. J. G., and Good, R. A.: Immunological restitution in lymphopenic immunological deficiency syndrome. *Lancet* **I**:503–506, 1968.

13. Polmar, S.H., Stern, R.C., Schwartz, A.L., Wetzler, E.M., Chase, P.A., Hirschborn R.: Enzyme replacement therapy for adenosine deaminase deficiency and severe combined immunodeficiency. *N. Engl. J. Med.* **295**, 1337–1343, 1976.

Characteristics of S-Sulfonated Gammaglobulin and Its Restored Form

K. Tomibe,* Y. Masuho,* T. Watanabe,* Y. Fukumoto,* A. Ohtsu,*
E. Yamagami,* N. Ohtomo,** and A. Tashiro**

ABSTRACT

GGS (human S-sulfonated gammaglobulin) prepared by treating GG (human gammaglobulin) with sulfite and tetrathionate, showed a reduced ability to bind with complement, but retained sufficient antibody activities. The conversion of the S-sulfonated group in GGS to disulfide bond occurred in rabbits judging from the fact that the original molecular weight of GG was observed in SDS disc electrophoresis and from the restoration of hemolytic activity. The participation of the Fc portion (Fc fragment of gammaglobulin) of GGS *in vivo* might be advantageous in intravenous clinical use.

INTRODUCTION

Intravenous administration of gammaglobulin is desirable for achieving a rapid increase in the antibody level, but the ideal preparation has yet to appear. The commercialized preparations have partly eliminated the Fc portion in order to avoid anaphylactic reactions.[1] Another preparation is suspected of inducing a new antigenicity.[2] However, the Fc portion plays an important role in binding with macrophages and in initiating phagocytosis.[3,4]

GGS in which the original interchain disulfide bonds were converted to S-sulfonated group, has a reduced ability with complement. Conversion of the S-sulfonated group of a peptide to a disulfide bond has been reported *in vitro*.[5] S-sulfonation of gammaglobulin has been developed by Franek *et al.*,[6] but some more experiments are required before it can be applied to human gammaglobulin for intravenous use. We reported[7] that the conversion of this group in GGS was observed *in vivo*. This experimental conclusion was supported not only by change of molecular weight,[8] but by the restoration

---

* Teijin Institute for Biomedical Research, Tokyo, Japan
** The Chemo-Sero-Therapeutic Institute, Kumamoto, Japan

291

of Fc activity as assayed by passive hemolysis of anti-tetanus GGS, which was done by using tetanus toxoid coated SRBC and complement in rabbits.

The scheme for the interconversion of S-sulfonated groups and a disulfide bond is as follows:

$$R\text{-}S\text{-}S\text{-}R' \xrightarrow{\ SO_3 \ , \ S_4O_6\ } R\text{-}S\text{-}SO_3^- + {}^-O_3S\text{-}S\text{-}R'$$

$$R\text{-}SH + HS\text{-}R'$$

[O]   [H]

GGS was preapred by treating GG with sodium sulfite and sodium tetra-thionate. The interchain disulfide bonds were selectively cleaved to the S-sulfonated group. The anticomplementary activity of GGS was about 10%. This is one of the most important properties in intravenous administration of gammaglobulin derivatives, because high anticomplementary activity of GG has been considered the main cause of anaphylactic reactions in intravenous administration of GG. After administration, the disulfide bonds were gradually formed from S-sulfonated groups of GGS *in vivo* in 24 hours. Then the normal Fc activity of the injected GGS was restored, just like that of GG. The half-life of GGS was as long as GG.

EXPERIMENTAL PROCEDURE

GG was prepared from human plasma collected from more than 500 donors according to Nitsman's method.[9]

GGS was generally prepared by the following standard method. GG (final volume 7.5%) was treated with sodium sulfite (final volume 162 mM) and sodium tetrathionate (final volume 41 mM) in PBS (phosphate buffered saline) for 4.5 hours at 45°C. Then the mixture was dialyzed against saline. For our labeled experiment, ^{35}S-labeled sodium sulfite with an initial specific activity of 3 mCi/mole was purchased from the Radiochemical Center in England.

Assay of anticomplementary activity. 0.5 ml of diluted guinea pig serum containing 50 CH_{50}, 0.5 ml of 5% gammaglobulin derivative solution and 1.5 ml of gelatin-veronal buffer (added Ca^{++}, Mg^{++}) were mixed. After incubation for 60 minutes at 37°C, the remaining complement activity was assayed by Mayer's method.[10] The results were expressed in percentages of the complement consumed by gammaglobulin derivatives.

RESULTS AND DISCUSSION

GGS had no covalent bonds among 4 peptide chains, but the conformation of GGS was preserved, similar to that of GG in normal circumstances as shown in Fig. 1, because of having ionic and hydrophobic bonds. The ultracentrifugal pattern of GGS was almost the same as that of GG in 0.15 M NaCl. The sedimentation constant of the main peak was 7S. In Sephadex G-200 column chromatography with PBS the flow pattern of GGS was also similar to that of GG.

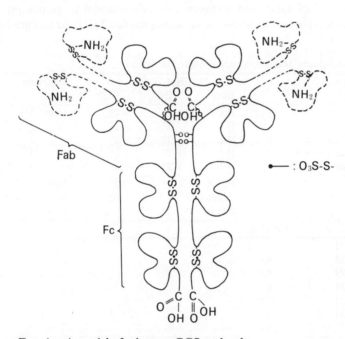

FIG. 1.   A model of a human GGS molecule

However, in the presence of perturbator GGS was separated to 4 single chains, but GG was not. In Sephadex G-200 column chromatography with 6 M urea and 1 N propionic acid the labeled GGS, which was prepared by treating GG with $Na_2{}^{35}SO_3$ and $Na_2S_4O_6$, mainly dissociated to H and L chains, in which the average numbers of incorporated labeled sulfite groups were 3.1 and 0.9, respectively. These results agreed well with those of reduction alkylation of GG.[11] IgG 1, the population of which is more than 70 % in human immunoglobulin, has 1 interchain disulfide bond per one L chain and 3 interchain disulfide bonds per one H chain. These facts supported the assumption that selective cleavage was introduced only at the interchain disulfide bonds in our treatment for S-sulfonation.

Antibody and anticomplement activities. Though the anticomplement activity of GGS almost dropped below 10%, antibody titers against toxins and viruses were selectively preserved as shown in Table 1. But the PHA titer of GGS against HBs decreased to a quarter of that of GG (See Fig. 5.). This decrease was recovered *in vivo* when GGS was restored to GG.

Serum complement level after intravenous administration of GGS to guinea pig. When 2 ml of GGS was intravenously administered to guinea pig, the complement level in the blood decreased within the first half hour and gradually

TABLE 1.   Antibody and anticomplementary activities

Antibody against		Antibody value		Comment
	assay	GG	GGS	
rubeola	H.I.	2^5	2^5	conc 3%
rubella	H.I.	2^7	2^7	3
mumps	H.I.	2^3	2^3	3
para influenza 1 (HVJ)	H.I.	2^6	2^4	3
para influenza 3 (HA-1)	H.I.	2^9	2^9	3
diphtheria	P.H.A.	2^9	2^9	0.04%
diphtheria	rabbit skin	1.1	0.9	NIH unit (10%)
tetanus	P.H.A.	2^4	2^3	conc 5%

Lot No.		$C[CH_{50}]$
XAO	231	0. %
	232	8.4
	233	8.0
	234	6.2
YKO	233	12.8
	234	3.4
	235	6.3

Anticomplementary activity

$$C(\%) = \frac{B - A}{B} \times 100$$

(A) Complement titer $\begin{cases} \text{guinea pig serum containing } 100CH_{50} & 1.0\text{ml} \\ 5\% \text{ GGS} & 1.0\text{ml} \\ \text{gelatin-veronal buffer pH7.4} & 3.0\text{ml} \\ \text{after 60 mins at } 37°C \end{cases}$

(B) Complement titer $\begin{cases} \text{guinea pig serum containing } 100CH_{50} & 1.0\text{ml} \\ \text{gelatin-veronal buffer pH7.4} & 4.0\text{ml} \\ \text{after 60 mins at } 37°C \end{cases}$

regained its previous level in 24 hours. The degree of this decrease occurring with GGS was almost same as that with albumin and much smaller than that with GG (See Fig. 2.). Furthermore, GGS was intravenously administered to five healthy adults, three times in doses of 500 mg, 1,000 mg and 1,000 mg, respectively. The complement levels were assayed by Mayer's method. No considerable decrease (less than 10%) of the complement level was observed after administration.

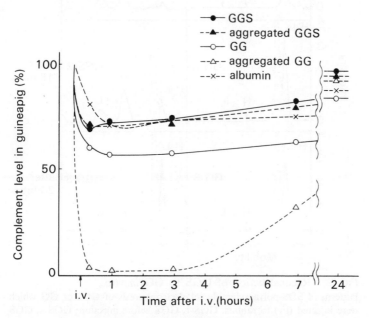

FIG. 2.   The complement level in guinea pigs after the injection of GGS or GG.
The complement titers before the injection were $120 \sim 220 \; CH_{50}/ml$ serum.
Aggregated condition was 63°C—10mins. Mean values of 3 guinea pigs.

Antigenicity. Antigenicity was examined in the homologous system using monkeys and rabbits. The PHA method was adopted in this experiment for detecting antibody against GGS. And it was proven that GGS did not elicit any modified immunogenicity.

Restoration of GGS to GG. GGS, which was treated with dithiothreitol and subsequently air-oxidized by dialysis with air-bubbled solution *in vitro*, showed the same SDS pattern as GG. The reconstructed GG regained the binding activity with complement and RPCA activity[12] to the level of GG. Figure 3

296   K. Tomibe *et al.*

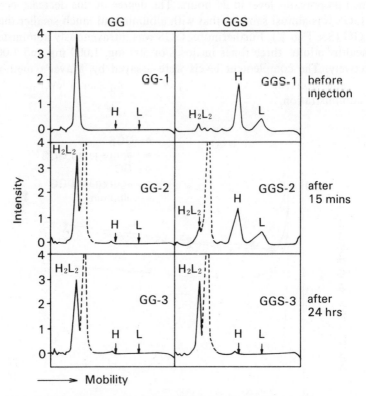

FIG. 3. Reconstruction of GGS to GG *in vivo*.
Patterns of SDS-polyacrylamide gel electrophoresis of GGS or GG which
were injected (i.v) to rabbits. GGS-1, GGS before injection; GGS-2, GGS
after 15 min; GGS-3, GGS after 24 hr. GG was injected to rabbits as the
control GG-1, GG-2, GG-3.
A broken line indicates a peak of rabbit IgG anti [human F(ab')₂].

shows the restoration of GGS to GG *in vivo*. These are the patterns of SDS
disc electrophoresis which were scanned with a chromatoscanner. In the
presence of SDS as a perturbator, GGS gave the pattern mainly separated to
H and L chains. GGS or GG was intravenously administered to rabbits,
and they were bled at 15 minutes and at 24 hours after the injection. In Fig.
3, the broken lines indicate a peak of rabbit IgG anti-human F(ab')₂ which
was added to recover the human gammaglobulin derivatives from rabbit sera.
In the 15 minutes' sample of GGS, there were large peaks at H and L. But
in the 24 hours' sample only H₂L₂ band was observed and almost nothing was

recognized at the position of H and L. As demonstrated, the S-sulfonated groups of GGS were electrophoretically restored to the disulfide bonds *in vivo*.

Restoration of Fc activity in GGS. The passive hemolysis activities of GGS, GG and F(ab')$_2$ (pepsin digested F(ab')$_2$ fragment of human gammaglobulin), and anti-tetanus antibody were examined by using tetanus toxoid-coated SRBC and complement. The activities of GGS and F(ab')$_2$ were negative *in vitro*. The anti-tetanus GGS or GG was intravenously administered to rabbits. Hemolytic activity of GGS, negative *in vitro*, gradually increased *in vivo*, and reached the level of GG 24 hours after administration, as shown in Fig. 4.

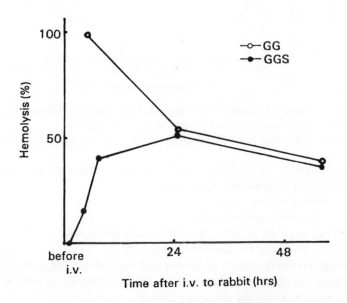

FIG. 4. Passive hemolysis of SRBC coupled with tetanus toxoid by the rabbit serum obtained after i.v. injection of human GGS or GG.

Turnover of human antibody. GGS, GG or F(ab')$_2$ anti-tetanus immunoglobulin was intravenously administered to rabbits. The turnover rate was estimated by means of passive hemagglutination. F(ab')$_2$ decreased rapidly to 1 % after 24 hours, however, GGS did so more slowly, as did GG. Further, the turnover rate was examined in the homologous system. One gram of anti-HBs GGS or GGP was intravenously administered to two healthy adults. The titers were assayed by PHA at intervals. The half-life of GGP was very short.[13] But that of GGS was more than 2 weeks (see Fig. 5).

298 K. Tomibe et al.

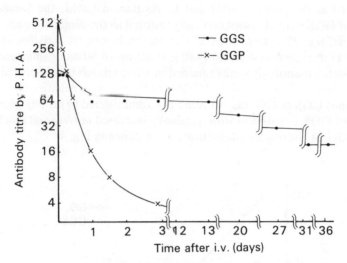

FIG. 5. One g of human antibody anti-HBs was intravenously administered to humans. The titer was assayed by P. H. A.
in vitro titer; GGS = 16,000, GGP = 128,000

As demonstrated, GGS has several interesting characteristics as a GG derivative for intravenous administration:

1. Long lasting activity *in vivo*;
2. Low anticomplementary activity;
3. Restoration of Fc activity after administration *in vivo*;
4. Freedom from any modified immunogenicity.

At present passive immunity of human immunoglobulin plays an important role in the prophylaxis and therapy of infectious diseases as well as in the treatment of immunological deficiency diseases.

We believe that the participation of the Fc portion of GGS *in vivo* might prove advantageous in intravenous clinical use.

Acknowledgements
The authors wish to thank Dr. T. Noguchi, Dr. S. Tsunoda and Mr. S. Ishimoto, of the Teijin Institute for Biomedical Research, for their helpful suggestions.

REFERENCE

1. Barandum, S., Castel, V., Makura, M.F., Morell, A., Plan, R. and Skvaril, F.:

Clinical tolerance and catabolism of plasmin-treated gammaglobulin for intravenous application. *Vox Sang.* **28**:157, 1975.
2. Stephan, W.: Undergraded human immunoglobulin for intravenous use. *Vox Sang.* **28**:422, 1975.
3. Mannik, M. and Arend, W. P.: Fate of preformed immune complexes in rabbits and rhesus monkeys. *J. Exptl. Med.* **134**:19s, 1971.
4. Reynolds, H. Y. and Thompson, R. E.: Pulmonary host defences. II. Interaction of respiratory antibodies with *Pseudomonas aeruginosa* and alveolar macrophages. *J. Immunol.* **111**:369 1973.
5. Katsoyannis, P. G., Tometsko, A., Zalut, C., Jahnson, S. and Trakattellis, A. C.: Studies on the synthesis of insulin from natural and synthetic A and B chains. *Biochemistry* **6**:2635, 1967.
6. Franek, F. and Zikan, J.: Limited cleavage of disulfide bonds of pig gammaglobulin by S-sulfonation. *Collection Czech. Chem. Commun.* **29**:1401, 1976.
7. Masuho, Y., Tomibe, K., Matsuzawa, K., Watanabe, T., Ishimoto, S., Tsunoda, S. and Noguchi, T.: Reconstruction of intact gammaglobulin from S-sulfonated gammaglobulin *in vivo. J. Biochem.* **79**:1377 1976.
8. Weber, K. and Osborn, M.: The reliability of molecular weight determination by dodecyl sulfate-polyacrylamide gel electrophoresis. *J. Biol. Chem.* **244**:4406, 1969.
9. Kistler, P. and Nitsman H.: Large scale production of human plasma fraction. *Vox Sang.* **7**:414, 1962.
10. Mayer, M. M.: Complement and complement fixation, *in*: Exp. Immunochemistry, and edition (E. A. Kabat and M. M. Mayer, eds.), C. Thomas Charles, Pub., Springfield, Ill., 1961.
11. Gall, W. E., Cunningham, B. A., Waxdal, M.J. and Edelman, G. M.: The covalent structure of a human γG-immunoglobulin IV. The interchain disulfide bonds. *Biochemistry* **7**:1973, 1968.
12. Herbert, W. J.: Passive hemagglutination with special reference to the tanned cell technique, *in*: Handbook of Exp. Immunology, and edition (D. M. Weir, ed.), Blackwell Scientific Publications, Oxford, England, 1973.
13. Koblet, H.: Turnover of standard-gammaglobulin, pH 4-gammaglobulin and pepsin digested gammaglobulin and clinical implication. *Vox Sang.* **13**:93 1967.
14. Masuho, Y., Tomibe, K., Matsuzawa, K. and Ohtsu, A.: Development of an intravenous γ-globulin with Fc activities. I. Preparation and characterization of S-sulfonated human γ-globulin. *Vox Sang* **32**: 175, 1977.
15. Masuho, Y., Tomibe, K., Watanabe, T. and Fukumoto, Y.: Development of an intravenous γ-globulin with Fc activities. II. Reconversion of S-sulfonated human γ-globulin into the original γ-globulin. *Vox Sang* **32**: 290, 1977

DISCUSSION

Dr. GOOD: Well, I just want to congratulate you, on what may be an extremely important contribution, since one of the main things we would like to do with intravenous gammaglobulin in the immunodeficiency state, or in infected patients, is to attack the encapsulated bacterial pathogenes by a process that requires complement activity. The question is, after reassembly or restoration of the immunoglobulin *in vivo*, does it then fix complement? Can it then opsonize effectively the encapsulated organisms like pneumococcus?

Dr. TOMIBE: We checked hemolysis activity.

Dr. OHTOMO: I am one of the colleagues of this group. And we have done the setup, the making of the experiment of the therapeutic effect of the GGS; comparing the GG and the GGP in mice mothers, using the pneumococcus. And we have not yet done the final analysis of the result, but so far we have the result that GGS treated the mice pneumococcal infection, as well as GG and GGP at certain times. I mean, when we add, when we treat the mice simultaneously with GG preparation and microorganisms, they cured the mice almost similarly in three instances. But when we changed the time course between the challenge and the treatment, the result appeared significantly different, but I have no exact answer to the question of Dr. Good on the presence of capsule.

Dr. HITZIG: As far as I know, clinically one of the most important features is the preservation of the Fc portion, and you have very convincingly shown that this is the case. So it should be expected that these preparations can activate complement. One word of warning. You have infused these materials to healthy persons, and have shown that there is no complement activation. However, unfortunately, in patients with agammaglobulinemia this is not necessarily so. Before you infuse it to agammaglobulinemics you should be very careful and use slow infusion starting with small amounts only and then slowly increase them. Because we have seen with another preparation which was very well tolerated by healthy people very severe reactions in an agammaglobulinemic subject.

Treatment of Immunologic Deficiency
States with Dialysable Transfer Factor

Shuzo Matsumoto,* Yukio Sakiyama,* Hideki Minami,* Takehiro Togashi,*
Hiroyoshi Itoh,** and Susumu Ohmura**

ABSTRACT

To date, transfer factor has been administered to 28 patients with a variety of immunodeficiencies and disseminated infections. A total of 108 units was used. Most patients have received multiple doses of transfer factor, ranging from 1 unit given every 3 months to 1 unit every week for 3 months.

The clinical benefits in chronic mucocutaneous candidiasis and Wiskott-Aldrich syndrome were clearly demonstrated. In the patients with those immunologic deficiency disorders, the response to TF was generally rather slow in clinical conditions and in DTH, and the duration of the effect also rather short. Therefore it appeared that repeated injections of TF in one to four (or eight in some cases) weekly intervals were required to maintain the beneficial effect of TF in those disorders.

But in primary tuberculosis, clinical improvement by TF was remarkable in combination with adequate antituberculosis chemotherapy. At the same time, DTH or LMIF to PPD were converted in less than 24 hours after injection. Doses required to obtain the beneficial effects, also, are thought to be rather small in this case (one to two units may be sufficient).

Transfer factor (TF) was originally described by Lawrence[1] in 1955. Cell free leukocyte extracts that had been taken from PPD sensitive donors were capable of transferring skin reactivity of a delayed type to recipients who had previously failed to react to PPD. Since dialysable transfer factor was first used successfully in 1970 by Levin et al.,[2] it has been administered by many doctors to patients with a number of disorders related to defects in cell-mediated immunity, such as immunodeficiency diseases, chronic progressive infectious diseases, and sometimes malignant diseases.

---

*   Department of Pediatrics, Hokkaido University School of Medicine, Sapporo, Japan
** Red Cross Hokkaido Blood Center, Sapporo, Japan

This paper presents our experiences with dialysable transfer factor administration to patients with immunodeficiency diseases and progressive infectious diseases.

I. PREPARATION AND ADMINISTRATION OF TRANSFER FACTOR

The method for preparation of leukocyte dialysates was essentially the same as Lawrence's original preparation of dialysable transfer factor (TF).[3] Briefly, the leukocytes from healthy adult donors were disrupted by 12 cycles of freezing and thawing, digested with deoxyribonuclease and then dialysed against distilled water. The dialysate was lyophilized and then reconstituted with sterile distilled water so that the extract from 10^9 cells (one unit) was contained in two ml. The final products were passed through a $0.22\,\mu$ micropore filter and tested for sterility. One unit of transfer factor corresponds to the extract of buffy coat originating from 400 ml of blood donations (Table 1).

TABLE 1.   Preparation of transfer factor

500 ml venous blood
$\downarrow$ added plasmagel for 1 hr at 37°C
sedimented
$\downarrow$
buffy coat (3–4 $\times$ 10^9/ml)
$\downarrow$
Lysed by 12 cycles of freezing and thawing
$\downarrow$ incubated with DNASE and $MgSO_4$ for 30 min at 37°C
dialyzed against distilled water for 48 hrs, at 4°C
$\downarrow$
filtrated with micropore filter
$\downarrow$
lyophilized
$\downarrow$
reconstituted with distilled water

As shown in Fig. 1, expecting the pooled immunologic reactivities from many donors would cover most of the potential pathogens in the patient's environment, fifteen units of TF at a time were prepared from thirty adult donors having a histories of good health. These procedures were carried out in the Red Cross Hokkaido Blood Center, using the white cell residue which remained after the separation of packed red blood cells and platelet-rich plasma.

Administration of transfer factor was done with hypodermal injections,

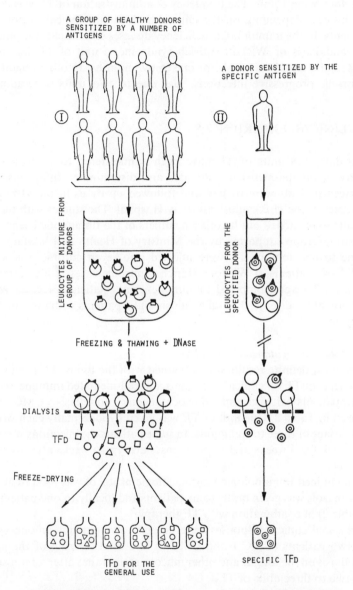

FIG. 1.   Method of preparation of transfer factor from mixed white cells of healthy adult donors or from leukocytes of specifically sensitized donors.

each dose being 1 unit. The frequency of administration of TF was determined case by case depending on the clinical and immunological responses of the recipients. In the immunologic deficiency diseases such as chronic mucocutaneous candidiasis or Wiskott-Aldrich syndrome, a unit of TF was repeatedly injected at a weekly intervals for one to two months. In other conditions such as chronic progressive infections, just one to two units were administered.

II. CLINICAL EXPERIENCES

To date, 108 units of TF have been administered to 28 patients with a variety of immunodeficiency diseases and disseminated infections in Japan. Fourteen patients were treated and followed up by us in the Department of Pediatrics of the Hokkaido University Hospital. The studies with the other 14 patients were carried out by other members of the Immunodeficiency Diseases Research Group supported by the Ministry of Health and Welfare of Japan.

One to ten units of TF were injected into seven chronic mucocutaneous candidiasis patients, 4 Wiskott-Aldrich syndrome cases, 2 ataxia telangiectasia cases, 3 severe combined immunodeficiency patients, 4 cases of chronic granulomatous disease, 3 of tuberculosis and 5 patients with disseminated viral infections.

1. Chronic mucocutaneous candidiasis

The most definite results were obtained with the use of TF in this disorder. The effects of TF on clinical symptoms and cell-mediated immune responses in seven patients with chronic mucocutaneous candidiasis (CMC) are summarized in Table 2. One unit of TF was given hypodermally each week with a total dosage of three to eight units. In some patients the injections were repeated each week for 3 weeks and in other cases every two weeks after that injection schedule.

A combined immunologic-pharmacologic protocol was used in all patients. Clotrimazole was given orally to six patients and locally to one patient (CMC-4 in Table 2) in combination with TF therapy.

Beneficial clinical responses were noted in five patients among seven. The first two patients (CMC-1 and CMC-2) had total clearing of the patches of candidiasis on the tongue and other mucous membranes after administration of only two to three units of TF.

In one case (CMC-1), a 7-year-old boy, white exudates with monilia were noted throughout the oral cavity and at both corners of the lips. This feature persisted almost from his birth. Amphotericine B or clotrimazole alone was

TABLE 2. Clinical results of TF therapy in chronic mucocutaneous candidiasis

Disease & Patient	Age(yr.) and Sex	Units of TF_D used	DTH[3]		L-stimulat.[4]		in vitro test MIF		E-RFC[5]		Other therapy	Clinical improvement
			bef.	aft.	bef.	aft.	bef.	aft.	bef.	aft.		
CMC-1[1]	7 M	3	+	+	−	+(c)			N	N	Clotrimazole	‡
−2	1.3 F	6	−	+	−	−			→	N	Clotrimazole	‡
−3	14 F	6	−	+	−	−					Clotrimazole	−
−4	5 F	6	−	+	+PHA +		−				local Ampho-B Clotrima.	+
−5	15 M	8	±	±							Clotrimazole	−
−6	1 F	5	−	±	−		−		→	N	Clotrimazole	‡ ECZ+[6] Slow.[7]
−7[2]	50 F (a γ-gl, & thymoma)	8	−	‡	±	‡					Clotrimazole γ-gl. (i.m.)	‡ Slow.[7]

[1] chronic mucocutaneous candidiasis
[2] immunodeficiency with thymoma
[3] delayed-type hypersensitivity to candida antigen
[4] lymphocyte stimulation in vitro with candida antigen
[5] E rosette forming cell
[6] improvement of eczema
[7] slow response to transfer factor therapy
(required repeated injections of multiple doses of TF for improvement)

(1976 April)

not effective on these lesions. So on this patient we used 1 unit of transfer factor once a week in combination with clotrimazole for 3 weeks. Oral thrush completely disappeared after the treatment. The proliferating granulomatous inflammations of candida of his fingernails and on the scalp were also resolved. Although this patient has had chronic mucocutanous candidiasis since his infancy, DTH to candida and to DNCB was positive and the response of the patient's lymphocytes *in vitro* after stimulation with phytohemagglutinin was also normal. But the stimulation index of the lymphocytes with candida sonicate antigens was very low. It was 1.3 before the use of transfer factor. But after the administration of transfer factor on 3 occasions, the stimulation index went up to 4.0 as shown in Table 3.

The second patient (CMC-2) was a 1-year-old girl and she had been repeatedly infected by candida at her neck and her buttocks since one month of age. Extensive thrush was always observed in her oral cavity. At 10 months of age, ulcerative necrotic lesions developed rapidly in her buttocks and she was admitted to Hokkaido University Hospital. Infected pathogens were *Staphylococcus aureus* and *Candida albicans*.

Precipitating antibodies against candida in the patient's serum were elevated to 1:16 by counterimmunoelectrophoresis. And the lymphocyte's response *in vitro* to candida antigen was also normal, but delayed-type skin reactivity to candida was not detected. So we used 1 unit of transfer factor every week in combination with clotrimazole and MPI-penicillin. Inflammations on the buttocks were diminished, the extent of the ulcer was getting smaller by 7 days after the TF therapy, and skin transplantation was successfuly performed 2 weeks after the TF administration. All candida lesions of the mucous membranes also disappeared after the administration of 2 units of transfer factor.

CMC-6 also had a disappearance of the mucocutaneous lesions of candida and an improvement of eczema, but beneficial responses were noted later than in the course of TF therapy for CMC-1 and -2. For the improvement of the extensive raised, scaling skin lesions with erythema on the forearms, four weeks' treatment (4 units) was needed, and for oral thrush it required five successive injections of TF at weekly intervals.

CMC-7 was also late in response to TF therapy. She was fifty years old and had immunodeficiency (agammaglobulinemia) with thymoma of the spindle cell type. She was admitted to the dermatology ward of Hokkaido University Hospital for the first time at fifty years of age because of persistent candida infections of the skin and the mucous membrane, and recurrent diarrhea since forty-six years of age. White plaques were present on the buccal mucosa, tongue both corners of the lips and on the vaginal ostium. On the surface of the tongue, granulomatous lesions were seen. There were also erythematous raised scaling

TABLE 3. Laboratory response to TF therapy in patient CMC-I (CMC with progressive pulmonary tuberculosis)

Date TF given		4.26 1974		3.31, 4.6, 4.16 1975	
Date of testing	4.8 1974	6.26 1974	3.24 1975	4.23	5.8
Skin tests					
PPD	0 × 0	17 × 12	18 × 14		
Candida	12 × 16		14 × 17		
DNCB	(+)	(╫)	(+)		
Lymphocyte transformation*					
PHA		22.889(140)			
Candida		225 (1.3)		282(1.2)	7.513(4.0)

*c.p.m. (S.I.)

lesions of the limbs and extremities, including the interdigital spaces, the palms and soles. The nails were pitted and there were several paronychia. Cultures of the mucous membrane lesions yielded *Candida albicans*. Diagnosis of thymoma was made after an X-ray had detected an anterior mediastinal mass. There were recurrent episodes of infection, especially bronchopneumonia, bronchitis and cystitis during the two years prior to admission. Specific immunoglublin concentrations were: IgG, 130 mg/100 ml; IgA, $<$ 5 mg/100 ml; and IgM, $<$ 5 mg/100 ml.

After the patient recieved replacement therapy with human immune serum globulin, she was protected against repeated sinopulmonary infections and diarrhea. But mucocutaneous candidiasis persisted in spite of local amphotericin B and systemic clotrimazole administration. Three units of transfer factor were injected over 3 weeks in combination with clotrimazole, but no change was observed in the candida lesions. After the fifth dose of TF injection the lesions had begun to resolve considerably. During the next few weeks clearing of lesions could be induced with the exception of those on the two fingernails and a toenail.

According to the results of TF therapy with those 7 patients, it's considered to be beneficial in 5 patients, as shown in Table 2. In all five patients in this group in whom transfer factor tended to be effective, delayed-type skin reaction with candida converted from negative response to positive after the treatment. The lymphocyte's response *in vitro* to candida sonicate antigen became positive in 2 patients (CMC-1 and -7) after TF administration. There are 2 cases (CMC-2 and -6) in whom an increase of E rosette forming cells was noted. According to these results and the observations by other authors,[4-7,14] chronic mucocutaneous candidiasis could be considered to be the most important indication for transfer factor treatment.

2. *The other immunodeficiency diseases*

Among the immunodeficiency diseases of other types, there were many reports[5-13,16] in the United States and western Europe including Levin's or Spitler's original descriptions.[2] Our clinical studies and the results of the other members of Immunodeficiency Diseases Research Group of the Ministry of Health and Welfare of Japan also show similar results in response to transfer factor.

As shown in Table 4, in two cases of Wiskott-Aldrich syndrome (WAS-3 and -4) the response to transfer factor therapy was striking. Infections were controlled, eczema was also cleared up. But those beneficial effects after the TF injections were not continued so long, only one week in WAS-3 and 2 to 3 weeks in WAS-4.

TABLE 4. TF Therapy for other immunodeficiencies

Diseases	Age and Sex	Units of TF	DTH bef.	DTH aft.	L-stimul. bef.	L-stimul. aft.	MIF bef.	MIF aft.	E-RFC bef.	E-RFC aft.	Other therapy	Clinical improvement
WAS –1	1.7M	1	—	—	—	—					GM, CER, MPI, ABPC	—
–2	6 M	6	—	+	—			+PHA	→	N	CER	+
–3	0.7M	3	—	—							antibiotics	‡ ECZ+
–4	1.0M	4	—	+							antibiotics	‡ ECZ+
Ataxia	6 M	3	—	++DN	—			+PHA	→	N	CER	+
	19 M	3	—	—CB	—						CER, ABPC	–?
SCID	1.7F	2	—	—	—				→	N	GM, CER, MPI	—
	0.8M	3	—	—	—				N	N	MPI, CER, SBPC	—
	1 M	3	—	—	—						SBPC, γ-gl, Penta, GM, KM	—
CGD	5 M	3	—	— (+asp)							antibiotics	—
	3 M	3	—	— (+asp)							—	—
	2 M	4	—	—							antibiotics	—
	11 M	4	—	—							antibiotics	—

WAS: Wiskott-Aldrich syndrome
Ataxia: Ataxia telangiectasia
SCID: Severe combined immunodeficiency
CGD: Chronic granulomatous disease
asp: aspergillus antigen
penta: pentamidine isethionate

(1976 April)

One of the other cases (WAS-2) was late in responding to TF (responded after using 3 units of TF in 3 weeks) and its effect was transient (three weeks' duration). In one patient, there was no apparent benefit.

In the patients of WAS, who showed clinical improvement, there were also conversion of skin reactivities to specific antigens (WAS-2 and WAS-4), lymphocytes' response to PHA and an increase in the number of E rosette forming cells (WAS-2).

Secondly, in ataxia telangiectasia, a patient, 6 years old, showed good clinical improvement in respiratory infections after TF therapy. This patient had complications of bronchiectasis as evidenced by recurrent sinopulmonary infections; however, the volume of sputum in the morning was markedly diminished and the chest X-ray findings returned to almost normal after administration of 3 units of TF. At the same time delayed skin reactivity or lymphocyte response to phytohemagglutinin converted to positive in this patient. The patient who was DNCB negative before therapy developed a marked hyperreactivity to this chemical after the treatment. As the donors were not previously sensitized to DNCB, this finding raised the question of the specificity of TF activities. We cannot exclude the effect of repeated testing on the development of contact sensitivity to DNCB, but this finding might possibly suggest that TF may also act by inducing nonspecifically the peripheral mainfestation of a cellular hypersensitivity already acquired but not expressed.

But the other patient (19 years old) with ataxia did neither respond clinically nor show conversion of skin reactivity from the administration of TF. No effect was observed on neurologic symptoms in either ataxia patients.

On the other hand, in 3 cases of severe combined immunodeficiency diseases no effect was noted on either delayed hypersensitivity or clinical course. E rosette forming cells were also extremely small in number both before and after the administration of TF. In 4 cases of chronic granulomatous disease, there was no improvement in clinical conditions.

3. Disseminated infections

There are some patients with infectious diseases in whom a deficient cell-mediated immune response to the infecting agents is detected. In this sort of field, TF therapy is thought to be indicated for patients in whom cell-mediated reactivities such as DTH are decreased although humoral antibody production is hyperactive. Disseminated coccidioidomycosis[6,17,18] is considered to be such an example. Lepromatous leprosy[19] is also an infection in which the clinical benefit of TF has been proven.

To a group of patients with a similar pattern of infection, we administered transfer factor to three patients with progressive primary tuberculosis who failed to respond to conventional antituberculous chemotherapy and in whom defects in cellular immunity to tuberculous infection were shown. The therapeutic experiences obtained in those cases are summarized in Table 5, together with the clinical observations on TF therapy in several disseminated viral infections.

Figure 2 shows the clinical course of the first patient (Tbc-1 in Table 5). This patient was a two-year-old girl without prophylactic immunization by BCG. Measles eruptions appeared on June 5th. Four weeks after measles, the chest X-ray film revealed disseminated miliary shadow. A high fever of more than 40° C also continued during this stage. She had no moist rale in her chest but liver and spleen were enlarged. So she was given KM, Rifampicin, isoniazid, PAS and SM, due to suspicion of disseminated miliary tuberculosis in measles anergy. Her uncle was diagnosed as having active pulmonary tuberculosis at that time. But high temperature persisted, WBC, ESR were also elevated, and X-ray findings progressed to some extent. So on August 5th, that is, about 2 months after measles, we tried to use one unit of transfer factor on two occasions. Ten days after transfer factor therapy the high fever dropped, gradually at first; WBC decreased and 3 weeks after the first injection of transfer factor, X-ray findings were much improved, and at the same time delayed hypersensitivity to PPD became definitely positive.

The second case is a 3-year-old boy (Tbc-2 in Table 5) who had no history of

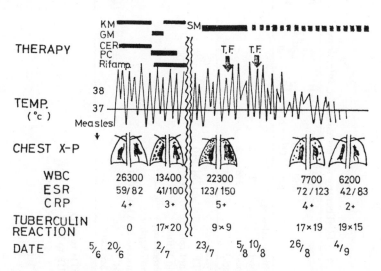

FIG. 2. Clinical course of patient (TBC-I): Miliary tuberculosis during measles anergy.

TABLE 5. TF Therapy for disseminated infections

Diseases	Age and Sex	Units of TF	DTH* bef.	DTH* aft.	L-stimul. bef.	L-stimul. aft.	MIF** bef.	MIF** aft.	E-RFC bef.	E-RFC aft.	Other therapy	Clinical improvement
—bacterial—												
Tbc-1	2F	2	–	+			–	+			SM, PAS, IHMS	++
Tbc-2	3M	2	–	+			–	+			SM, PAS, IHMS	++
Tbc-3	7M	1	–	+				+		N →	SM, PAS, IHMS	+
—viral—												
SSPE	12M	10										±
Giant cell pn. in Wilms	6F	2	–	–							anticonvulsants	–
Herpes zoster in lymphoma	14F	2	–	–								+
Varicella in AML	10M	2			+	+PHA						+?
Chr. act. hepatitis	6M	3	–								prednisolone	+?

* DTH to PPD
** MIF to PPD

(1976 April)

BCG immunization, and a cousin of the first case. As Fig. 3 shows, the onset of measles was on July 26. After one week, high fever reappeared; a chest X-ray revealed bilateral perihilar infiltrations and a massive shadow on the left. Although skin reaction to PPD was negative, intensive treatment with isoniazid PAS and SM in combination was given in consideration of our experience in the first case. In spite of these treatments, chest X-ray findings appeared to be slightly progressed. So the dialysable transfer factor was injected two times. This was 10 weeks after the onset of measles. At first delayed-type hypersensitivity to PPD converted from a negative to a normal response, and at the same time temperature went down to a normal range and the X-ray shadow began to be smaller. It almost disappeared one month after the transfer factor treatment. Both cases are now completely well.

The last case (Tbc-3) was a 7-year-old boy with chronic mucocutaneous candidiasis. Candida infection of the patient had continued from 1 month of age. His serum γ-globulin level was quite normal. The absolute number of peripheral lymphocytes was 3000/mm². Although DTH to candida was positive, that to DNCB was only weakly responsive and that to PPD was completely negative. Lymphocyte transformations to PHA *in vitro* were in the normal range, but no reaction to candida sonicate antigen was seen. His father suffered from pulmonary tuberculosis and had been receiving chemother-

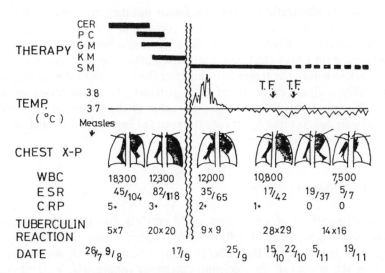

FIG. 3. Clinical course of patient (TBC-2): Progressive pulmonary tuberculosis during measles anergy.

314   S. Matsumoto *et al.*

apy for several months. An abnormal chest X-ray had been noted in this boy too almost at the same time. He had been receiving antituberculous chemotherapy for 6 months, but chest X-ray findings were becoming worse and he had high fever frequently in spite of this treatment. Therefore he was given transfer factor in conjunction with antituberculous chemotherapy. After the transfer factor administration skin reaction to PPD changed to normal in just 24 hours. The chest X-ray film taken 4 weeks after TF therapy showed striking improvement of lung lesions.

As summarized in Table 6, in all these cases, DTH to PPD were negative

TABLE 6.   Laboratory response to TF therapy in all 3 patients with primary tuberculosis

	TBC-1		TBC-2		TBC-3	
	Before	After	Before	After	Before	After
Skin Test						
PPD	0 × 0	18 × 15	5 × 7	23 × 22	0 × 0	26 × 21
Candida	ND	ND	ND	ND	12 × 16	12 × 24
PHA	ND	11 × 11	8 × 8	ND	10 × 10	22 × 23
LMIT	−	+(63%)	−	+(74%)	ND	+(51%)
Clinical Effect		+		+		+

before the administration of transfer factor but they became clearly positive after transfer factor injections and this conversion was going so fast within 24 hours. With the PHA skin test, there were no differences before and after treatment. With LMIT (leukocytes migration inhibition test), they were mostly non-reactive before the treatment. But after the treatment a definitely positive response was observed in all of these patients. These observations would possibly suggest that TF has a clinical value in the treatment of persistent tuberculosis due to some defects of cell-mediated immunity if used in combination with effective antibiotics.

III. DISCUSSION

Our observations of TF therapy in 28 patients with immunodeficiency or infections are summarized briefly in Table 7. Clinical improvement occurred in more than two-thirds of the patients (9 in 13 cases treated, with 60 units in total) in the groups of chronic mucocutaneous candidiasis, Wiskott-Aldrich syndrome, and ataxia telangiectasia. Most of these patients (8 of 12 cases tested) also showed conversion of skin test reactivity from negative to positive and

TABLE 7. Summary of the results of TF therapy

Diseases	No. of Patients	TF units	Conversion DTH	Conversion L-stimul.	Conversion E-RFC	Improvement (%)
CMC	7	40	5/7	2/4	1/2	5/7 (71)
WAS	4	14	2/3	1/2	1/1	3/4 (75)
Ataxia	2	6	1/2	1/1	1/1	1/2 (50)
SCID	3	8	0/3	0/2	0/3	0/3 (0)
CGD	4	14	0/4			0/4 (0)
TBC	3	5	3/3	MIF2/2	1/1	3/3(100)
viral	5	19	0/3	1/1		2/5(40)
	28	108				(1976 April)

more than half of the patients tested (4 of 7 cases) became responsive to lymphocyte stimulation by antigens or phytohemagglutinin. Further, it was found that some patients (3 of 4 tested) showed an increase in the number of E rosette forming cells after TF administration.

The results of the study with progressive pulmonary tuberculosis in anergy states led us to evaluate the effects of TF therapy more clearly. All three patients responded well to TF therapy and at the same time they showed rapid conversion of delayed-type hypersensitivity to PPD and also showed LMIF production to PPD.

It should be pointed out that the dosage of TF required to cause clinical or immunological improvement is different between immunodeficiency diseases and infectious disease. Larger amounts of TF were apparently needed for the same effect in patients with primary immunodeficiency syndrome compared with dosages for infectious diseases.

We are currently evaluating TF from healthy adult donors in patients with a variety of immunodeficiency syndromes; however, there is an obvious need for a controlled clinical trial with TF to clarify its role in the treatment of these disorders. Besides this, many questions remain before one can properly assess the value of TF in treatment of persistent infections in immunodeficient patients.

The first problem to be resolved is that of specificity.[20] It is still unclear whether TF with immunologic specificity is essential for favourable clinical responses in immunodeficiency states. We used TF derived from a candida positive donor for most patients with chronic mucocutaneous candidiasis and favourable effects were noted. Results of Kirkpatrick[4] with chronic candidiasis were evaluated by using nonspecific TF and similar results were obtained.

The second important problem to be resolved may be a purification of active components in human TF. *In vitro* studies of TF have shown that there are

316   S. Matsumoto et al.

some components having inhibitory effects on lymphocyte stimulation.[24] Thus it seems to be more reasonable to use isolated active material without inhibitory effects. In preparing this kind of component, identification and purification of both the active and inhibitory material of TF should be facilitated.

And the third problem in TF therapy is the difficulty of establishing a reliable in vitro assay of TF activities. It has greatly hampered understanding of the mode of action of transfer factor. It reflects also the difficulty of checking the immunological activities of TF preparations. From a practical point of view preparations of the same potency must always be available for general use. An in vitro assay system has proved very difficult to establish, although Asher et al.[21] reported some success in the use of antigen-specific TF in the conversion of nonimmune to immune responsiveness, as measured by antigen-mediated lymphocyte transformation, and Hamblin et al.[22,23] demonstrated that dialysable human transfer factor in tissue culture medium augments lymphocyte transformation to PPD or phytohemagglutinin.

According to our results on lymphocyte stimulation in vitro mediated by candida antigen or phytohemagglutinin, no augmenting activity of TF preparation could be detected either specific or nonspecific stimulation. Sporadic reports of successful results in the past, therefore, have appeared to be difficult to confirm. But it is essential to establish a simple and reliable in vitro assay system of TF activities for preparation of TF of a uniform immunological potency.

Acknowledgments

The authors would like to express their appreciation of the support of the Ministry of Health and Welfare of Japan. We especially thank Dr. Noboru Kobayashi, Chief of IDS Research Group of M.H.W., for his advice and encouragement. We wish to thank the following physicians who participated in this study either by referring patients to us or by treating the patients with transfer factor supplied by our laboratory and performing studies: T. Oura, T. Tonooka, N. Itoh, F. Kaneko, Y. Terayama, H. Murase, S. Miyazaki, T. Matsumoto, D. Amano, Y. Kobayashi, C. Hara, J. Yata, K. Hoshina, T. Kanno, M. Hori, H. Mikawa, T. Hirao, and M. Kubata.

REFERENCES

1. Lawrence, H. S.: The transfer in humans of delayed skin sensitivity to strepto-

coccal M substance and to tuberculin with disrupted leukocytes. *J. Clin. Invest.* **34**:219, 1955.

2. Levin, A. S., Spitler, L. E., Sites, D. P., *et al.*: Wiskott-Aldrich syndrome, a genetically determined cellular immunologic deficiency. Clinical and laboratory responses to therapy with transfer factor. *Proc. Nat. Acad. Sci.* (Wash) **67**: 821, 1970.

3. Lawrence, H. S.: Transfer Factor. *Adv. Immunol.* **11**:195, 1969.

4. Kirkpatrick, C. H. and Smith, T. K.: Chronic mucocutaneous candidiasis: Immunologic and antibiotic therapy. *Ann. Intern. Med.* **80**:310, 1974.

5. Kirkpatrick, C. H.: Restoration of cell-mediated immune responses with transfer factor. Birth Defects Original Article Series. Vol. XI, No. 1 (D. Bergsma, R. A. Good and J. Finstad, eds.), The National Foundation—March of Dimes, New York, 441, 1975.

6. Spitler, L. E., Levin, A. S., and Fudenberg, H. H.: Transfer Factor II: Results of therapy. Birth Defects Original Article Series. Vol. XI, No. 1, (D. Bergsma, R. A. Good, and J. Finistad, eds.), The National Foundation—March of Dimes, New York, 449, 1975.

7. Rocklin, R. E.: Use of transfer factor in patients with depressed cellular immunity and chronic infection. Birth Defects Original Article Series. Vol. XI, No. 1, (D. Bergsma, R. A. Good, and J. Finstad, eds.), The National Foundation—March of Dimes, New York, 431, 1975.

8. Griscelli, C.: Transfer factor therapy in immunodeficiency. Birth Defects Original Article Series. Vol. XI, No. 1, (D. Bergsma, R. A. Good, and J. Finstad, eds.), The National Foundation—March of Dimes, New York, 462, 1975.

9. Spitler, L. E., Levin, A. S., and Fudenberg, H. H.: Transfer Factor in Clinical Immunology, Vol. 2, (F. H. Back and R. A. Good, eds.) Academic Press, New York, 154, 1974.

10. Kirkpatrick, C. H., Rich, R. R., and Smith, T. K.: Effect of transfer factor on lymphocyte function in anergic patients. *J. Clin. Invest.* **51**:2948, 1972.

11. Basten, A., Croft, S., Kenny, D. F., *et al.*: Uses of transfer factor. *Vox Sang.* **28**:257, 1975.

12. MacKie, R. M.: Transfer Factor 1975. *Brit. J. Dermatol.* **94**:107, 1976.

13. Good, R. A., Varco, R. L., Aust, J. B., and Zack, S. J.: The use of leukocyte dialysate in combined immunodeficiency. *Ann. N. Y. Acad. Sci.* **64**:882, 1967.

14. MacKie, R. M., Cockran, R., de Sousa, M., *et al.*: Chronic mucocutaneous candidiasis treated with transfer factor. *Brit. J. Dermatol.* **94**:79, 1976.

15. Good, R. A.: Transfer Factor. *Cell Immunol.* **3**:1, 1972.

16. Spitler, L. E., Levin, A. S., Sites, D. P., Fudenberg, H. H., Pirofsky, B., August, C. S., Stiehm, E. R., Hitzig, W. H., and Gatti, R. A.: The Wiskott-Aldrich syndrome. Results of transfer factor therapy. *J. Clin. Invest.* **51**:216, 1972.

17. Stevens, D. A., Pappagianis, D., Marinkovich, V. A., *et al.*: Immunotherapy in recurrent coccidioidomycosis. *Cell. Immunol.* **12**:37, 1974.

18. Graybill, J. R., Silva, J., Alford, R. H., *et al.*: Immunologic and clinical improvement of progressive coccidioidomycosis following administration of transfer factor. *Cell. Immunol.* **8**:120, 1973.

19. Bullock, W. E., Fields, J. P., and Brandriss, M. W.: An evaluation of transfer

factor as immunotherapy for patients with lepromatous leprosy. *New Engl. J. Med.* **287**:1053, 1972.

20. Salaman, M. R. and Valdimarsson, H.: Specificity of transfer factor. *Nature* **259**:250, 1976.
21. Ascher, M. S., Schneider, W. J., Valentine, F. T., *et al.*: *In vitro* properties of leukocyte dialysates containing transfer factor. *Proc. Nat. Acad. Sci.* (Wash.) **71**:1178, 1974.
22. Hamblin, A.: The effect of transfer factor on cultured lymphocytes. Behring Inst. Mitt. No. 57, 25, 1975.
23. Hamblin, A. S., Dumonde, D. C., and Maini, R. N.: Human transfer factor *in vitro*, I & II. *Clin. Exp. Immunol.* **23**:290, 303, 1976.
24. Burger, D. R., Vandenbark, A. A., Daves, D., *et al.*: Nicotinamide: Suppression of lymphocyte transformation with a component identified in human transfer factor. *J. Immunol.* **117**:797, 1976.

DISCUSSION

Dr. GOOD: In the transfer factor preparations that you used that seemed to be effective in your patients, was there any difference whether the patients had sensitivity to the agent you were concerned with, or not? Our studies, and I think they agree with those of Seligmann, seem to indicate that in what we call transfer factor, which is a very crude material, there is something that enhances the capacity to be sensitized to very low concentrations of antigen, and that the original concepts of transfer factor as conferring sensitivity of a specific type perhaps are not so urgent now as they once seemed. And in our own work, we seem to have as good effects in chronic mucocutaneous candidiases of transfer factor from patients who are not obviously sensitized as we do from patients who are sensitized to candida antigens. Furthermore, we can transfer capacity to express sensitivity to 2-4-dionitrochlorobenzene in doses below the threshold that will bring about this expression in normal individuals. It seems to me that the critical issue with transfer factor is that it does not work in experimental animals, but maybe we have just been asking the wrong question. We have been asking for it to be specific. Now, our results with transfer factor in chronic mucocutaneous candidiasis have been with about fifty per cent of them. It does not seem to relate whether they are granulomatous form or flat form. We seem to get benefit from very persistent transfer factor therapy, and Wiskott-Aldrich syndrome has been a problem. These patients with Wiskott-Aldrich syndrome do have a propensity to develop autoimmune manifestations, but we have seen shortly after transfer administration the development of hemolytic anemia in two of our patients.

Dr. AIUTI: I would like just to present this data because it is similar to the data obtained and presented now by Dr. Matsumoto. Also, it has been done with different transfer factor preparations in different countries.

The transfer factor was given to several patients with different immunodeficiency diseases. This was the first patient who had chronic mucocutaneous candidiasis since the sixth month of age. Now she is 35 years old. She has suffered throughout her life with severe pulmonary infection from candida. When she was admitted to the hospital, she was treated with all the serial, anti-candida drugs without any effect. And after treatment with transfer factor the tongue became white, but there was no candida at all. After one week this starts to disappear. And this is the son of this patient. He developed chronic mucocutaneous candidiasis at the same age as the mother, at six months, exactly the same age. So he is a familial case. We treated these patients with transfer factor preparation, and we noted the clinical improvement with the conversion of the delayed activity sensitivity reaction against candida. However, after four months, after several injections, the candida reappears in the skins, and after one year, he developed a chronic, aggressive hepatitis documented by a liver biopsy. So we do not know if this depends on the transfer factor, or not. It was HB antigen positive.

This is also another patient. This is the best result after transfer factor. This is before, this was when he was seven years old, and then ten years old. And this is after transfer factor therapy. And this patient now, after two years of treatment, has had no relapse of candidiasis. This is after transfer factor therapy for three years. This is another patient who suffers from tuberculosis with a very high fever, four months with severe miliary tuberculosis. She was four years old, and she also had associated IgA deficiency, so we treated her with four doses of transfer factor, and we observed the decrease of fever, clinical improvement, weight improvement and also conversion from negative to positive from the serum immunological barometer, but we noted that the PPD skin test became positive before the transfer factor, just three days before, so we must be very careful in this skin reaction. This is just a summary of all the four cases of chronic mucocutaneous candidiasis that we treated, these were the two that we represented. We noted clinical improvements, but now after six months, and after one year, they have both relapsed.

Dr. BLAESE: I hope we will have some definitive answers on transfer factor. There is a multi-center combined double-blind cross-over study going on at the moment that has approximately 35 patients entered into the study. We received transfer factor prepared by Lynn Spittler under a code I do not know. We have treated seven patients with it and I see no difference between the two groups but I do not know which they are getting. But so far our results have not been impressive. It is a real problem, I think, particularly with this disease, that it has such a variable clinical course. The patients can be very ill, and then be well, and you will not see them for two or three years, and then they will have very severe episodes of infection again.

Dr. SOOTHILL: I want to suggest that that very important point Bob has raised is open to us. Of course, we have no idea whether we are usng this for a specific or a nonspecific purpose, but I think that results should only be presented in those individuals in whom positive cell skin responses have been transmitted, or at least they should be analysed separately because different batches of this material have a different level of effectiveness. We can use the antigen nonspecific transmission of capacity to respond to an antigen as a test. I told you earlier that we have now, five times out of six, turned off cytomegalovirus in the urine of patients with congenital infection. We need common conditions so that we can do control trials, and mucocutaneous candidiasis is not common enough probably. That is the reason why I think that that provides a useful possibility.

Dr. HITZIG: It has been mentioned that the great difficulty is that there is no reliable test to prove transfer factor activity in animals, or *in vitro*. The deficiency of Lawrence's experiments is that he used adult recipients. We have therefore used neonatal lymphocytes *in vitro* and this study, which was a very long study, turned out to show essentially an unspecific activity of transfer factor, and I would formulate it like this: it shifts the reactivity of lymphocytes, or it might lift it to a higher level. If you do those response curves with these lymphocytes, you see that the response is shifted to a higher level of sensitivity, and that might explain the action in patients. But if there is no reactivity at all you cannot achieve anything with transfer factor, and I think this explains the conflicting results in different patients. So it certainly does something in patients who have already the possibility to react, but it does not cure patients who do not have this possibility.

Dr. GOOD: This case, I think, illustrates so well the problem of evaluating those hemolytic anemias which we have seen after transfer factor therapy because they can occur in patients with a Wiskott-Aldrich syndrome without any transfer factor in the picture. And in this instance the transfer factor seemed to make matters better. However, I do think there is an approach to the hemolytic anemia associated with cytomegalovirus infection, and the way to treat that, although everyone is complaining that we do not have material to give out, I think we have shown conclusively the way to treat that virus in humans, and in humans with immunodeficiency, is with interferon. We have repeatedly seen a complete disappearance from the secretions, and ultimately from the blood and secretions of immunodeficiency patients who have been treated with interferon. It works as well with the cytomegalovirus as it works with the herpes virus, on both of them, it works in both situations. But I think that we are going to have to define our interferon, just like we have to define our transfer factor because in these preparations that we call interferon, there are many other substances, and all the substances that are there are biologically highly active and present in tiny amounts, and the problem of their purification, identification and molecular analysis is a very real one.

Induction of T Cell Functions in Nude Mice by a Thymus Factor Extracted from Calf Thymus

Tohru MASUDA,* Susumu IKEHARA,** and Yoshihiro HAMASHIMA**

It is clearly established that the thymus plays an important role in the induction of T cells from precursors of T or stem cells.[1] Several investigators have prepared a variety of thymic humoral factors which can restore some immunological functions either in thymectomized mice *in vivo* or in normal bone marrow cells *in vitro*.[2] Thymus grafts into nude mice work very well in restoring T-dependent immunological functions,[3] in contrast, the humoral factors have had little success in generating T cells or T-dependent functions in nude mice.[4] The humoral factors reported so far are summarized in Table 1; thymosin by A. Goldstein,[5] thymopoietin by G. Goldstein,[6] THF by Trainin,[7] thymic factor by Bach,[8] *etc*. These humoral factors are all proteins or polypeptides and their molecular weights lie between 1,000 and 12,000. In 1974, a symposium concerning biological activities of thymic hormones was held in Rijswijk, Holland and the activities of these factors were tested by a variety of bioassay systems.[9] Most of the assays were performed by using spleen, bone marrow or thymus cells derived from ordinal mice, but some used nude mice.

TABLE 1. Physical and chemical properties of thymic hormones

Thymic Hormones	Laboratory	Chemical Class	Molecular Weight
Thymosin	A. Goldstein	Protein	12,000
Thymopoietin	G. Goldstein	Protein	5,562
Thymic Humoral Factor (THF)	N. Trainin	Polypeptide	3,220
Thymic Factor (TF)	J. Bach	Polypeptide	1,000
Lymphocyte-Stimulating			LSHh 17,000
Hormone (LSH)	T. Luckey	Protein	LSHr 80,000

* Institute for Immunology, Faculty of Medicine, Kyoto University, Kyoto, Japan
** Department of Pathology, Faculty of Medicine, Kyoto University, Kyoto, Japan

We hoped to get evidence proving that thymus humoral factors induce T-dependent immunological functions in nude or thymectomized mice, rather than generate Thy-1 bearing cells. However, results on both induction of Thy-1 antigen and responsiveness to T cell mitogens were inconclusive in this experiment.

We initiated our study by preparing a humoral factor from calf thymuses according to the method of A. Goldstein.[5] However, the procedures were oversimplified intentionally, as shown in Fig. 1, in comparison with the original method. The thymus factors which can restore T cell functions, that

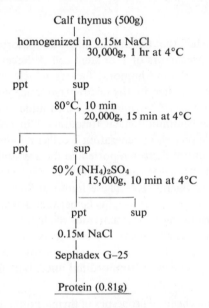

FIG. 1.   Preparation of a thymus factor.

is, which can induce maturation of stem or precursor T cells, would consist of many components. Some of them might be lost in the process of purification. This is the reason why we used crude materials. Briefly, saline extract from calf thymuses was heated at 80°C for 10 min., then saturated ammonium sulfate was added to a concentration of 50% saturation. The precipitate, dissolved in saline, was passed through Sephadex G-25 to remove free ammonium sulfate. The protein fractions were combined and diluted with saline. The same fractionation procedure of calf spleens was carried out as a control.

The bioassay systems for the thymus factor (TF) are shown in Fig. 2. Four-week-old athymic nude mice, backcrossed with BALB/c mice, were injected

EXPERIMENTAL SCHEDULE

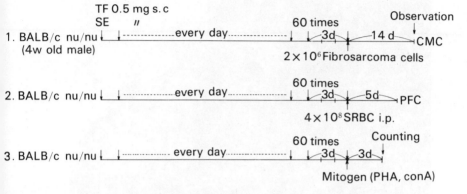

FIG. 2.

subcutaneously with 0.5 mg of TF or SE (spleen extract) once a day for 60 days. By using these mice we were able to test: (1) capability for rejecting allografted tumors and the killer activity of spleen cells in the mice with transferred allogeneic tumor cells; and (2) antibody production against T-dependent antigen, sheep red blood cells (SRBC), the proportion of Thy-1.2 positive cells in the spleen and the spleen cells, mitogen responses to PHA (phytohemagglutinin-P) and ConA (concanavalin A).

In the first experiment, 2×10^6 allogeneic fibrosarcoma cells originating from methylcholanthrene-treated C3H/He mice were transferred into 5 nude mice, one day after their last injection of TF or SE. No tumors were detected in the group pretreated with TF, whereas no rejection took place in the nude mice treated with SE. Histological findings showed a remarkable accumulation of lymphocytes in T-dependent areas around postcapillary venules of lymph nodes in the TF-treated group (Fig. 3a). In contrast, no lymphocyte accumulation in this area was observed in mice pretreated with SE (Fig. 3b). TF can also restore the capability to reject allografts in neonatally thymectomized mice (not shown). By using the spleen cells of these mice which were transplanted with allogeneic tumor cells, microcytotoxicity tests were performed according to the method of Takasugi.[10] It is demonstrated in Table 2 that killers of sarcoma cells are generated only in the spleens of either TF-treated nude or neonatally thymectomized mice. Further, the killer cells are eliminated by anti-Thy-1.2 and C treatment of the spleen cells. These results suggest that the TF induces killer T cells, which have a major role in the rejection of allografted

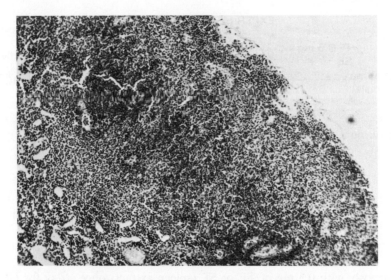

Fig. 3a.   Axillary lymph node after TF-treatment.
Lymphocyte accumulation is observed in T-dependent area around post-capillary venuli.

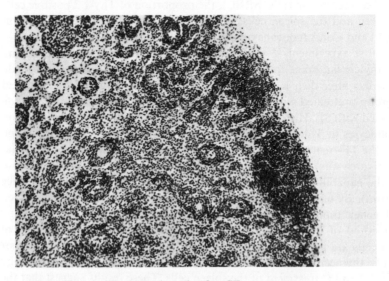

Fig. 3b.   Axillary lymph node after SE-treatment.
No lymphocyte accumulation is observed in the T-dependent area.

tumors, in both nude and thymectomized mice. It can be seen in Table 3 that Thy-1.2 bearing cells, whose existence was proved by the trypan blue exclusion test using anti-Thy-1.2 antiserum and guinea pig C, appear in the spleens or lymph nodes of nude mice pretreated with TF, but not with SE. Their proportion in the spleens is almost comparable to that of nu/+ spleens (23% and 28%, respectively).

The second step was to consider whether helper T cells could be induced by TF in nude mice or not. Three days after the last injection of TF or SE, nude mice were immunized with 4×10^8 SRBC intraperitoneally. The other two control groups were nu/+ and nude mice which were injected with antigen, but

TABLE 2. *In vitro* cytotoxic effects of spleen cells from thymectomized A/J and *nu/nu* mice subjected to long-term injections of either thymus factor (TF) or spleen extract (SE) on allogeneic tumor cells

Mouse**			Injection			Tumour rejection	% Cytotoxicity (mean ± s.e.m.) Cell-mediated cytotoxicity* (at 48 hr)	Treatment with anti-θ serum + C (1:12)
T	A/J	(5)	SE	(0.5 mg × 20)		no	6.3 ± 2.2	1.2 ± 0.5
T	A/J	(5)	TF	(0.5 mg × 20)		yes	89.4 ± 8.3	1.8 ± 0.3
nu/nu		(3)	SE	(0.5 mg × 60)		no	1.8 ± 0.4	ND
nu/nu		(3)	TF	(0.5 mg × 60)		yes	62.5 ± 6.3	2.1 ± 0.6

A microcytotoxicity assay was performed by using spleen cells from both thymectomized and nude mice which had rejected tumor allografts following TF-treatment, and also from those which had shown no tumor rejection.
* Effector cells/Target cells = 50/1
** Numbers in parentheses indicate the number of mice in the group. ND, not done.

TABLE 3.   Evidence for T-cell induction by a thymus factor in athymic nude mice

Mouse*	Injection	Cell source	Cytotoxic index (%)
nu/nu(3)	SE (0.5 mg × 60)	Spleen	0.5 ± 0.1
		Lymph node	0.7 ± 0.1
nu/nu (2)	TF (0.5 mg × 60)	Spleen	23 ± 2
		Lymph node	39 ± 3
nu/+(2)	no	Spleen	28 ± 3
		Lymph node	58 ± 4

On the third day after the last injection of TF or SE, the mice thus treated and *nu/+* control mice were sacrificed. Pooled spleen and lymph node cells from each group were used in the cytotoxicity test with anti-Thy 1.2 serum and guinea pig complement. Cytotoxic index was evaluated by the trypan blue exclusion technique.
* Numbers in parentheses indicate the number of mice in the group.

not treated with TF. Five days after the antigen stimulation, the plaque forming cell (PFC) response to SRBC was determined by Cunningham's technique. The results are shown in Fig. 4. Both direct and indirect PFC response of the TF-treated nude mice was increased to 9.5 × 10⁴ and 9.2 × 10⁴, respectively. These numbers are almost comparable to the results in nu/+mice. The responses of the SE treated or untreated nude mice, on the other hand, were very poor, approximately 200 direct and 1200 indirect PFC in both groups. These findings imply that the TF can induce helper T cells in nude mice.

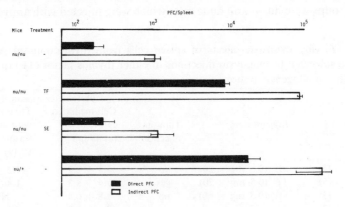

FIG. 4. Helper induction in *nu/nu* mice by TF.
On the third day after the last injection of TF or SE, all 3 mice in each of the 4 groups shown were immunized intraperitoneally with 4 × 10⁸ SRBC. After 5 days, the number of PFC in the spleens was determined by Cunningham's method. Indirect PFCs were developed by polyvalent rabbit anti-mouse Ig serum. The columns represent the mean ± standard of error.

The next experiment was to determine the capacity of TF to restore responsiveness to T cell mitogens, PHA and ConA. Pooled spleen cells of nude mice, which had received 60 injections of TF were used in this experiment. Age-matched and sex-matched controls consisted of untreated nude and ordinal BALB/c mice. Figure 5 shows dose responses to the mitogens. A half million of each cell in 0.2 ml of RPMI 1640 medium supplemented with 5% fetal calf serum was cultured with or without various amounts of PHA or ConA for 3 days in a CO_2 incubator by using micro-culture plates (Falcon) and the reactivity of each spleen cell was determined by measuring the uptake of ³H-TdR which was added to each well 24 hours before termination of the culture. It can be seen that spleen cells from untreated nude mice respond neither to PHA nor to ConA. On the other hand, spleen cells from nude mice

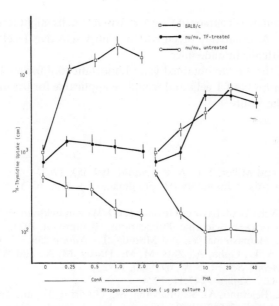

FIG. 5. Effect of TF on the responsiveness to PHA and ConA of *nu/nu* spleen cells.
Two 4-week-old male *nu/nu* mice were subcutaneously injected every day with 0.5mg of TF for 60 days. Three days later, the mitogenic reactivity of their spleen cells was determined by measuring the uptake of ³H-thymidine into DNA. □————□, BALB/c mice; ●————●, *nu/nu* mice treated TF; ○————○, untreated *nu/nu* mice. Each point and bar represents the mean ± standard of error.

treated with TF show a remarkable response to PHA. The level of the response is almost the same as that given by the spleen cells of BALB/c mice. In contrast with the response to PHA, the nude spleen cells treated with TF respond poorly to ConA, although they do show a statistically significant difference from that of the untreated nude spleen cells.

Our present studies have demonstrated that the thymus factor is capable of preferentially restoring PHA responsiveness, helper and killer functions in athymic nude mice. It has been reported by several investigators that there are two kinds of T cell subsets; the one responds relatively well to ConA, the other relatively well to PHA.[11,12] It is unclear whether our TF regulates the first step of differentiation of stem cells to precursor T cells, or induces functionally mature T cells from precursor T cells. Further, the TF is still crude and its biochemical character has not been determined. It might turn out to be a mixture of a few active components of the thymus. A factor which can

328 T. Masuda *et al.*

effectively stimulate precursor of ConA-sensitive T cells might not be contained in our sample. Alternatively precursors of ConA-sensitive T cells may be lost or decrease with age in nude mice.

Either way, the TF we obtained is an important tool for analyzing the differentiation pathway of T cells and would be applicable for use in some clinical disorders in the future.

REFERENCES

1. Osoba, D. and Miller, J. F. A. P.: *Nature* **199**:653, 1963.
2. Thymus Factors in Immunity (H. Friedman, ed.), Ann. N. Y. Acad. Sci., 1975, p. 249.
3. Biological Activity of Thymus Hormones (D. W. van Bekkum and A. Kruisbeek, eds.), Kooyker Scientific Publications, Rotterdam, 1975.
4. Ikehara, S., Hamashima, Y., and Masuda, T.: *Nature* **258**:335, 1975.
5. Goldstein, A. L., Guha, A., Zats, M. M., Hardy, M. A., and White, A.: *Proc. Nat. Acad. Sci.*, U.S.A., **69**:1800, 1972.
6. Goldstein, G.: *Nature* **247**:11, 1974.
7. Trainin, N., Bejerano, A., Strahilevitch, M., Goldring, D., and Small, M.: *Israel J. Med. Sci.*, 2:549, 1966.
8. Bach, J. F., Dardenne, M., Pleau, J. M., and Bach, M. A.: *Ann. N. Y. Acad. Sci.,* **249**:186, 1975.
9. Proc. of 1st International Workshop on Nude Mice (J. Rygaad and C. O. Povlsen, eds.), Gustav Fischer Verlag, Stuttgart, 1974.
10. Takasugi, M. and Klein, E.: *Transpl.* **9**:219, 1970.
11. Stobo, J. D. and Paul, W. E.: *J. Immunol.* **110**:362, 1973.
12. Stout, R. D. and Herzenberg, L. A.: *J. Exp. Med.* **142**:611, 1975.

DISCUSSION

Dr. GOOD: This is a very impressive accomplishment, especially in the face of so many failures in attempting to reconstitute the nude mice and to reconstitute the neonatally thymectomized mice especially after they have lost their post-thymic cells. If you use thymus in a milipore chamber you can very nicely reconstitute mice if you get them when they have still got some post-thymic, but incompletely differentiated, cells. I think the key to your very convincing demonstration is the 60, all of those many, many injections, because most of us did not keep it up that long. I think that using purified thymopoietin, which is fully defined in terms of its amino acid sequence and its active site, has not only been identified, but synthesized, this material readily induces in the nude mouse the differentiation of the surface markers of the T-lymphocytes, which in the initial experiments did not reconstitute. But now that Goldstein and Schide are really hammering at the animals in the same way that you have, they have induced ConA, PHA,

MILC responses and they have not yet done the tumor immunity which you demonstrate. The way I interpret this, the way all of the failures in the past, is that it takes really two concentrations of thymopoietin, or thymic factor, you do not have yours identified yet, but I think it is probably the same, to do two different jobs. One of those jobs is to induce the start of the differentiation phenomena, and this really requires very high concentrations. Another is to carry this further, which requires much lower concentrations. Have you conducted any experiments to possibly dissect that characteristic? If it were possible to induce peripheral differentiation without going through the thymus with low concentrations, I think we might have a very chaotic situation in that these concentration differentials may be the key to the control differentiation and thus the reason we need to have a special site.

Dr. MASUDA: Thank you very much, Dr. Good. I think also we need to analyse the dose dependency for inducing T-cells in nude mice, but I have never used doses of TF so far. The reason is an economic reason; nude mice are so expensive, so we are now making an *in vitro* system. It is a little bit successful. Perhaps by using an *in vitro* system I will look at the dose problem.

Dr. COOPER: Dr. Masuda, I would like to continue the line of discussion that Dr. Good raised. There seems to be still a controversy over whether or not a stem cell, a multifocus stem cell, must go to the thymus in order to begin that pathway of T-cell differentiation, or if it can do so outside, before it gets there. I realise that a lot of people have strong opinions about what may happen. What I would like to know is, can you, using your factor, take what everyone would accept as a stem cell, or a source tissue for stem cells, which has not had any opportunity to travel to the thymus, such as the yolk sac, or the liver from a mouse fetus let us say 11 or 12 days of age, and cause that cell, *in vitro*, to assume a T-cell function, markers, *etc.*?

Dr. MASUDA: I have no direct evidence about your question, but I think there would be at least two types of pre-T-cells. One can skip the thymus and migrate into, perhaps, the spleen and differentiate into a helper. Another pre-T should be required to pass through the thymus, and thereafter, maybe, migrate out into the spleen. The former may be circulating too, and the latter may be a pool of suppressor, or something with a forming pattern. This is just speculation.

Dr. COOPER: I like your idea, and I think it would fit the data. But, we also just heard yesterday that the nude mouse does have lymphoid cells. Your thymic factor could therefore be influencing those cells that have left the thymus when you begin treatment at four weeks. So your data does not prove that a cell can by-pass the thymus in order to become a T-cell, it does not seem to me. So I am asking if you can do *in vitro* experiments, have you done *in vitro* experiments, showing that you can take a true multi-potent stem cell, or a source containing these, before the thymus could have influenced them directly, and make them become a T-cell?

Dr. MASUDA: I think so.

Thymic Transplantation and Thymic Hormone Therapy in Patients with T Cell Deficiency

F. Aiuti,* M. Fiorilli,* P. Ammirati,* R. D'Amelio,*
and L. Businco**

ABSTRACT

Thymus transplant and thymic hormone therapy are the most investigated attempts to correct T cell defects. In this paper we summarized our experience. Two patients with severe T cell deficiency were immunologically reconstituted by fetal thymus transplant. One is dead, two years after transplant, owing to a B cell lymphoma. Twelve patients with various forms of immunodeficiency were treated with a thymus extract capable of increasing immune functions in mice and also in humans *in vitro*. Five out of 6 T cell deficiency patients improved clinically and immunologically after thymosin therapy. Two infants with SCID, 3 with GVH and one with Wiskott-Aldrich syndrome did not show any clinical benefit or immunological modification. We underline the various pathogenetic mechanisms behind these syndromes which make therapeutic approach difficult. We suggest that some patients with T cell defect have an absence of thymic hormone, as shown by clinical and experimental trials, and that this defect can be corrected by a substitutive therapy.

In this paper the background of clinical and immunological data on T cell deficiencies is summarized, and some perspectives on the therapy for these forms given.

Some investigators have tried to separate the T cell deficiencies (in which there is evidence of some immunoglobulin and antibody synthesis) from classical SCID.[1,2] In T cell deficiency syndrome group are included patients with DiGeorge syndrome, Nezelof, sporadic or familial T cell defects and normal Ig, nucleoside phosphorylase deficiency. Other forms manifesting thymic aplasia and functional T cell defects in chronic viral diseases have been described.[3,4] The possible inheritance patterns, the onset of clinical signs,

---

* Department of Internal Medicine III, University of Rome, Italy
** Department of Pediatrics, I, University of Rome, Italy

and the pre-eminent clinical signs of the T cell deficiency syndrome are summarized in Table 1. All these forms also present a different pathogenetic
mechanism and different degrees of immunological abnormalities, as reported
in Table 2.

TABLE 1. Inheritance patterns and clinical findings in patients with primary T cell
deficiency

Syndromes	Possible Inheritance Patterns	Onset of Clinical Signs	Prominent Clinical Signs
Thymic hypoplasia hypoparathyroidism (DiGeorge: partial and complete)	Unknown (familiar)	Birth	Facial and cardiac abnormalities Ipocalcemic convulsions Infections
Thymic hypoplasia with Ig synthesis (Nezelof)	Autosomal recessive	Birth	Infections (viral and fungal) Failure to thrive Diarrhea
T cell defect with NP absence	Hereditary Possibly autosomal recessive	First month of life	Anemia Infections
Other forms not classifiable at present	Familiar Sporadic	After one year of age. At birth	Severe infections Failure to thrive Diarrhea
Thymic hypoplasia with normal T cells	None (?)	Birth	Infections (viral)

The approach to therapy is still difficult because the exact pathogenetic
mechanism of these syndromes is not known. Thymus transplantation, transfer
factor and thymic hormones have been used to correct T cell deficiency patients. Table 3 reports the results of thymus transplantations performed by
several investigators over the last 8 years. Maximum success has been achieved
in DiGeorge syndrome. Six out of 7 infants in whom thymus transplantations
were performed are living; conversely, only 9 out of 38 non-transplanted
patients are alive.

In primary T cell deficiency patients the results are worse, but recently
optimistic data were obtained by Ammann[5] performing thymus transplantation within 6 hours of abortion, giving thymus intraperitoneally, plus several
doses of transfer factor before the transplantation. The mechanism by which
thymus transplantation restores immunity is not clear. However, the very rapid
response of cellular immunity (several hours or a few days), and the absence of
chimerism, lead to the hypothesis that a humoral factor is inducing already-

TABLE 2. Possible etiopathogenesis and immunological defect of primary T cell deficiencies

Syndromes	Possible Etiopathogenesis	Immunological Defect
Thymic hypoplasia hypoparathyroidism (DiGeorge)	Absence or reduction of epithelial thymus for dysmorphogenesis (absence of thymic hormones)	Complete T cell defect since birth (absence of E rosettes; absence of mitogenic and allo-geneic response; defect of some immune response against thymus-dependent antigens)
Thymic hypoplasia with Ig synthesis (Nezelof)	Thymus absence	Complete severe T cell defect
T cell defect with NP absence	NP absence in red cells and NP inducing I. deficit	Severe T cell defect
Other forms	Thymic involution (Genetic mechanism?) Viral infections (CMV)	Partial or complete T cell defect
Thymic hypoplasia with T cells	CMV or other viral infections inducing involution of thymus and T-D system	Functional T cell defect (?)

present prethymic precursors to mature, or is inducing stimulation of a possible rudimental epithelial thymus present in some of these patients. Levels of thymic hormone measured pre- and post-thymus transplantation would appear to support this hypothesis.[6] However, spontaneous recovery of depressed immune functions was observed by some investigators.[7,8] The prompt recovery of T cells we observed[9] in two patients with severe infections and T cell defect favors thymus therapy. In these patients, following thymus transplantation, we noted an improvement of the clinical signs (infections, diarrhea, autoimmune hemolytic anemia) and of the laboratory data (normalization of Ig-E level and decreasing titers of antibody against Epstein-Barr virus which were consistently elevated for months before transplantation). In addition there was an increase of E rosette forming cells, a prompt response to PHA always absent before transplantation. One of these patients is still alive and normal after 3 years, the other developed a malignant B cell lymphoma and died after 2 years. We believe that high mortality in the non-transplanted patients, together with the low risks and recovery observed in most patients undergoing thymus transplantation, lead one to favor this approach.

Another approach for patients with T cell deficiency is therapy with thymic hormones. This therapy is justified by numerous experimental data. Several polypeptide factors have been isolated in the last ten years by A. Goldstein (thymosin),[10] G. Goldstein (thymin),[11] Trainin (thymic humoral factor),[12]

TABLE 3. Characteristics of immunological reconstitution after fetal thymus transplant (1968–1976)

Type of Deficiency	No. of Cases (alive)	P	NP	Partial	Total	Possible Mechanism	Methods	Onset of Immunity	Observ.
Di George	7 (6)	6	1	2	5	Thymic factor inducing maturity of thymic cells (?)	3 im 4 ip	Hours or few days	3 with Transfer Factor
Thymic hypoplasia with Ig (T cell deficit)	7 (5)	2	5	1	6	Thymic factor inducing maturity of T precursor cells (?)	4 im 3 ip	Hours few days or weeks	3 with Transfer Factor 1 BM
SCID	2 (2)		2	2	2	Cellular repopulation	ip	Weeks months	GVH, 1 Transfer Factor

P = permanent reconstitution
NP = not permanent
im = intramuscularly
ip = intraperitoneally
BM = Bone Marrow

and J. F. Bach (circulating thymic factors).[13] These factors were capable of restoring cellular immunity in thymectomized mice or modifying from − to + the mitogen and the MLC responsiveness and GVH-inducing capacity, or inducing in mice and in humans the appearance of theta or T cell markers in precursor T cells incubated with some of these extracts.[10,13,14,15,16,17]

However the mechanism by which T cell differentiation occurs and cellular immunity is restored is still obscure. A few preliminary clinical trials have been made recently in various centers using A.L. Goldstein thymosin, by Goldstein[10] and Wara.[17] The most clearcut effects bear on the *in vivo* correction of low E rosette values, similar to what has been shown in *in vitro* experiments. In some patients there was also clinical benefit.

Because we observed several patients with primary T cell deficiency and severe infections, and because of the good results obtained *in vitro* in inducing T cell differentiation,[18] we treated patients seriously ill with T cell deficiencies. Calf thymus extract was given at 1 mg/kg/day for one week and then twice a week for several months. The thymus extract was prepared in the laboratory of Serono Institute, Friburg, as follows. The crude precipitate obtained by ammonium acetate and ammonium sulphate was purified by gel filtration on Sephadex G-50, and the fractions were desalted and lyophilized. Upon electrophoresis on polyacrylamide gel at pH 8.3, one of the active fractions revealed two characteristic bands: one with an Rf of 0.22 and the other with an Rf of 0.42. Their molecular weights, evaluated by gel filtration on Sephadex G-50, were less than 10,000. The thymus extract was capable of stimulating cord blood lymphocytes to form rosettes, of modifying mouse spleen lymphocytes' reactivity to mitogen stimulation, and of stimulating immature lymphoid cells to induce an *in vivo* GVH reaction in mice.[19] The extract did not cause any acute toxic effects when administered to mice in doses of up to 100 mg/Kg, and did not alter the neuromuscular transmission.[19]

We treated six infants with T cell deficiency and severe infections of respiratory and gastrointestinal tracts, diarrhoea and failure to thrive with this extract. In all these patients a deficit of T cell markers as detected by E rosette forming cells and absence of or reduced response to PHA were present. After thymosin therapy marked clinical improvement and regression of infections were observed in 5 of these patients. One infant died, however, with acute pneumonia after three months of immunotherapy. In all six treated patients, we documented an increase of T peripheral blood lymphocytes (absolute number and percentage of E rosette forming cells) and in 4 of 6 children a conversion from − to + of the PHA response *in vitro*. The immunological parameters of one of these patients are reported in Fig. 1.

The therapy was performed in 5 patients for six months. After 4–5 months

336   F. Aiuti *et al.*

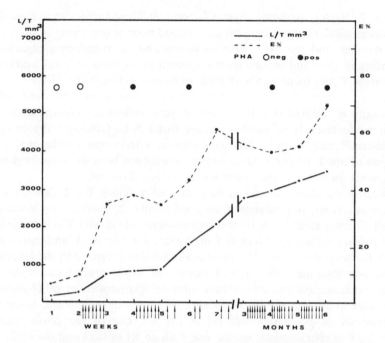

Fɪɢ. 1.   Represents the immunological parameters of a patient with
T cell deficit before, during and after therapy with thymic-extract.
L = lymphocytes/mm³ in peripheral blood; E% = percentage of
lymphocytes forming E rosettes; PHA = response *in vitro* of lymphocytes
to PHA. In these experiments we consider the response negative when the
stimulation index is less than 5 and positive more than 10; ↑ indicate
thymosin injection (1 mg/kg/day)

of interruption, the clinical situation as well as the immunological data were
normal. On two occasions we observed that interruption of the therapy for
two weeks during the first two months was followed by a decrease of all immunological parameters which promptly reconstituted after thymosin re-
injection.

Our clinical and experimental trial suggests that some patients with T cell
deficiency have an absence of thymic hormone that can be corrected by
substitutive therapy.

Against these positive results, thymosin therapy was found useful neither
clinically nor immunologically in two patients with SCID, in three with
common variable hypagammaglobulinemia, and in one with Wiskott-Aldrich
syndrome (Table 4).

TABLE 4. Results of treatment with thymosin of patients with various forms of immunodeficiencies

Type of ID	No. of patients	Clinical benefits	Immunological improvement
SCID (ADA + with B cell)	1	no	none
SCID (ADA + without T and B cell)	1	no	none
Common variable hypogammaglobulinemia (1 with associated T cell defect)	3	no	none
Wiskott-Aldrich	1	?	yes
T cell deficiencies	6	yes in 5	yes in all

These negative data obtained in several immunodeficiency syndromes using thymosin therapy have shown the possibility of biological factors other than thymosin exerting influence on the development of lymphoid stem cells.

In conclusion, due to the scarce preliminary clinical data in our and other centers, it is too early to interpret these results or to consider them conclusive. It is necessary to obtain other data from random trials using standardized preparations of thymosin with a well-defined half life. Additional knowledge of the chemistry of the various samples of thymic hormones is still required as far as the clinical utility of recognizing and defining variants of SCID and related syndromes are concerned.

Abbreviations

SCID = severe combined immunodeficiency
GVH = Graft versus host reaction
PHA = phytohemaglutinin
NP = Nucleoside phosphorylase
CMV = Cytomegalovirus
T-D = Thymus-dependent
CVH = Common variable hypogammaglobulinemia
ADA = Adenosine Deamirase
NP = Nucleoside Phosphoribose

REFERENCES

1. Lawlor, G. J., Ammann, A. J., Wright W. C., et al.: The syndrome of cellular immunodeficiency with immunoglobulins. J. Pediat. 84:183, 1974.
2. Aiuti, F., Businco, L., Griscelli, C., et al.: Improvement in methods for identifying patients with severe combined immunodeficiencies and related syndromes. Z. Immun. Forsch. 153, 95, 1977.

338 F. Aiuti et al.

3. Groshong, T., Horowitz, S., Lovchik, J., et al.: Chronic cytomegalovirus infection, immunodeficiency and monoclonal gammopathy-antigen-driven malignancy. J. Pediat. 88:217, 1976.
4. Businco, L., Rezza, E., and Aiuti, F.: Thymic aplasia with T lymphocytes. in preparation.
5. Ammann, A. J., Wara, D. W., Doyle, N. E., et al.: Thymus transplantation in patients with thymic hypoplasia and abnormal immunoglobulin synthesis. Transplantation 20:457, 1975.
6. Bach, J. F.: Thymic hormones. Immunol. Immunopathol 5:iii, 1976.
7. Gatti, R. A., Gershanik, J. J., LevKoff, A. H., et al.: DiGeorge syndrome associated with combined immunodeficiency. J. Pediat. 81:920, 1972.
8. Aiuti, F. and Calvani, M.: unpublished observations.
9. Aiuti, F., Businco, L., and Gatti, R.: Reconstitution of T cell disorders following thymus transplantation. Birth defects: Original Article Series, Vol. XI, No. 1, p. 370, 1975.
10. Goldstein, A., Thurman, G. B., Cohen, G. H., et al.: Biological Activities of Thymic Hormone (D. W. Van Bekkum ed.), p. 173, 1975.
11. Goldstein, G.: Isolation of bovine thymin: A polypeptide hormone of the thymus. Nature 274:11, 1974.
12. Trainin, N., Small, M., Zipori, D., et al.: Biological activities of thymic hormone. (D. W. Van Bekkum ed.), p. 117, 1975.
13. Bach, J. F., Dardenne, M. and Salomon, J. C.: Studies on thymus products. Absence of serum thymic activity in adult NZB and (NZB-NZW) mice. Clin. Exper. Immunol. 14:247, 1973.
14. Incefy, G. S., L'Esperance, P., and Good, R. A.: In vitro differentiation of human marrow cells into T lymphocytes by thymic extracts using the rosette technique. Clin. Exper. Immunol. 19:475, 1975.
15. Touraine, J. L., Touraine, F., Outruge, J., et al.: T lymphocytes precursors and T lymphocyte differentiation in partial Di George syndrome. Clin. Exper. Immunol. 21:39, 1975.
16. Komuro, K. and Boyse, E. A.: In vitro demonstration of thymic hormone in the mouse by conversion of precursor cells into lymphocytes. Lancet 1:740, 1973.
17. Wara, D. W., Goldstein, A. L., Doyle, N. E., et al.: Thymosin activity in patients with cellular immunodeficiency. N. Engl. J. Med. 292:70, 1975.
18. Aiuti, F., Schirrmacher, V., Ammirati, P., et al.: Effect of thymus factor on human precursor T lymphocytes. Clin. Exper. Immunol. 20:499, 1975.
19. Falchetti, R. Bergesi, G. and Caprino, L.: Isolation, partial characterization, and biological effects of a calf-thymus factor. IIIrd European Immunology meeting, Copenhagen, 1976.

DISCUSSION

Dr. SELIGMANN: I think your results are very interesting, but what I would like to ask you more precisely is where you try to draw the borderline between T-cell deficiency with immunoglobulin, and combined immunodeficiency? It is well known that in Nezelof's syndrome, if you look for humoral immunity, you find a very important defect of humoral immunity for various antigens which, of course, might be just the consequence of the absence of helper T-cells and so on, but this is not absolutely sure. There is really, in the few patients with the so-called Nezelof syndrome who have been well studied, one was by Hitzig's group and others, there was an important defect in humoral immunity after vaccination and so on. On the other hand, in SCID, we have cases with B-lymphocytes, and cases of B-lymphocytes and IgM, and cases of B-lymphocytes and IgM and some IgG and IgA, and so I think it is very important, especially in view of what you show about the effect, the *in vivo* effect of thymic factors which seem to operate only in one category. On the other hand if you could explain to us where you put the borderline for what you call T-cell deficiency, or pure T-cell deficiency with Ig.

Dr. AIUTI: This is the same question that I have put yesterday to another speaker about the confusion in the classification of severe combined immunodeficiency. I think that we must now start to differentiate patients with classical severe combined immunodeficiency in whom there is no evidence of antibody synthesis, in whom there is no evidence of, at least, normal immunoglobulin production. In patients that we presented in the first table, 10 patients, we observed low T-cell number, absence of blastogenic response or MLC response, but with normal immunoglobulin level, normal B-lymphocytes and with normal antibody production after injection with typhoid antigen and with tetanus, while we have never found in patients with severe combined immunodeficiency. In addition, we also had other details from a histological point of view and we think that in patients with T-cell deficiency the depletion of lymph nodes, the B area, is not so severe as in severe combined immunodeficiency. We have done extensive study with Baroni and we found in almost all of the cases the presence of follicles, and plasma cells in lymph nodes and tonsils, contrarily to the disorganisation of the lymph node architecture in severe combined immunodeficiency. Of course, I agree with you that the distinction is very, very difficult.

Dr. SELIGMANN: I am sorry if you spoke about that on Monday and I asked you again today, because I was not here on Monday, but I would agree with you, and I understand it perfectly except probably for putting the so-called Nezelof's syndrome in your list of purity cell deficiencies. I think this may be confusing because as far as I know in these cases the histology is not the one you describe in your purity cell deficiencies, and I think it can get confusing to put Nezelof's syndrome in the same bag.

Dr. AIUTI: I put severe combined immunodeficiency with related syndromes, but I put in parenthesis also some patients who have demonstrated some B-cell functions, some defect in antibody synthesis, but I agree, I think we could wait to speak tomorrow about this.

The Use of Lymphoblastoid Cell Lines
for DW Typing
Primed Lymphocyte Testing
and Biased Responders*

Richard A. GATTI,** Nancy REINSMOEN,*** Erik A. J. SVEDMYR,† and
Wolfgang LEIBOLD†

INTRODUCTION

We have shown that DW typing can be accomplished by utilizing lympho-blastoid cell lines (LCL) from HLA-D homozygous persons to replace conventional peripheral blood lymphocyte (PBL) typing cells in mixed leukocyte cultures (MLC).[1,2] By this method, typing responses are comparable in strength to that of autologous responses whereas non-typing responses are much stronger.

LCL cells can also be utilized in primed lymphocyte (PL) experiments, either as primary[3] or secondary stimulators. When LCL cells are utilized for secondary stimulation of primed lymphocytes, an autologous stimulation of the primed lymphocyte is not observed (unless priming was against an autologous cell) and responses to LCL cells of third parties are very low or absent unless they share a pertinent antigenic determinant with the primary stimulator cell.[4] In this report, we present data utilizing an HLA-D homozygous cell panel for DW typing with primed lymphocytes.

The methods used in these studies have been published elsewhere.[3,4] When not specified, primed lymphocyte cultures were terminated after 48 hours' incubation. All cultures were pulsed for 18 hours prior to termination.

*   This work was supported by the Amie Karen Cancer Fund, NCI Grant No. R01 CA18892–01 and USPHS Grant 5P01-CA-16042/02.
**   Cedars-Sinai Medical Center, Department of Pediatric Hematology, Oncology and Immunology, Los Angeles, California, U.S.A.
*** University of Minnesota Hospitals, Department of Laboratory Medicine, Minneapolis, Minnesota, U.S.A.
†   Karolinska Institute, Department of Tumor Biology, Stockholm, Sweden
†   Institut für Pathologie der Tierarztlichen Hochschule, Hannover, West Germany

RESULTS

1. Priming with LCL cells versus PBL cells

As can be seen in Table 1, priming with LCL cells gives results comparable to priming with PBL cells from the same typing donor. In this experiment, PBL and LCL cells from a homozygous DW2 donor were used to prime two persons. The primed lymphocytes were then restimulated with six HLA-D homozygous LCL cells, including the positive control, LCL–17. The strongest responses (cpm) observed for both donors were to LCL–17. Note also that primed cells from both donors appeared to cross-react with LCL–18 (DW8) and LCL–21 (DW?). Such cross-reactions do not appear to be any more or less common when LCL cells are utilized for priming than when PBL cells are used.

TABLE 1.   Comparison of primary stimulation by PBL vs. LCL cells*

Secondary		$R_1 \times 17m$		$R_2 \times 17m$	
Stimulators	DW	PBL–17m	LCL–17m	PBL–17m	LCL–17m
LCL–17	2	22035(3.80)	17191(1.19)	19024(2.56)	20473(2.57)
18	8	7766(.97)	12875(1.70)	5241(.41)	NT
19	?	1567(.30)	2057(.45)	1179(.17)	1724(.35)
20	?	512(.18)	645(.27)	NT	NT
21	?	16992(2.93)	13402(1.03)	8641(.69)	13019(1.38)
24	7	8026(.51)	12986(.70)	2344(.04)	10087(.63)

* Results given in cpm with Interaction Indices in parentheses

2. Absence of "autologous stimulation" after priming

Figure 1 depicts the responses of two responders (ES and RG) primed against third party cells. Note that when autologous LCL cells were utilized as secondary stimulators, almost no response was observed (arrows). This fact is of utmost importance in attempting to define specificities and allelic splits by restimulating with HLA-D homozygous LCL cells.

3. Kinetics of primed lymphocyte responses

When primed lymphocyte (PL) testing is limited to cultures terminated at one point only (usually 48 hours) results may be misleading. Three types of curves are commonly observed: 1) a peak at 48 hours, usually the most specific of PL reactions; 2) a peak at 72 hours, often to a cross-reacting specificity (but not always; as evidenced in B of Figure 2 by the 72 hour peak of an anti-DW1 PL to a DW1 line, LCL–15) and 3) a peak at 48 hours followed by an upswing of the response curve: This probably represents the beginning of a second primary response (*e.g.* Fig. 2: the responses in A) to LCL–11 and in

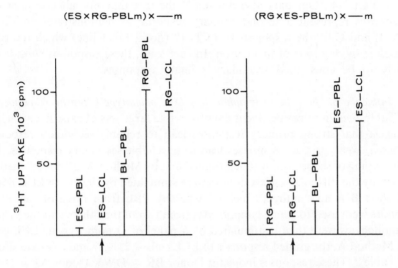

FIG. 1. Bar graphs represent responses of two primed lymphocyte combinations against PBL and LCL cells from autologous, pertinent and non-pertinent donors.
Note that autologous LCL cells do not stimulate autologous primed lymphocytes (arrows) as they would stimulate non-primed lymphocytes.

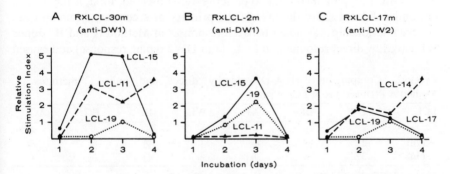

FIG. 2. Three combinations of primed lymphocytes were restimulated with LCL cells carrying pertinent and non-pertinent alleles.
Cultures were terminated on days 1, 2, 3 or 4 of incubation. Several types of curves were observed. See text for discussion.

C to LCL–14.) Our data also document the fact that not all cross-reacting responses represent a second primary response as demonstrated in Figure 2A, B and C by the responses to LCL–19 (not a DW1 line) which return to baseline by day four of incubation. In each case, these responses subside too early to be considered secondary primary responses.

4. Influence of the primed lymphocyte's DW phenotype ("biased responders")

Table 2 summarizes pertinent data from two large sets of experiments which suggest that strong primary responses lead to reliable secondary responses whereas weak primary responses lead to unreliable secondary responses. The DW typing of six persons was determined first by Method A, a "direct" method whereby the PBL of these six donors were stimulated by the entire LCL panel. Method B is an "indirect" method whereby PBL from three of the above donors were used to prime lymphocytes from two of the others and the primed lymphocytes were then restimulated by a panel of D homozygous LCL cells. In Method A, the graded responses to LCL cells −2, −17 and −14 are shown in Table 2. These responses indicate: Donor BR = DW3, Donor AJ = DW1, Donor WL = DW2 and Donor IL = DW1. The DW typing of EG and AJ was not apparent and did not appear to be DW1, 2 or 3. (These DW types were confirmed by more extensive testing using conventional and LCL typing methods).

When the above results were compared to those obtained using Method B, the "indirect" typing method, two patterns were observed. First, if the primed responder did not share the DW of the primary or secondary stimulator, an inverse relationship was noted between responses in Method A and B: donor WL gave low direct responses to LCL–17 (a DW2 typing response) and caused

TABLE 2. Comparison of HLA-D typing by "direct" and "indirect" methods
Method A ("Direct") R × LCLm panel

LCL	DW	BR	AJ	WL	IL	EG	AG
—2m	1	⫴	+	⫴	⧺	⫴	⧺
—17m	2	⫴	⫴	+	⫴	⫴	⫴
—14m	3	+	⫴	⫴	⫴	⫴	⫴

Method B ("Indirect") Q × Rm   10 days (Q × Rm) × LCLm panel

LCL DW		(BR × WLm)	(BR × ILm)	(BR × EGm)	(AJ × EGm)	(AJ × AGm)	(AJ × ILm)
— 2m	1	6278	19645	3468	9276*	14332*	10625*
—17m	2	16458	3840	3408			
—14m	3	23628*	10086*	4461*	26820	20625	23147

* primed lymphocyte was biased?

high responses of [BR × WLm] × LCL–17m in Method B. Similarly, Donor IL gave low responses to LCL2 in Method A and caused high responses of [BR × ILm] × LCL−2m in Method B. Conversely, WL gave high direct responses to LCL–2 (a non-typing response for DW1) and caused low indirect responses of [RB × WLm] × LCL−2m in Method B. IL gave high direct responses to LCL–17 and was associated with low indirect responses of [BR × ILm] × LCLm.

A second pattern was observed when the responding cell shared the DW allele of either the primary or the secondary responder. In general, this reaction was difficult to interpret, unreliable and showed no concordance between Methods A and B. Note, for example, the failure of AJ, who was DW1 by "direct" testing, to identify IL as DW1 by "indirect" testing. Note also that BR, who gave only a weak direct response to LCL–14, responds in Method B with a pattern which suggests that WL is DW3: This was contrary to WL's typing by Method A (as well as by conventional methods). These data suggest that AJ and BR were "biased responders" in the two above examples.

In another set of experiments, the specificity of primed lymphocytes again seemed to depend to some degree upon the genetic background of the cells being primed. Two donors, neither of which was DW1 or 2 by conventional testing, were primed against three homozygous LCL cells: LCL–30 and LCL–2 were DW1; LCL–17 was DW2. The responses are summarized in Figure 3.

When R1 was primed with LCL–30, the anti-DW1 primed lymphocyte recognized the positive control and the other two DW1 lines in the panel. They also responded somewhat to LCL–34, a homozygous typing cell which may be DW3. They failed to respond to five other LCL cells representing DW alleles 2 and 3. In the same experiment, another donor was primed against the same LCL–30 line. These anti-DW1 primed responses were less discriminatory in that they failed to recognize the positive control (LCL–30) and cross-reacted to some extent with DW3. Nonetheless, the strongest response was still against a DW1 line. When these same donors were primed against another DW1 line (LCL–2), the results were similar. R1 gave better discrimination than R2; however, R1 failed to recognize one DW1 line (LCL–30), suggesting that the DW1 allele of primary stimulator (LCL–2) may be "shorter" than the DW1 of LCL–30.

These same donors were also primed against a DW2 homozygous line (LCL–17). In this case, discrimination of both donors' primed lymphocytes was very good. It is not clear why neither primed responder recognized LCL–26, which is thought to be DW2 and possibly homozygous at this locus. Taken together, these results suggest that while both responders R1 and R2 were capable of being primed against a DW2 allele, priming against DW1 alleles

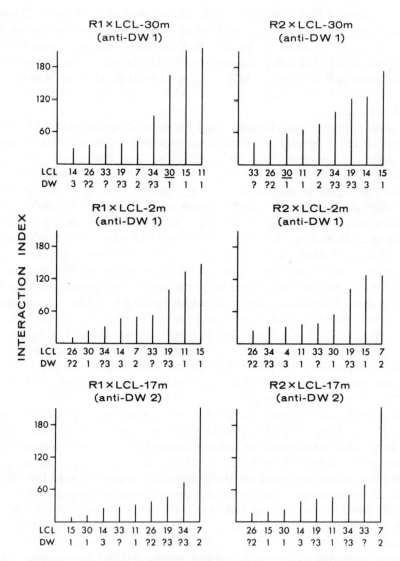

FIG. 3.   Six combinations of primed lymphocytes were re-stimulated with a panel of LCL cells containing pertinent and non-pertinent DW alleles.
See text for discussion.

was more definitive with R1 than with R2. R2 may represent another example of a "biased responder" for priming against DW1-related specificities.

DISCUSSION

In preliminary investigations with primed lymphocytes, we have demonstrated that LCL cells derived from HLA-D homozygous typing donors provide a valuable tool with which to further define HLA-D alleles. The LCL cells can be utilized either for primary or secondary stimulation or both. The supply of these cells for such experiments is unlimited. The absence of autologous secondary stimulation to primed lymphocytes allows for discrimination to DW alleles. Since LCL cells for primary or secondary stimulation are stored directly in culture plates, it is not a difficult task to test each responder primed against a large LCL typing panel, thereby minimizing problems with "biased responders." Our panel presently consists of over 40 homozygous lines and for "direct method" typing we require 6×10^6. Similar experiments can be performed in other laboratories by shipping the LCL typing plates. In fact, experiments reported herein were performed jointly between Minneapolis and Los Angeles by shipping either fresh LCL cells for primary stimulation or the LCL typing plates for secondary stimulation.

Theoretically, by this approach it should be possible to: 1) DW type, 2) define allelic splits and 3) characterize new alleles. In fact, when PL results have been compared to those of conventional "negative response" typing, previously excluded DW alleles have been noted in some persons typed by conventional methods.[5] R2 in Fig. 3 may be a case in point since PL data suggest that she shares a DW1 allele while conventional testing concludes that she is not DW1. In addition, when negative response typing is performed with PBL and LCL cells from the same typing donors, occasional typing responses are noted with LCL typing cells, but not with comparable PBL typing cells.[6] Cross-reactions have also been noted by most investigators. While the basis of these cross-reactions is as yet unclear, several factors appear to influence the specificity of primed lymphocyte reactions. First, the length of secondary incubation appears important, as described in Section 3 above. Termination of cultures at only 48 hours can be misleading, although this appears to be the time for best discrimination if only one point is to be measured. PL reactions have very dynamic kinetics.[3]

A second factor which influences the specificity of the PL reaction is the genetic background of the lymphocyte population to be primed. Stated another way: If there has been no primary response, a secondary response should not be expected. For this reason, we include direct "negative response" testing against our LCL Panel as a control for the lymphocyte to be primed. Persons who give weak responses to a particular line give secondary responses to that line which are unreliable and bear little or no relationship to the known DW alleles of the primary stimulating cell. We suggest that such donors represent "biased responders" for the pertinent allele. Conversely, persons showing strong (non-typing) primary responses to a particular line give secondary responses which clearly define pertinent DW alleles on the primary stimulator cells.

When typing is performed by both the "direct" (R × LCLm) and "indirect" ([Q × Rm] × LCLm) methods, an inverse relationship in the responses is noted, provided that "biased responders" are excluded: if R responds strongly to a particular LCL, [Q × Rm] responds poorly to that same LCL; whereas if R responds weakly in the "direct" method (i.e., a typing response), in the "indirect" method [Q × Rm] responds strongly to that LCL (i.e., again, a typing responder). The "indirect" typing approach may be especially useful in typing patients with severely depressed or absent T lymphocyte function, such as patients with severe combined immunodeficiency disease. When used in conjunction with a large LCL typing panel, the combined data of "direct" and "indirect" typing methods may provide for more reliable DW typing than with conventional methods alone. However, because the "indirect" method must include more than one primed responder for each person to be typed (we prefer three responders), it does not appear to be a practical approach for large family or population studies and is probably best reserved for defining "allelic splits."

REFERENCES

1. Svedmyr, E. A. J., Leibold, W., and Gatti, R. A.: Possible use of established cell lines for MLR locus typing. Tissue Antigens. 5:186, 1975.
2. Gatti, R. A., Leibold, W., Netzel, B., and Svedmyr, E. A. J.: The use of lymphoblastoid cell lines for HLA-D locus typing. Proc. First HLA Workshop of the Americas (R. J. Duquesnoy, ed.), J. C. Fuller, Publ. DHEW Publication No. 76-1064, pg. 160, 1976.
3. Reinsmoen, N., Yunis, E. J., Bach, F. H., and Bach. M. L.: Lymphoblastoid cell lines of homozygous typing cells used for sensitization in PLT. Tissue Antigens. 9:11, 1977.
4. Svedmyr, E. A. J.: Long-term maintenance in vitro of human T cells by repeated exposure to the same stimulator cells. Scand. J. Immunol. 4:421, 1975.
5. van Rood, J. J., van Leuwen, A., Persijn, G. G., et al.: Transplant. Proc. 9:459,1977.

6. Gatti, R. A., Svedmyr, E. A. J. and Leibold, W.: Dissociation of MLC responses to peripheral lymphocytes versus established cells from an HLA-D homozygous typing donor. *Vox Sanguinis* (submitted).

DISCUSSION

Dr. COOPER: I would just like to ask for my own edification whether the antibody that reacts with B-cell determinants and monocyte determinates is directed toward the products of the D-locus. Do they not block the MLC response, and how do they correlate with this kind of typing?

Dr. GATTI: The evidence suggests that many of the B-cell alloantigens are similar to DW alleles, but by no means all of them. Anti-HLA antisera would inhibit MLC. We have sera that are wholly against B-cell alloantigens (they merit antisera) and do not contain HLA-A and-B antibodies: they inhibit MLC markedly. What we do not know is whether the original studies that told us HLA-A and-B antisera inhibit MLC are still valid, or do those sera contain antibodies to B-cell antigens as well, and was that what was blocking the MLC? No one has really answered that question yet.

Experimental Models for Prevention of Graft-versus-Host Reaction in Bone Marrow Transfusion

Sumio MIYAZAKI, Kikuo NOMOTO, Ataru KUROIWA, Nagahide GOYA, and Kenji TAKEYA

ABSTRACT

Induction and suppression of splenomegaly and cytotoxicity against C57BL/6 cells were studied in ABF1 hybrid adult mice after the transfer of AKR lymphoid and bone marrow cells.

1) Splenomegaly and cytotoxicity were dissociated in the developmental stages of GVH reaction. When lymphoid and bone marrow cells of normal AKR mice were injected into F1 recipients, splenomegaly was prominent on days 5 and 7, but cytotoxicity of spleen cells was not detected. Splenomegaly became less prominent but the cytotoxicity became detectable on day 14 after the injection.

2) Cytotoxic activity of spleen cells of F1 recipients was suppressed by treatment of AKR donors with C57BL/6 lymphoid cells in FCA. Splenomegaly, however, was substantially enhanced by such treatment of the donors. On the other hand, induction of cytotoxic activity was facilitated by treatment of donors with C57BL/6 skin grafts.

3) F1 hybrid mice could be protected from GVH reaction by the injection of AKR anti-C57BL/6 serum or pretreatment of AKR donors with sonicated cellular antigens of C57BL/6.

4) When AKR donors were obtained 12 hours after treatment with C57BL/6 cells in FCA or later, splenomegaly was augmented but cytotoxicity was suppressed. When the transfer was carried out at stages as early as 3 or 6 hours, cytotoxicity was enhanced but splenomegaly was suppressed. Some irreversible differentiation of lymphocytes appears to occur 12 hours after such treatment.

Departments of Pediatrics and Microbiology, Faculty of Medicine, Kyushu University, Fukuoka, Japan

INTRODUCTION

Transfusion of the bone marrow cells from donors carrying serologically-defined and lymphocyte-defined histocompatibility antigens identical with those of the recipients seems to be one of the best ways to prevent graft-versus-host (GVH) reaction. However, selection of such histocompatible combinations of donors and recipients may not be possible in every case. In many cases, bone marrow may become available from donors carrying some histocompatibility antigens which are non-identical with those of the recipients. Experimental models suitable for establishment of methods to prevent GVH reaction in such a situation may be useful.

One of the prominent features in systemic GVH reaction is splenomegaly.[1] It has been assumed to depend not only upon the proliferation of donor cells but also accumulation of host cells.[2] Another prominent feature is runt disease, which consists of reduction in body weight or retardation of growth and other systemic illness in the host. In order to efficiently suppress GVH reaction in bone marrow transfusion, relationships between these cellular events have to be understood as precisely as possible. The experimental models capable of selectively suppressing or augmenting these individual events shown in this paper may be valuable tools for this purpose.

MATERIALS AND METHODS

Animals.   Inbred mice of AKR and C57BL/6 strains were obtained from the breeding unit of Kyushu University School of Medicine. Fl hybrids between AKR and C57BL/6 (ABF1) were raised in our laboratory. Female AKR mice 8 weeks of age were used as donors and ABF1 mice 6 weeks of age were used as recipients.

Preparation of cell suspensions.   Spleens and cervical, axillary, inguinal and mesenteric lymph nodes were removed and squeezed with 2 glass slides in Hanks' balanced salt solution (HBSS) in petri dishes. The femurs were removed and both ends were cut by scissors. The marrow was flushed out with HBSS using a syringe equipped with a Mantoux needle. Cell suspension of methylcholanthrene (MCA)-induced sarcoma of C57BL/6 origin was prepared by trypsinization of small fragments according to the conventional method.

Preparation of anti-C57BL/6 serum.   AKR mice were subcutaneously injected with 3×10^7 lymphoid cells of C57BL/6 mice in Freund's complete adjuvant (FCA). Intraperitoneal injections with 1×10^7 lymphoid cells in saline were carried out 6 times daily every 4 days with an interval of 2 weeks from the primary immunization. The blood was harvested 5 days after the last immunization.

Conditioning of donors. Normal Fl mice were used as donors in control groups. AKR donors included the following 4 groups: a) Non-treated AKR mice; b) AKR mice intravenously injected twice a week and intraperitoneally twice a week with sonicated cellular antigen of C57BL/6 mice; c) AKR mice transplanted with skin grafts from C57BL/6 mice and used as donors 7 days later when the development of cytotoxicity proved to reach a plateau; and d) AKR mice with lymphoid cells 2×10^6 of C57BL/6 mice in FCA subcutaneously injected into both sides of the flank and used as donors 3, 6, 12, 24 and 72 hours later.

Splenomegaly. Donor cells were the mixed cell population consisting of 1.5×10^7 lymphoid cells and 1.0×10^7 bone marrow cells. Donor cells were intravenously injected into ABFl recipients and spleens were removed 5, 7 and 14 days later. The spleen index represented the ratio of the spleen weight (relative to body weight) of the treated animals to the spleen weight (relative to body weight) of the controls treated with an equivalent number of syngeneic Fl lymphoid cells.[1]

Cytotoxicity test. Spleens were removed from the recipients 5, 10 or 14 days after the injection of donor cells. Cell suspensions were prepared as described above. Spleen cell suspensions were treated with 1/4-diluted anti-C57BL/6 serum and rabbit complement at 37°C for 30 min in order to eliminate the recipient cells carrying $H-2^b$ antigens. After washing, 1.25×10^7 viable spleen cells were added to 5×10^5 MCA tumor cells of C57BL/6 origin and the mixture was subcutaneously injected into the AKR mice exposed to 500 R of whole-body irradiation. Tumor growth was measured 7 days after the injection and tumor size was recorded as an area (mm^2) of the largest diameter times the smallest diameter.

RESULTS

Suppression and augmentation of splenomegaly by various treatments.

Spleen indices were determined 5, 7 and 14 days after the injection of mixed AKR cells into Fl recipients (Table 1). Splenomegaly was detected on days 5, 7 and 14 after the injection of mixed cells from normal AKR mice, although it was more remarkable on days 5 and 7 than on day 14. When 0.1 ml of of antiC57BL/6 serum was intravenously injected, together with normal AKR cells, splenomegaly was not detectable on days 5, 7 and 14. When AKR donors had been pretreated with sonicated cellular antigens of C57BL/6 mice, spleens

354 S. Miyazaki *et al.*

TABLE 1. Suppression and augmentation of splenomegaly by treatment of donors or recipients

Treatment of Donors	Treatment of Recipients	Days after Transfusion	Spleen Index of Recipients FI[a]	Number of Recipients
Syngeneic F1	None	5	1.00 ± 0.07	10
		7	1.00 + 0.09	10
		14	1.00 ± 0.08	10
Normal AKR	None	5	1.42 ± 0.27	10
		7	1.53 ± 0.28	35
		14	1.25 ± 0.24	25
Normal AKR	Anti C57BL/6 Serum 0.1 ml	5	1.02 ± 0.10	10
		7	1.06 ± 0.11	15
		14	1.07 ± 0.15	15
AKR Pretreated with Solubilized C57BL/6 Cells	None	5	0.98 ± 0.11	10
		7	0.96 ± 0.10	15
		14	0.97 ± 0.09	10
AKR Grafted with C57BL/6 Skin	None	5	1.03 ± 0.12	10
		7	1.01 ± 0.12	20
		14	0.86 ± 0.10	10
AKR Pretreated with C57BL/6 Cells in FCA	None	5	1.59 ± 0.29	10
		7	1.74 ± 0.32	15
		14	1.46 ± 0.21	10

a) Average values of 10 to 35 animals ± standard error

of recipients did not enlarge on days 5, 7 and 14. Splenomegaly was also suppressed by pretreatment of AKR donors with C57BL/6 skin grafts. However, splenomegaly was augmented when AKR mice pretreated with C57BL/6 cells in FCA were used as donors 3 days later.

Suppression and facilitation of cytotoxic activity of spleen cells by various treatments. Cytotoxic activity of spleen cells against the host antigens (H–2^b) was assessed by *in vivo* neutralization test on days 5 and 14 after injection of donor cells (Table 2). In the presence of cytotoxic activity, growth of indicator tumors was suppressed. When mixed cells of F1 hybrid were injected into F1 recipients, their spleen cells did not exibit cytotoxicity and indicator tumors grew progressively. When mixed cells of normal AKR mice were injected into F1 recipients, cytotoxic activity of spleen cells was detected on day 14, but not on day 5. Cytotoxic activity was not raised on days 5 and 14 in the recipients who received normal AKR cells and anti-C57BL/6 serum or mixed cells from the AKR mice pretreated with sonicated cellular antigens of C57BL/6 mice. Cytotoxic activity of spleen cells was suppressed by treatment of AKR donors with C57BL/6 lymphoid cells in FCA in the presence of

TABLE 2. Suppression and facilitation of cytotoxicity by treatments of donors or hosts

Treatment of Donors	Treatment of Recipients	Cytotoxicity of Spleen Cells in FI Recipients	
		5 days after injection	14 days after injection
Syngeneic FI	None	35.4 ± 27.9(−)[a]	33.4 ± 11.6(−)[a]
Normal AKR	None	38.4 ± 26.6(−)	10.6 ± 5.2(+) (p < 0.01)
Normal AKR	Anti C57BL/6 serum 0.1 ml	34.4 ± 13.5(−)	33.9 ± 19.5(−)
AKR pretreated with solubilized C57BL/6 cells	None	35.7 ± 19.5(−)	33.6 ± 18.2(−)
AKR grafted with C57BL/6 skin	None	2.3 ± 2.0(+) (p < 0.01)	3.5 ± 3.0(+) (p < 0.01)
AKR pretreated with C57BL/6 cells in FCA	None	41.5 ± 13.5(−)	40.0 ± 21.1(−)
Control		38.2 ± 18.5	42.0 ± 22.1 (controls inoculated with tumor cell alone)

a) Growth of indicator tumors expressed as areas of the largest diameter times the smallest diameter (mm²). The values represent average values of 10 to 15 animals and standard error.

remarkable splenomegaly. On the other hand, induction of cytotoxic activity was facilitated by treatment of AKR donors with C57BL/6 skin grafts.

Kinetics of irreversible differentiation of lymphocytes to effectors of splenomegaly. When donor cells were obtained from AKR mice at 3, 6, 12, 24 and 72 hours after treatment with C57BL/6 cells in FCA, the development of splenomegaly and cytotoxicity were modified as shown in Table 3. The development of cytotoxicity was enhanced when AKR donor cells were transfused 3 or 6 hours after the treatment. When AKR donor cells were transfused 12 hours after the treatment or later, cytotoxicity was not raised but splenomegaly was augmented.

DISCUSSION

The occurrence of splenomegaly precedes the appearance of cytotoxicity,

TABLE 3.   Enhancement and suppression of cytotoxicity and splenomegaly by treatment of donors with antigen in FCA at various times before cell transfer

Time after pretreatment of AKR with C57BL/6 cells in FCA	Spleen index of recipients Fl[a]		Cytotoxicity of spleen cells in Fl recipients[b]		
	5 days after injection	10 days after injection	5 days after injection	10 days after injection	Controls inoculated with tumor cell alone
3 hours	1.13 ± 0.12	1.15 ± 0.14	$12.2 \pm 6.1(+)$ $(p < 0.01)$	$14.5 \pm 6.5(+)$ $(p < 0.01)$	38.0 ± 10.2
6	1.17 ± 0.15	1.14 ± 0.13	$17.4 \pm 5.2(+)$ $(p < 0.01)$	$15.9 \pm 5.3(+)$ $(p < 0.01)$	30.0 ± 6.9
12	1.47 ± 0.26	1.32 ± 0.18	38.8 ± 12.5 $(-)$	42.5 ± 13.9 $(-)$	36.5 ± 8.9
24	1.61 ± 0.28	1.47 ± 0.25	45.5 ± 13.5 $(-)$	38.1 ± 11.5 $(-)$	43.9 ± 12.6
72	1.59 ± 0.29	1.60 ± 0.31	39.2 ± 10.8 $(-)$	45.8 ± 12.0 $(-)$	42.0 ± 15.5
Normal AKR	1.42 ± 0.27	1.49 ± 0.25	38.4 ± 26.6 $(-)$	12.0 ± 5.1 $(+) (p < 0.01)$	42.0 ± 22.1

a)   Average values of 5 to 10 animals $\pm$ standard error
b)   Growth of indicator tumors expressed as areas of the largest diameter times the smallest diameter (mm^2).
    The values represent average values of 5 to 10 animals and standard error.

when donor cells are obtained from normal AKR mice, as shown in Tables 1 and 2. Some portion of splenomegaly may depend upon proliferation of donor cells preceeding the appearance of cytotoxic lymphocytes, since elimination of dividing cells in early phases in mixed lymphocyte culture abolishes subsequent cytotoxic activity, as described by Cantor and Jandinski.[3]

Cytotoxic activity against host antigens is detectable at a relatively late stage after the injection of normal AKR cells, although no mortality is shown in this system. The cytotoxicity may be ascribed largely to cytotoxic T lymphocytes of donor origin. However, the possibility of contribution of host cells to nonspecific cytotoxicity cannot be excluded, as described by Singh, Sabbadini, and Sehon[4] and Ptak, Hanczakowska, and Skowron-Cendrzak.[5]

When the donors have been treated with skin grafts of C57BL/6 mice, cytotoxic activity becomes detectable at an early stage in Fl recipients in the absence of preceding splenomegaly. This may be due to the fact that a proliferative phase has already been achieved in the donors during the interval between skin grafting and transfusion of cells. However, another possibility which cannot be excluded is that skin grafting stimulates differentiation of a T cell subpopulation destined to be cytotoxic lymphocytes, but not proliferation of other T cell subpopulations, since cellular immune responses against allogeneic antigens have proved to be contributed to by distinct T cell subpopulations.[6,7,8,9]

Splenomegaly is augmented by 3-day immunization of donors with C57 BL/6 cells in FCA as shown in Table 1. This augmentation may be ascribed not only to an enhanced proliferation of primed donor cells but also to an accumulation of macrophages as an expression of a delayed hypersensitivity reaction. In such recipients exhibiting augmented splenomegaly, cytotoxicity was not detectable. In this experimental model, however, cytotoxicity was induced if pretreated AKR cells were transfused at stages as early as 3 or 6 hours after immunization as shown in Table 3. Within 6 hours after such stimulation, lymphocytes may be in the transitional state from which they can differentiate to killer cells in the presence of stimulation by viable cells in the recipients. After 12 hours of differentiation lymphocytes may be irreversibly destined to become the effector cells of splenomegaly.

Tigelaar and Gorczynski[10] have reported that delayed hypersensitivity and cytotoxicity are mediated by distinct subpopulations of T cells, and Henney, Gaffney, and Bloom[9] have reported that T cell-mediated cytolysis and production of chemical mediators can be dissociated by the use of inhibitors of protein synthesis.

Isoantibodies have been known to suppress the rejection of tumor allografts[11,12] or skin allografts.[13,14,15] This enhancement has been applied to protect the Fl recipients from GVH reaction by the transfer of parental lymphoid cells, as reported by Voisin, Kinsky, and Maillard,[16] and Jose, Stutman, and Good.[17] In the present study, splenomegaly and cytotoxicity do not occur in Fl recipients, when AKR donors have been immunized with sonicated cellular antigen of C57BL/6 mice as shown in Tables 1 and 2. The protective effects in our studies may be due to passive transfer of antibody-producing cells as described by Fink et al.[18]

In the systems presented herein, splenomegaly and cytotoxicity are selectively augmented or suppressed. Such systems may be useful for analytical studies on cellular traffic in GVH reaction and establishment of new methods to prevent GVH reaction from occurring in histo-incompatible recipients.

REFERENCES

1. Simonsen, M.: Graft-versus-host reactions. Their natural history and applicability as tools of research. *Progr. Allergy* **6**:349, 1962.
2. Howard, J. G., Michie, D., and Simonsen, M.: Splenomegaly as a host response in graft-versus-host disease. *Brit. J. Exp. Pathol.* **42**:478, 1961.

3. Cantor, H. and Jandinski, J.: The relationship of cell division to the generation of cytotoxic activity in mixed lymphocyte culture. *J. Exp. Med.* **140**:1712, 1974.
4. Singh, J. N., Sabbadini, E., and Sehon, A. H.: Cytotoxicity in graft-versus-host reaction. I. Role of donor and host spleen cells. *J. Exp. Med.* **136**:39, 1972.
5. Ptak, W., Hanczakowska, M., and Skowron-Cendrzak, A.: Cytotoxic macrophage in graft-versus-host reaction. *Transplantation* **19**:12, 1975.
6. Bach, F. H., Segall, M., Zier, K. S., *et al.*: Cell mediated immunity: Separation of cells involved in recognitive and destructive phases. *Science* **180**:403, 1973.
7. Cantor, H. and Asofsky, R.: Synergy among lymphoid cells mediating the graft-versus-host response. III. Evidence for interaction between two types of thymus-derived cells. *J. Exp. Med.* **135**:764, 1972.
8. Matter, A.: The differentiation pathway of T lymphocytes. Evidence for two differentiated cell types. *J. Exp. Med.* **140**:566, 1974.
9. Sabbadini, E.: Regulation of cell-mediated cytotoxicity. II. Synergism of two types of thymus dependent cells *in vivo*. *Cell Immunol.* **18**:76, 1975.
10. Tigelaar, R. E. and Gorczynski, R. M.: Separable populations of activated thymus-derived lymphocytes identified in two assays for cell-mediated immunity to murine tumor allografts. *J. Exp. Med.* **140**:267, 1974.
11. Kaliss, N.: Immunological enhancement of tumor homografts in mice: A review. *Cancer Research* **18**:992, 1958.
12. Snell, G. D., Winn, H. J., Stimpfling, J. H., *et al.*: Depression by antibody of the immune response to homografts and its role in immunological enhancement. *J. Exp. Med.* **112**:293, 1960.
13. Benkö, S., Lázár, G., Troján, I., *et al.*: Prolongation of skin graft survival using immune serum. *Nature* **226**:451, 1970.
14. Brautbar, C. H. and Nelken, D.: Passive immunological enhancement of skin allografts in rats. *Transplantation* **11**:135, 1971.
15. Nelson, D. S.: Immunological enhancement of skin homografts in guinea-pigs. *Brit. J. Exp. Pathol.* **43**:1, 1962.
16. Voisin, G. A., Kinsky, R., and Maillard, J.: Protection against homologous disease in hybrid mice by passive and active immunological enhancement-facilitation. *Transplantation* **6**:187, 1968.
17. Jose, D. G., Stutman, O., and Good, R. A.: Inhibition of graft-versus-host reactions in mice by host-directed antibody. *Transplantation* **17**:211, 1974.
18. Fink, M. P., Cloud, C. L., and McCarthy, K. F.: Local graft-versus-host reaction suppressed by immuno-blocking antibody secreted by antibody-forming cells transferred with the graft. *Cell Immunol.* **11**:74, 1974.

DISCUSSION

Dr. GOOD: How do you feel you can use this to obviate the GVH? It has long been known that if you have antisera in the system against the cells that you introduce, you will block the GVH, but the problem is, then you also destroy the stem cells, so you must have an antisera that dissects the population and will not attack the stem cells which have the alloantigens on their surface. The way we have approached this and have been getting around it has been to identify antigens that recognise this specific differentiation state.

Dr. MIYAZAKI: If you apply this experiment clinically, I will have very much difficulty in using it because as you pointed out the antiserum kills the normal cells.

V. GENERAL DISCUSSION AND SUMMARY

General Discussion

Dr. SELIGMANN

If Dr. Kobayashi agrees, maybe we could have a little general discussion now before going to some specific presentations on some of these topics which are planned for this morning and early afternoon. So that I think if we keep it as it stands here on the board, what I would like first to discuss is the very practical points raised by Dr. Hitzig about gammaglobulin therapy, and staying very practical, I think the first thing raised by him we could discuss would be the problem of treatment, or absence of treatment, of patients with selective IgA deficiency, and severe, rather severe, infections of the respiratory tract, for instance. I think this is a very important practical problem, and as he said, there are many drawbacks to treatment by gammaglobulins, and probably still more by rather more purified IgA preparations. It is mainly in these cases that therapy with plasma has been done by several groups, and I think it would be interesting to know what you think and what the group thinks about it. And especially, who are those who would treat rather easily patients with selective IgA deficiency, and of course, relatively serious infections of the respiratory tract, and of those which are asymptomatic? So I think that this would be the first point for discussion. Who wants to discuss this point?

Dr. COOPER

I have no answer to that problem. We have assiduously avoided giving any form of serum treatment to patients with IgA deficiency because of the occurrence in the past of anaphylaxis when serum was given containing IgA. So we have considered it important not to sensitize such patients to the possibility of anaphylaxis on exposure to IgA, and have not taken an open-minded view toward this question. It strikes me that that view is, as you pointed out, no longer satisfactory. One has to begin to consider other possibilities. Some of these patients do indeed have very severe infections, frequent ones; although they are not always life-threatening, some are. I think that it has been demonstrated, at least to my satisfaction in a few patients, that these patients were not always just deficient in their ability to make IgA antibodies; that is just the most striking deficit. Some of them have been shown not to make antibodies of their IgG class as well as normals following immunization, and conceivably, if one gave them antibodies of other classes when they were deficient, those patients would not do much better. It would be interesting to know how susceptibility to infection correlates with deficits extending to other classes of antibodies or production of them among those patients who have a striking deficit of IgA in their serum.

Dr. SELIGMANN

Now, I must confess that I have given a few times to such patients crude gammaglobulin injections. Theoretically it should not be active because you do not give IgA, and even if you give IgA, one should say that it should not go in the secretory system where the infection is, so for scientific man in the laboratory it should be useless. And I must confess in fact that even in patients without proof of impairment of systemic antibody formation in other classes, you can get some clinical improvement. However, my position is to avoid, as much as possible, such treatment in these patients.

Dr. SOOTHILL

It depends on what you mean by a scientist. I think a scientist is someone who doubts, and I think there is very good reason for doubt because IgG injection is so effective in patients with panhypogammaglobulinemia.

I have used IgG injections in patients with isolated IgA deficiency, like everyone else. I have used them not very frequently. Last week we had a new patient with both IgA deficiency and thrombocytopenia who reacted through the IgA system to a platelet infusion before she was known to be IgA deficient. How common are these reactions is a question I want to ask the audience because I have not seen them in the patients I have treated.

Next point is that this general idea is a very important one for planning future treatment, not only in the field of IgA deficiency, but also in the field of isolated IgM deficiency. We know that the patients with panhypogammaglobulinemia do not get meningitis when we put them on effective IgG treatment, and that seems to be, according to Hobbs and according to our findings, the thing for which IgM really matters. I can see no convincing evidence that there is a need for any parenterally administered immunoglobulin other than IgG, and I see no evidence that IgA can be got to where we think it matters most, namely in the secretions. I think we ought to take a rather firm view that unless someone can provide convincing evidence that something other than effective IgG therapy is needed, then money and effort are not wasted for serums.

Might I raise one other point earlier on Walter's list? I would like to ask people if anyone else has tried rifamycin in chronic granulomatous disease? We have shown that it does kill the organisms inside the polymorphs of these patients, we have seen it produce good therapeutic effects. Has anyone else tried it *in vivo*? It certainly worked *in vitro*, and I think it has a special role *in vivo*.

Dr. GOOD

I want to speak about both of these. We have not used rifamycin in chronic granulomatous disease because with granulocytes in good health and good vigor we cannot kill organisms within the polymorphonuclear leukocytes or within the monocytes with rifamycin. If we damage the cells with toxic concentrations of rifamycin then we can kill organisms within the cells. It is exactly the same story as with sulphur drugs, chloramphenicol and the other potentially toxic antibiotics. So we do not use it clinically. I would be interested in some serious data on its effectiveness because it is an antibiotic that does not need to act within the cell, and to get within the cell in chronic granulomatous disease, we know now, is not absolutely essential to effective interrupted therapy or effective antibiotic therapy in this disease.

Dr. GATTI

I for one would like clarification on whether or not the IgA immunoglobulin positive cells in the IgA patients have been documented to be truly IgA now that we know that there is a ladder that is C-binding, a non-specific binding in the work of Winchester. If you use an Fab for IgA, are those cells still IgA positive in the IgA deficient patient?

Dr. SELIGMANN

I think the answer is yes, and also if you look at synthesis of membrane bound IgA in such patients after stripping, it is there. So it is an actual cell product, it is not an Fc.

Dr. GATTI

Then I think the next set of questions would be directed to this mysterious phenomenon of the patients with anti-IgA antibodies. We have been hearing about this now since Valasquez reported, in 1968 I think it was, somewhere around then. It comes, it goes, it seems to be a definite phenomenon and yet we do not have any further information on it. I have been asking at various places around the world what the incidences of these patients are. How many of the IgA deficient patients have anti-IgA antibodies, because if this is a disease which is so common then there are a lot of presumably normal people walking around in every country who not only have IgA deficiency, but have anti-IgA antibodies, and then are subject to anaphylactic shock when given transfusions. I think this is a whole situation that needs to be clarified because it has far-reaching clinical implications. So I would ask the following questions of the people that have these large series of IgA patients whom they have studied. What is the real incidence of antibodies to IgA in these patients? Secondly does the incidence of IgA antibodies correlate at all with trace levels of IgA, or are these the patients, or are the patients without the antibodies the ones with the higher levels of IgA? Thirdly, are the patients with the antibodies to IgA those that have been treated with gammaglobulins and products that might contain IgA, or are those antibodies there before treatment as well? And finally, we should define which brands of gammaglobulin have IgA in them, because I know that some gammaglobulin has virtually no IgA, at least the batches that I happened to see these runs on. And some of them are not.

Dr. SELIGMANN

Now just before we leave the problem of gammaglobulin therapy, there is another very important practical question that was raised by Dr. Aiuti.

When you have a patient with any hypogammaglobulinemia who has severe shocks after giving gammaglobulin in whom you cannot demonstrate antibodies, in whom you are not able to prove you have complement activation and aggregates in the preparation, what is your practical attitude for further treatment? Do you go on, and if you go on, do you go on under cortisone? I think this is a very important point. Our attitude is not to stop the treatment after one shock because you may see no shock for the next ten injections even if you were not able to prove what was the mechanism of the shock, and I think this is an important practical question to which we should have a quick answer.

Dr. HITZIG

We have the same attitude, and at the beginning we gave a slow infusion of gammaglobulin, or small quantities of intramuscular injection and we waited for the shock to proceed and then we could give large amounts. Now we know that probably what is going on is the formation of large complexes of gammaglobulin together with complement, and I think the danger of producing antibody-antigen complexes and insuring disease is big. And I think this is not safe anymore and it should not be done. I am rather of the opinion that shocks have to be avoided and if they occur the treatment has to be stopped and another preparation of gammaglobulin should be tried.

Dr. GOOD

We have a few such patients who, after each injection, get a reaction and in some of these we have been able to demonstrate activation of the complement system; in some we have not. In those patients, if you spin down the gamma-globulin for that particular administration, you avoid the reaction, so it probably is the absorption of the aggregated material. But those are the exceptions. Our experience has been more like Maxime's experience, and we have continued carefully in giving small amounts of gammaglobulin and then later large amounts of gammaglobulin, and we are able to treat most of our patients who have had sinkable reaction with gammaglobulin therapy. But we have recently been concerned that we might produce vascular injury this way, and so for most of these now when we have a reaction, it is repeated once, and if a sinkable reaction is repeated once, we switch over to a body therapy.

Dr. SELIGMANN

If I may I would like to make a comment which will be more on the theoretical than the practical side about these transplantations in the patients with SCID and B-cells, and this is the following. I think it is of some general interest, but it may have been covered on Monday.

We can learn something about what is happening in the pathogenesis of the disease in some of these patients who have been completely, or partly, reconstituted by compatible bone marrow grafts. There is one such patient whom we studied with Riscelli in Paris several years ago who is completely reconstituted after bone marrow grafts of an HLA - and HLAG-compatible sibling, and this patient was one of the first ones to be shown to have a normal number of B-cells in a severe combined immunodeficiency. Now, it has been proven in this patient, who is fully reconstituted both on the B and on the T immunity, that the T-cells are from the donor and the B-cells are from the recipient, as shown by analysis of the chromosomes with special techniques, and this seems to be really true. From this we would like to infer that in this patient the fact that he was able to have a T-cell reconstitution brought out the possibility of the terminal differentiation of the patient's B-lymphocytes which were there, and which were unable to become plasma cells, and therefore possibly the main defect was a lack of helper T-cells which seems to be a good possibility, and that it was not a stem cell defect.

Now, it is interesting to note Gier's case. In this case the patient had bone marrow transplantation with an HLA-compatible sibling, and we were able to show by the same techniques that after bone marrow transplantation, the T-cells were from the donor, whereas the B-cells were from the patient. But, although the patient's B-lymphocytes were there, they were unable to become plasma cells and there was no reconstitution of humoral immunity. And in his paper he concluded that this meant that he was dealing with a stem cell defect and not with a defect of helper T-cells, since when the T-cells were there the B-cells were still unable to further differentiate. And I think this conclusion is possibly not right since, for instance, he did not look for suppressor T-cells in this patient, and if suppressor T-cells were there, they could be responsible for the inability of the B-cells to differentiate further. I think that this kind of analysis of patients with marrow grafts can help us to understand what is going on, but it is really necessary to know for each patient for whom we had a success or failure of grafts, if B-cells were there before, or if suppressor cells were there before, and so on, otherwise we cannot understand. But I thought this might open a short discussion about what we can learn from cellular engineering about the mechanism involved in cellular combined immunodeficiency, and the heterogeneity of mechanics which are present. I may add that something which I think is important is that inside adenosine deaminase deficiency, you have some patients with B-cells and some without B-cells. So that if you look at the heterogeneity of severe combined immunodeficiency, which was one of the topics I wished to cover in my lecture on Monday, we cannot put on the same level for heterogeneity, for instance, presence or absence of B-lymphocytes and presence or absence of adenosine deaminase, because we know that there is no correlation between these two kinds of findings. So will there be some comments that we can learn about the nature of the defect by cellular engineering?

Dr. GOOD

Unfortunately, I think your case does not really get at the question that Tada and Cooper were concerned with on the first day of this meeting, whether or not you can get cooperation between T and B when there is a majoristic compatability mismatch. We know that you can, when you have just a part in experimental systems, when you just have part of the majoristic compatibility system matched, and your patient was a matched donor. So that I think that the issue of the suppressor cell in bone marrow transplantation is a very crucial one. We have on two occasions found that suppressor cells were present. We could demonstrate that *in vitro*, and when we used very large doses of cyclophosphamide to get rid of those suppressor cells, then we got a full reconstitution. So what I would do in Gier's case is transplant from the same donor after cyclophosphamide treatment.

Summary of an International Conference
Primary Immunodeficiency Disease Still a Great Teacher*

Robert A. Good

As we come to the end of a very long and very productive symposium on the immunodeficiency diseases, it is appropriate that we take a few moments to reflect on our deliberations and consider what we have said and what we have learned in this conference.

The first thing we learned was a new word, coined for the occasion by Professor Kobayashi. This word, "*nanbyō*," stands for all those chronic and sometimes devastating diseases we still understand too poorly. Such diseases are disseminated lupus erythematosus, rheumatoid arthritis, autoimmune diseases, anemias, aplastic anemias, leukemias, and cancers. They are the very diseases which study of the primary immunodeficiency diseases promises to help us understand because they occur so frequently in conjunction with certain of the primary immunodeficiencies.

I believe many of these diseases will turn out to represent persisting or continuing infection, probably with viruses, made possible by one or another immunodeficiency, be it general or lacunar. I agree with Professor Kobayashi that an appropriate approach to the understanding of at least some of them will be to concentrate on analysing, treating, and preventing the "*nanbyō*" by analysing, treating, and preventing the primary, generally genetically determined immunodeficiencies. It is in this way that we can answer the challenge flung to us by Dr. Torrigiani of the World Health Organization that we should be sure to bring from our deliberations understanding that will be helpful in coping with the common diseases of man, especially as these are expressed in the developing nations. Prior to this conference, many of us considered immunodeficiency diseases of man to be rare diseases and thought that

President and Director, Sloan-Kettering Institute, for Cancer Research, New York, New York, U.S.A.

*The original work by Dr. Good and associates referred to has been aided by grants CA-08748, CA-19267, AI-11843, NS-11457 and AGOO541 from the National Institutes of Health; by the National Foundation-March of Dimes; by the Zelda R. Weintraub Cancer Fund; and by the Judith Harris Selig Memorial Fund.

justification for putting so much effort into their study derives from the fact that they have been and are continuing to be such effective teachers of immunology. In this conference, we have seen once again how often the patients with the primary, generally genetically determined, diseases can raise the critical question and can challenge our developing knowledge as it appears. Indeed, patients with the primary immunodeficiency diseases are often unique sources of critical new information and crucial tests of the reality of our best notions that often derive from the insights suggested by our animal and test tube experiments. Thus, we have too often justified the study of the primary immunodeficiencies alone by what we learn of immunology in general from their analysis. But the cold reality is that the primary immunodeficiencies themselves are common diseases, and that the immunodeficiencies, in a sense represented by them, are among the most common diseases of mankind. Indeed, I consider immunodeficiency to be man's most frequent life-threatening disorder. Let me explain this statement for one minute. The primary, genetically determined, immunodeficiencies in childhood occur with a frequency at least equivalent to that of leukemia plus the lymphomas. Perhaps, when isolated IgA deficiency is included, they are as frequent as all hematological cancers. However, immunodeficiencies are a regular concomitant and consequence of nutritional deficiency, Hodgkin's disease, leukemias, carcinomas, sarcomas, so-called autoimmune diseases and, if Soothill is correct, many or all allergies, aging, virus infections, persistent parasitic infestations, persisting bacterial infections like leprosy, fungus infections, and some forms of tuberculosis. The lessons to be learned from study of the patients with primary immunodeficiencies are often directly relevant to these so-called secondary immunodeficiency diseases and disorders of man.

Next, we looked at the thymus and the lymphoid tissue in morphological terms with Dr. Landing. The morphological definitions of the X-linked infantile, the severe combined immunodeficiency, and the Di George Syndrome, presented by Peterson et al. as prototypes, were well supported by his analysis. However, he added new ways of defining thymus deficiency in morphological and histochemical terms that sharpened his dissection. He spoke of a pinealoid appearance of the thymus and admonished us to pay greater attention to the epithelial stem of the thymus and to consider the special characteristics within the thymus, like the stem bud, cystosis, histiocytic infiltration, and eosinophilia. To me the most important contribution Landing made from this analysis was reflected in his statement that there are a number of diseases which have not previously been viewed as primary immunodeficiency diseases, which may so qualify from careful analysis of the morphology of their peripheral and central lymphoid tissues. This rather startling finding surely needs further analysis. However, Landing convinced me, for one, even though I thought at first that he was giving us a specialist's view of the multi-faceted features of accidental involution of the thymus. He pointed out very great differences in thymic and lymphoid histology in different diseases of equally prolonged and severe morbidity. The questions Landing raised in this conference should be a challenge to all of us in the years ahead, especially as we develop methods to reproducibly quantify the cellular and hormonal products of the thymus.

To become able to enumerate reproducibly the short-lived T lymphocytes separately from longer-lived ones, and to quantify thymic hormones, should provide opportunities to answer more critically the important questions Landing placed in clear focus. It is the historical role of the pathologist, never more important than today, to be the gadfly and to raise questions that challenge dogma as it develops, to stimulate other laboratory scientists to generate precise and unequivocal answers to his questions. These questions are frequently generated by skilled interpretation of morphological relationships. We will surely want to use the best methods we can generate to investigate the challenges Dr. Landing has given us.

From Dr. Landing's analysis as well as analyses of others, it seems especially pertinent to consider more precisely the influences of viruses on development of the thymus and, consequently, on the development of the rest of the lymphoid tissues. It has become commonplace to attribute abnormalities of lymphoid development to the rubella virus, which produces developmental abnormalities of many organs and tissues. But now we surely must pay equal attention to the influence of other viruses like the EB virus, cytomegalovirus, measles virus, oncogenic DNA and RNA viruses that are vertically transmitted, and many others. Such agents can certainly, through very direct or indirect influences on development, exert a profound influence on the immunological apparatuses available to the individual or to the tempo at which its components appear, function, and influence one another.

Tada, Blaese, M.D. Cooper, Yata, and my own discussions reflecting the analyses of S.Schwartz, F. Siegal, S. Gupta, J.W. Chiao, L. Shou, N. Berlinger, and others, focussed much appropriate attention on what has to be considered a major new departure in thinking about the primary and secondary immunodeficiency diseases of man. Until Gershon[1] introduced the concept of suppressor lymphocytes, and Waldmann[2] applied this concept to the consideration of the common variable immunodeficiency syndrome and proposed a pathogenetic significance for the suppressor cell, we were content to look always at what cells or what compartments of cells are lacking in immunocapacity. Now we must forever consider pathogenetic mechanisms that involve possibilities of excesses of specific or non-specific suppressor cell functions and complex interactions of positive and negative loops of the immunological network.[3] This complicates what was becoming a nice little world, but the elegant studies these investigators have presented in this conference will continue also to demand much consideration in the years ahead. It is important, as I repeatedly urged, to sort out carefully what is really a pathogenetic relationship and what is merely a camp-follower relationship, and not relate blindly the presence of suppressor cells of whatever class to pathogenesis. To relate the finding of suppressor lymphocytes in patients with Bruton's agammaglobulinemia, where abundant evidence links the disease to absence of B cells, to the pathogenesis of that disease might be as unwise as blaming the agammaglobulinemia of the bursectomized/X-irradiated chicken on the suppressors of B lymphocytes, which Blaese has demonstrated unequivocally in that circumstance.[4] On the other hand, I am absolutely certain that such cells will be found to play major roles in pathogenesis and maintenance of immunodeficiencies. In the studies of S.Schwartz et al.[5] in our Center, suppressors of B lymphocyte function were found, undoubtedly, to have played a role in inhibiting take or expression of function of the B lymphocyte line. Elimination of this adverse influence by high-dose cyclophosphamide in several instances permitted the B lymphocytes to flourish. I am sure that during the next 5–10 years, the literature on the lymphoid system, and even the monocyte-macrophage system, will abound in suppressor cells and suppressor influences taking many forms. It is amazing how rapidly new information about suppressor cells, their nature, relationship to helper cells, and basis of action is being generated. Even the knowledge of the molecular basis of their action seems now most proximal. The importance of the major histocompatibility relationships in the positive as well as the negative interactions of the lymphoid cell classes and subclasses was repeatedly stressed in this conference by Tada and others.[6] Thus, in negative interactions of lymphoid cells as in their positive interactions, stressed by Benacerraf and his associates[7,8] as well as McDevitt,[9] relationships at the major histocompatibility region demand much attention.

Tada insisted that such interactions regularly, if not always, reflect the influences of two separate genes in the MHR, the product and receptor for it being controlled by separate genes operating from locations quite close together. Ability to recognize and work with the lymphoid subpopulations in the mouse, which exert the different helper, suppressor, and killer influences, and that reflect different lines of differentiation, may permit much sorting out of the nature of the differentiative impulses as well as functional basis of the influences of the several subpopulations of lymphoid cells. The cell surface analyses carried out with the methods developed by Old and Boyse have been crucial to the realization of this potentiality, but I am certain, and our conference revealed it, that similar analyses will soon be available for human lymphoid cells as well. It will take much hard work to reach the sophistication provided by analyses using the Ly system in certain strains of mice, but it will be accomplished I am sure, since a start has already been made. I like what Dick Gatti is doing, because I think he and others will find isoantisera that will help us sort out not only compatibilities between individuals but subpopulations of T and B lymphocytes and their several developmental stages. Already our own studies with J.W. Chiao and S. Gupta, and those of Cooper, using receptors for IgM and IgG, show that one can define subpopulations of human T lymphocytes that contain cells acting predominantly as helpers or suppressors in the differentiation of B lymphocytes to plasma cells that synthesize and secrete immunoglobulin molecules. Further, our own studies with Touraine and Hadden[10,11] recognize several stages in the development of T lymphocytes that appear to occur in sequence. If one precursor stage is lacking, the subsequent step cannot be taken; thus, the sequential relations implied in differentiation and cellular development as well as the individual steps become absolutely crucial.

In further analyses, use of purified subpopulations and purified subsets of cells representing developmental stages will permit the much needed sorting out of influences that cannot be achieved when we study complex mixtures of cells. We need to make much more progress toward this goal. Ideally, T cells, B cells, monocytes, general T suppressors, specific T suppressors, T helpers, T suppressors of B cell function, adherent helper cells, and adherent suppressor cells, B precursors of several stages, and T precursors at various stages all must be obtained in pure form free of alternative influences before the influences of these cells on one another can be clarified. It is no wonder that we must develop a veritable army of cellular immunologists to clarify these vital issues.

Dr. Blaese described a much needed ingredient for these analyses of cell-cell interactions in man—namely a pure B-cell mitogen equivalent to LPS, which has been so useful in mouse systems. He then took away this useful reagent when he said that the Nocardia source no longer produced the mitogen. Such a reagent is much needed and would be most important.

The finding of Waldmann, which is also reflected in the work of Gupta et al.[12] and Siegal and Siegal,[13] that suppressor lymphocytes are susceptible to hydrocortisone, called to mind the dramatic experiment of nature of Soothill, published years ago. Soothill found one patient with common variable immunodeficiency who could be effectively treated using large doses of hydrocortisone. Following such treatment, the patient's hypogammaglobulinemia and antibody deficiency disease dramatically disappeared only to return following discontinuation of adrenal steroid therapy. F. and M. Siegal have found the suppressor cells to be highly susceptible to X-irradiation, and Schwartz showed, in the experiments described earlier, that establishment of B cell function in bone marrow and fetal liver transplantation may require reduction or elimination of suppressor cell influence. It is thus clear that the studies of specific and non-specific suppressor cell influence do not represent highly theoretical and confusing complexities but the most practical reality of modern immunobiology. The understanding of their function is essential if we are to cope with the primary and secondary immunodeficiencies of man.

Pursuing this theme, Blaese then gave the conference a real bombshell. He told of experiments in Waldmann's laboratory which *he* attributed to Krakauer,[14] in which production of SIRS—a soluble immune response suppressant— by treatment of the thymic cells of Balb/c mice with ConA could be used to prevent the progression and/or development of the lethal autoimmune and renal diseases of NZB/NZW mice. As I understood his description of these experiments, weekly injections of this fascinating new reagent will prevent the immunological damage that may be attributable to a deficiency of suppressor cells.[15] Further definition of this important material is mandatory. How it relates to the ability of people like Ann Gabrielsen, who prevented the B/W mouse's renal disease by treatment with actinomycin D,[16] and the work by Fernandes *et al.* which showed that this disease can be prevented[17-21] and even treated after its onset by dietary restriction[22] remains to be determined. There seems little question, however, that this finding represents an initial example of the potential usefulness of studying suppressor cells and the molecules that are responsible for their actions.

Max Cooper always looks at things in an original way. In this conference, he gave all of us several things to think about and to work on. From his work with Kincade in chickens, he came to recognize proto-B cells as smallish lymphocytes that contain small amounts of IgM in their cytoplasm, but which lack readily demonstrable surface Ig.[23] He now finds these proto-B cells to be present in the bone marrow but not in blood or peripheral lymphoid tissues of patients with Bruton-type agammaglobulinemia.[24] They are present, of course, in the marrow of normal persons but have been absent from marrow in patients with thymoma-agammaglobulinemia syndrome. This was a surprise to me, since it represents the first evidence that B lymphocytes are present in the X-linked agammaglobulinemic patients. One problem with this definition of a proto-B lymphocyte as I see it is that such a cell has not yet been identified as one of the cell types of the B lymphomas or leukemias. Perhaps, direct confirmation of Cooper's finding is needed, and I would urge careful search for a B lymphoma of this cell type. Maybe we haven't looked hard enough yet. Pathology of the lymphoid malignancies surely should contain monoclonal malignant deviations of each of the cell types reflecting the several stages of differentiation. Cooper also emphasized his studies with Webb[25] and, more recently, the development of the studies of Moretta and his associates[26] and Moretta in Cooper's laboratories.[24] Parallel experiments have for several years been done in my laboratory by J.W. Chiao,[27-30] who talked of double marker lymphocytes possessing T cell markers plus IgG or IgM receptors. S. Gupta in our laboratory, too, has worked with these subpopulations.[31-33] From Moretta and Cooper's work it looks as though the helper cell function may be exercised by cells contained in the subpopulation of T lymphocytes which has receptors for IgM, and the helper T lymphocytes in the subpopulation which has receptors for IgG. Cooper also insisted that the relationships of suppressor lymphocytes to B cells and helper T lymphocytes in immunodeficiency may be quite complex, containing forms in which B cells cannot be helped, variants with T cells that cannot help B cell differentiation properly, and variants where the suppressor influence may be paramount. Dr. Siegal's work also reflects similar complexities. To properly evaluate such complexities we do, indeed, need to be able to work with purified T helper cells, purified T suppressor cells, purified adherent cells of the monocyte-phagocyte series, and purified B lymphocytes. Further, it may be necessary to look at all of these cells at each of several stages of their differentiation. It is no wonder all this seems so complex right now. In addition, the complexities imposed by the influence of numbers of cells and vagaries of the analyses have made it possible for Platt-Mills to argue that the defect in common variable immunodeficiency is really located at the B cell level.[34] Thus far, I continue to find this view most attractive.

Hitzig gave us a very nice review of severe combined immunodeficiency disease (SCID) based on a collected series of 328 cases suffering from this nosologic entity. He showed that, genetically speaking, cases of SCID may be heterogeneous and, enzymatically speaking, they may be heterogenous, but they are appropriately gathered together in a generic framework of SCID. Certainly, one thing stood out from his analysis. If a member of a family succumbs to SCID, a subsequent child in the family who has immunodeficiency, even when studied shortly after birth, will usually be found to have severe combined immunodeficiency just like the first child. The functional defects and cellular defects described are thus certainly not secondary to the many infections and stresses of the disease. Rather they are an integral part of the syndrome. This finding does not mean that combined immunodeficiency cannot also be a secondary manifestation of other diseases; but it does mean that there are entities generally genetically determined, that are primary consequences of a maldevelopment in the two immunity systems. This justifies the classification SCID, which has been used to gather this group of patients together.

When Dr. Hitzig told us that the literature contained 2 cases of severe combined immunodeficiency from Japan, he probably reflected accurately the information available in the literature prior to this conference. This turns out to be a gross inaccuracy since from this conference we now know of at least 28 cases of SCID in Japan. These have been collected from the cooperative national Japanese study reported by Professor Kobayashi, Dr. Hayakawa, and colleagues. SCID occurs in Japan as it does in all countries where studies and medical care have been adequate to detect it. Even its relative infrequency in the industrially, and therefore immunologically, well-developed countries like England and America may be a gross underestimate of reality, as is suggested by the pathological analyses of Berry[35] and those stressed here by Landing. Hitzig's paper, I am sure, will make excellent reading and, as always, will place him right at the forefront of analysis of the disease he has done so much to define in years gone by.

K. Tamaoki of Tokai University broght evidence that much more study in modern immunologic perspective is needed for Down's syndrome. Even though a number of efforts to analyse the immunodeficiency in Down's syndrome has been presented, I have never been convinced that any of them have as yet given us a satisfactory explanation for the increased susceptibility to infection that characterizes this disease. Tamaoki associated Down's syndrome and congenital biliary atresia with strange cystic Hassall's corpuscles in the thymus. This type of Hassall's corpuscles has been associated in the past with certain forms of myasthenia and with thymic tumor. I believe they are also sometimes seen when the thymus is undergoing rapid accidental involution. A deficiency of Hassall's corpuscles observed by Tamaoki and also Landing in Down's syndrome and in congenital biliary atresia, perhaps linked to a temporal relationship by Landing's analysis of his cases of biliary atresia, suggests that whatever is leading to the maldevelopment in Down's syndrome and congenital biliary atresia may affect the thymus along with other organs and thus influence immunological development in an important way. Our improved methods for studying T cell subpopulations and thymic hormones, as reflected in my discussions and the published work of J.F. Bach and Dardenne,[36] Incefy et al.,[37] and Twomey et al.[38,39], should quickly be brought to bear upon further, more definitive explorations of these issues.

Kawai reported his studies of the human tonsils in disease and convinced us that much will be learned from further studies of these fascinating lymphoid organs. They are not just lymph nodes located in the throat but have a composition and pathology of their own, which may be closely linked to the pathology of the IgA and IgE local and systemic immunity systems. Further, these organs, being located near the surface, are readily available for assays that do not require the degree of invasion necessary when sampling of deeper lymph nodes, spleen, and other gut-associated lymphoid tissue (GALT) is desired.

Both Hitzig and I placed emphasis on progress made in defining the association of enzymatic disturbances with immunodeficiency diseases. A listing includes adenosine deaminase deficiency associated with SCID[40,41,42] and T cell deficiency syndromes, nucleoside phosphorylase deficiencies associated with T cell immunodeficiencies and combined immunodeficiencies.[43,44,45]

In addition, enzymatic deficiencies that are now linked inextricably with functional defects of the granulocytes and monocytes in several different forms of chronic granulomatous disease, extreme forms of glucose 6 phosphate dehydrogenase deficiency, glutathion peroxidase deficiency[46], and, perhaps, deficiencies of NADH-dependent oxidases in the cell membrane[47] that launch the oxidative metabolic burst yielding biochemical bases of halogenation of bacteria and the bactericidal singlet oxygen $'O_2$, superoxide O_2^- and hydroxyl radicals OH^- must be listed.[48] We still do not know for sure the exact enzymatic or peptide abnormality in the classic form of chronic granulomatous disease (CGD), but the recent discoveries of Marsh et al.,[49] defining an antigenic abnormality (absence of Kx) on the surface membrane of the leukocytes related to the Kell system could represent a finding that finally puts us on the right track toward defining just the enzyme or peptide that must be lacking or abnormal in this disorder. Nonetheless, the functional defect in the oxidative burst following phagocytosis and its associated deficiencies of generation of H_2O_2, the OH^- singlet oxygen $'O_2$, and superoxide O_2^- radicals so vital to killing of ingested organisms has been well defined, and that seems a big step.

Further, deficiencies or abnormalities of the complement components and their inhibitors and modulators represent other increasingly well defined enzymatic aspects associated with immunodeficiency.[50] Deficiencies of almost every one of the complement components can now be associated with human disease. After extensive study, each of them (not just C3 deficiency) has been associated with increased susceptibility to infection. Further, many of these defects are associated with increased susceptibility to the so-called autoimmune, mesenchymal or vascular and renal diseases. These findings represent major challenges to students of immunodeficiency diseases. We must understand their meaning completely if we are to develop the needed understanding of the pathogenesis of the mesenchymal diseases that make up such a big part of the nanbyō of which Dr. Kobayashi speaks.

Dr. Gatti shared with us his religious stories as well as his extensive new efforts to analyse the histocompatibility systems. I think it was terribly important for him to emphasize again the progressive neurological disease that can occur in patients with immunodeficiency. I have been well aware of this association for many years, having encountered 3 patients with this awful combination of diseases. I had not realized, however, even though I had seen each of the reports as they have come along, how many such cases have been observed. It is important to emphasize that the patients with apparently primarily B cell deficiencies, such as X-linked infantile agammaglobulinemia, may have a very high frequency of progressive, destructive neurological disease, undoubtedly in many instances due to persistent viral infection. In the patient Gatti described, he discovered a fascinating factor that was cytotoxic to B lymphocytes in the circulation. Such factors have been seen before in patients with immunodeficiency disease and they may be of pathogenetic significance. The factor Gatti is chasing, he thought, is not an antibody. If he can study that factor further and define it a bit better, it might be most revealing and could be an important immunoregulator. For the present, I recognize such factors are usually antibodies.

Seligman took us through his magnificent study of an antibody with specificity for a subclass of B lymphocytes that appeared to have a pathogenetic significance in his patient. Whether this antibody was also of pathogenetic significance in ulcerative colitis, which seems to me to be likely, or whether it produced an immunodeficiency which led to colitis on another basis of infection, is hard to establish right now. This antibody was surely cross-reactive with fibroblasts as well as with epithelial cells of the colonic mucosa. And I think that we must not, from this work and from Rosen's earlier work, overlook the possibility that an autoantibody (an autoimmune mechanism directed against the immunological system) may be pathogenetically important as a crucial mechanism in the development of some cases of immunodeficiency. Further, the possibility that there may be autoantibodies directed against many if not ultimately each of the components of the immunological system, could turn out to be of great pathogenetic significance. The immunity system, functioning as a means of interfering with immunity or with crucial controls on immunological function, raises again the issue first raised by the studies of Prausnitz and Kustner,[5] who prevented the expression of passively transferred allergy by what in retrospect seems like active immunization rather than desensitization. I think Dr. Seligmann's experiment of nature shows us how that mechanism—unwanted in this instance—worked in a particular patient. This unfortunate immune response, of course, gave rise to a pathological state in Seligmann's case, but I believe it gives us a glimpse of a potential scientific approach to immunization against immunity. Such truly effective immunologic control of unwanted immunity could have all manner of benefit. When I think this way, I am, of course, reflecting also on the promising work of Ishizaka, Kishimoto and their colleagues, who have been developing rapidly this approach to prevention of allergy. Already they have developed methods by which they can stimulate a helper mechanism for IgG responses to certain antigens in experimental animals, while stimulating suppressor influence on IgE production.[52,53]

We considered all too briefly neurological diseases in the perspective of immunodeficiency. Here I like to think of lacunar immunodeficiencies; but more general relationships to immunodeficiency, such as Gatti emphasized, must also be considered. A lacunar immunodeficiency is a state where the individual may be able to handle all but a single viral agent normally but is compromised by an immunological malfunction to that organism. Subacute sclerosing panencephalitis and multiple sclerosis may have such a basis.

We considered this possibility in relation to POL antigens with Dr. Kuroiwa. He showed us that in at least one circumstance, namely in progressive multifocal leukoencephalitis, where Papova viruses had been demonstrated, an immunodeficiency of rather narrow range could exist. The question that is always raised by such a relationship is that of a passenger virus versus a true pathogenetically important infection; but I think there will certainly be individuals who do not deal with DNA viruses like SV40 or Papova viruses normally, and this immunodeficiency might be crucial in permitting the type of infection that might lead to susceptibility to cancer. From Dr. Eisinger's efforts at the Sloan-Kettering Institute we can now work *in vitro,* at least to some extent, with the DNA tumor virus associated with warts.[54] This virus, of course is one that has a capacity for neoplastic transformation. Furthermore, recent studies have shown that patients with certain primary immunodeficiencies like Wiskott-Aldrich syndrome, and even members of their families, are excreting Papova viruses in their urine. Myeloma that produces a curious neurological clinical syndrome seldom seen in Europe or the United States seems rather frequent in Japan. This is something to pay attention to. One wonders, of course, whether or not such manifestations are not a consequence of the distribution of the particular immunoglobulin in the population or whether the myeloma has opened the door to the otherwise unusual disease by permitting infection or autoimmunity. There no longer seems a question that many neurological diseases have to be looked on in the perspective of immunological function and deficiency.

Dr. Kuroiwa showed us that in Japan multiple sclerosis does not have the same HLA type distribution that it does in America and Europe. The real question then would be what are the relationships vis à vis the HLA-, the D locus, or the recently defined locus determining the B cell alloantigens. Do Caucasians and Japanse with multiple sclerosis have the same D locus or B cell alloantigen locus associations? The possibility of definitive analyses of this question is very proximate with methodologies currently available. If a lacunar immunodeficiency based on genetic make-up really underlies multiple sclerosis, can cellular engineering, using mismatched marrow, be used to treat this dreaded disease? I think it likely.

Kano presented an extraordinary paper in which he talked about the isolated IgA deficiencies in Japan. He showed us that in Japan, as in the U.S. and Europe[55,56] an array of diseases are associated with IgA deficiency. The perfectly normal life that used to be claimed for patients with IgA deficiency must be challenged by data now from the East as well as the West. Certainly, in Japan, if Dr. Kano's evidence is representative, persons with IgA deficiency are susceptible to a whole variety of autoimmune diseases, respiratory and gastrointestinal infections, and even cancers. It was of interest that the cancers observed seemed especially to involve the stomach. Further studies of Grob and his associates[57] in Switzerland and of the British investigators cited by Soothill have revealed important associations of IgA deficiency with epilepsy. In addition, Soothill clarified that the hydantoins used to treat epilepsy can also be suppressive of the IgA production. But the situation is more complicated than this. It seems indicated, both by Soothill's studies and by the studies of Grob and his associates in Zurich, that a suppressed IgA occurs more frequently in patients with primary epilepsy (idiopathic epilepsy) and not in patients with secondary epilepsy. Therapy of the epilepsy with hydantoin seems to add to this deficiency.

John Soothill stimulates all of us. Sometimes I think he overstimulates me. His views seem often so iconoclastic. But they *are* extraordinarily creative. He challenges constantly what seem to be well-established perspectives to arrive at truly innovative notions. He presented two papers yesterday in which he raised issues about immunodeficiencies associated with common diseases, tonsillitis, allergies, and perhaps protein dietary deficiency. Indeed, I take his argument as saying, as I have so often recently, that the most common diseases of man may be associated with immunodeficiency. I think that concept is terribly important and cannot be overemphasized. Allergies and tonsillitis are surely widespread in the population; if these are indeed associated with immunodeficiency, then when we think of immunodeficiencies, we are certainly considering a huge population. Further, Soothill tried to persuade us, and I think he nearly persuaded me, that if you protect an allergy-prone patient from early exposure to allergens, *e.g.* by breast milk feeding, you may avoid subsequent allergic disease. He further related at least some allergic manifestations to the major histocompatibility system in terms which might define lacunar immunodeficiency. All of his observations represent an extraordinary display that we must digest ultimately with the challenge of either confirmation or rejection.

We also looked, with Kubo and B. Kobayashi, at specific forms of immuno-deficiency and obtained further encouragement for the view that individual cases, very carefully studied, still may be cornerstones to important advances in the field of immunology. Each of these questions, of course, must be taken to the laboratory for fundamental analyses.

With Nomoto, we witnessed a very beautiful demonstration of a fundamental approach that may be useful in defining which of the immune functions is important in the defense against which kinds of pathogens. He showed us how to analyse the influence of the non-immune phagocytes, T cell immunity, and even contributions of T-dependent and T-independent antibody responses in man. Such studies may yield methodologies for further dissection of the microbial universe.

Certainly, a major highlight of this symposium was to hear about the extraordinary nation-wide study the Japanese immunologists have made of the primary immunodeficiency diseases of man. I recognize this as an extraordinary administrative achievement as well as an important scientific achievement which also may reflect a splendid cooperative characteristic of the Japanese people. I submit that this characteristic is not very widely distributed in the world. The extraordinary accumulation of patients with primary immuno-deficiency disease, the analysis of these patients, and the development of a Registry that really works, are the patently important consequences of this effort. The allergies, malignancies and autoimmunity, which the Japanese team has found to be associated with immunodeficiencies, do not represent new associations. We have known them before; but it is nice to see that each of these associations holds also now for a very different population. We must be challenged by these findings and must continue to find the why and how answers for these vital relationships.

We were given fundamental new approaches to analysis of lymphoid cell differentiation that may help us understand better our immunodeficient patients. I was interested in the paper on the POL antigen, the polymerized flagellin. The concern I always have with each antigen introduced for study of primary immune responses in man is whether or not we are really studying the primary immune response when we *say* we are studying the primary immune response. POL seems to come as close to meeting the necessary stringent demands as any antigen available for general use. I still have reservations though and cannot accept this antigen as perfect for study of primary immunity until I see that this antigen behaves similarly with lymphoid cells of the developing embryo of pathogen-free swine in the system, which Kim continues to emphasize at the Sloan-Kettering Institute.

I will not review in detail the full day of presentations on therapy of primary immunodeficiencies. Hitzig reviewed this exhaustively in his summary and there is no need to repeat it here.

For details, his chapter in this book should be authoritative. Surely, the challenges Hitzig set down for us as therapists are beginning to be met. He asked for an intravenous preparation of gamma globulin which would not produce reactions and yet would be fully effective in bodily defense. Ohtomo, Tomibe and their associates then presented evidence for just such a preparation—a sulfonated gamma globulin that seems to be restored after absorption into the body—to be non-antigenic and not provocative of complement activation. This gamma globulin preparation must still be studied in agammaglobulinemic patients who are much more susceptible to the adverse influences of aggregated or partially aggregated gamma globulin. Indeed, many so-called unaggregated gamma globulin preparations have floundered on this shoal. The sulfonated compound proposed looks very exciting. In our country, Cutter uses a preparation of gamma globulin for intravenous administration. This one still contains enough aggregated gamma globulin to produce sometimes quite severe reactions upon intravenous injection in agammaglobulinemic patients. When large amounts of gamma globulin must be used intravenously, I believe we surely need a much better preparation. The Ph-4, pepsin-digested, papain-digested gamma globulin preparations which have been tried all have had serious drawbacks. Some still contain aggregates, others have been split to such small fragments that they are rapidly lost in the urine or they have been broken down in such a way that they have lost much of their ability to protect against infection by acting as antibodies capable of addressing the biologic amplification processes, e.g. the complement system.

We again talked about the use of transfer factor in therapy. Many problems considered in the past about transfer factor still plague us. But regardless of these problems, transfer factor is being used and it has had a beneficial influence on some of the most dreaded diseases of man, e.g. mucocutaneous candidiasis.[58–64] It seems to have some effects that are reproducible from clinic to clinic around the world. I am not convinced that it helps much in treatment of the Wiskott-Aldrich syndrome. Indeed, in some cases it may have been harmfully provoking autoimmunity.[65] I am, however, convinced that it helps in a significant proportion of patients with the worst forms of chronic mucocutaneous candidiasis. If we can identify the molecular basis of the action of this compound that can *enhance* cell-mediated immunity—rather than a compound that can *transfer* specific immunity, as we have been seeking—we may have in transfer factor a good drug for treatment of a variety of clinical conditions. Indeed, we were told in the presentations of the transfer factor work that even common diseases and progressive bacterial infections may be favorably influenced by transfer factor. We were also shown that one of the complications of transfer factor therapy, namely hemolytic anemia, may even be treatable with transfer factor. These observations are, of course, provocative. Michael Blaese sobered us very much by associating four cases of hemolytic anemia, eight cases of malignancy, and two cases of the nephrotic syndrome with transfer factor therapy. Some of these associations may not be related to transfer factor therapy, but others may, and they are serious complications. Nephrotic syndrome is not a frequent manifestation of Wiskott-Aldrich syndrome. Nonetheless, we must demand a better denominator if we are to be appropriately concerned. Certainly, Blaese's comments should keep us thinking about the possible untoward consequences of any new means that we are beginning to use to manipulate the immunologic system.

We also discussed several candidates for thymic hormones or thymic factors, which have been described, and I believe here we are also making rapid progress. We have well defined, even sequenced, the facteur thymique serique (FTS) of Bach,[66] thymopoietin, ubiquitin, and bursopoietin fully defined molecules of G. Goldstein,[67-70] thymosin and thymosin α_1 of A.Goldstein,[71,72] along with a veritable hoard of less purified extracts. We may not yet have one single hormone that can do the entire work of the thymus, and I think it would be amazing if we did. The possibility, however, that different concentrations of a single factor can initiate differentiation and expand an appropriately differentiated state of the T population still has to be considered. Studies over the next four or five years will yield much information about the way the thymus accomplishes its task, and we will soon have dissected in cellular and molecular terms, *in vitro* as well as *in vivo*, the several influences of this vital organ.

Thymic transplantation, fetal liver transplantation, and bone marrow transplantation are being enthusiastically pursued as approaches to therapy of the primary immunodeficiencies, and each has yielded spectacular results. We are, indeed, curing by this form of treatment many otherwise incurable diseases. The list of previously incurable diseases that have now been cured by cellular and macromolecular engineering grows longer each year. It includes four genetically separate forms of severe combined immunodeficiency diseases, Di George syndrome, Wiskott-Aldrich syndrome, fatal granulomatous disease, complement component deficiencies, several forms of aplastic anemia, and even some leukemias and lymphomas. The experimental approach to cellular and macromolecular engineering is also developing with amazing speed, and bone marrow transplantations, thymus transplantations, and fetal liver transplantations, along with macromolecular manipulations, will surely become major means of coping with diseases considered fatal up to now. When we get more skillful than we are now at avoiding or controlling the graft-vs-host reaction, many hematological diseases, diseases featured by persistent infection with viruses and bacteria, and even some of the malignant diseases will be treated by cellular and macromolecular engineering.[73]

In concluding, we all are confident we have had an extraordinary conference. The most important thing about this conference is that a large group of scientists and scholars from Europe and the Americas have had a real opportunity to get together with, learn the names of, and appreciate the thoughts and work of our colleagues in Japan. You have made great strides in taking leadership in this field of immunology in recent years. We have learned to think constructively with you, argue with you, occasionally even quarrel with you over scientific interpretations, and yet end up good friends. This is the essence of the scientific approach. We must always realize that the most valuable help we can give to one another is to criticise each other's work intensively. Each comes forward with what he considers his most brilliant ideas and approaches that he believes will prove most important relationships. But unless properly and incisively criticised, we will be short of the mark, or off the mark, much of the time. All of us from abroad are pleased that we have come to Tokyo for this conference. We are proud to have studied with you and learned from you and from your very special material on primary immunodeficiencies. We are pleased to visit your extraordinary and perfectly beautiful country. I am sure you will conclude that we do not understand you very well as yet, but I am equally sure that mutual understanding will derive very rapidly from meetings such as this one, and I am hopeful, from what I have heard in informal discussion, that many collaborations and ongoing exchanges have been launched. I wish to express my deep personal appreciation, and for the foreign guests our appreciation, for the organization and the financial support provided by our Japanese colleagues and the Japanese Government for this conference. Thanks are also due to the National Foundation-March of Dimes, the Allergy Foundation of America, and to the Department of Health, Education and Welfare for support of the travel of several of the American participants.

REFERENCES

1. Gershon, R. K.: T cell control of antibody production. *Contemp. Top. Immunobiol.* 3:1–40, 1974.
2. Waldmann, T. A., Broder, S., Krakauer, R., McDermott, R. P., Durm, M., Goldman, C. and Meade, B.: The role of suppressor cells in the pathogenesis of common variable hypogammaglobulinemia and the immunodeficiency associated with multiple myeloma. *Fed. Proc.* 35:2072, 1976.

3. Jerne, N. K.: Towards a network theory of the immune system. *Ann. Immunol.* (Paris) **125c**:373–389, 1974.
4. Blaese, R. M., Weiden, P. L., Koski, I. and Dooley, N.: Infectious agammaglobulinemia: transmission of immunodeficiency with grafts of agammaglobulinemic cells. *J. Exp. Med.* **140**:1097–1101, 1974.
5. Schwartz, S. A., Shou, L., Good, R. A. and Choi, Y. S.: Suppression of immunoglobulin synthesis and secretion by peripheral blood lymphocytes from normal donors. *Proc. Natl. Acad. Sci.* **74**:2099–2103, 1977.
6. Tada, T., Taniguchi, M. and David, C. S.: Properties of the antigenic-specific suppressive T-cell factor in the regulation of antibody response of the mouse. IV. Special subregion assignment of the gene(s) that codes for the suppressive T-cell factor in the H-2 histocompatibility complex. *J. Exp. Med.* **144**:713–725, 1976.
7. Katz, D. H. and Benacerraf, B.: The function and interrelationship of T cell receptors, Ir genes and other histocompatibility gene products. *Transplant. Rev.* **22**:175–195, 1975.
8. Kapp, J. A., Pierce, C. W. and Benacerraf, B.: Immunosuppressive factor(s) extracted from lymphoid cells of nonresponder mice primed with L-glutamic acid[60]-L-alanine[30]-L-tyrosine[10] (GAT). II. Cellular source and effect on responder and nonresponder mice. *J. Exp. Med.* **145**:828–838, 1977.
9. McDevitt, H. O. and Landy, M., eds.: Genetic Control of Immune Responsiveness. New York, Academic Press, 1973.
10. Touraine, J. L., Hadden, J. W. and Good, R. A.: Sequential stages of human T lymphocyte differentiation. *Proc. Natl. Acad. Sci.* **74**:3414–3418, 1977.
11. Touraine, J. L., Touraine, F., Hadden, J. W., Hadden, E. M. and Good, R. A.: 5-bromodeoxyuridine-light inactivation of human lymphocytes stimulated by mitogens and allogeneic cells: evidence for distinct T-lymphocyte subsets. *Int. Arch. Allergy Appl. Immunol.* **52**:105–117, 1976.
12. Gupta, S. and Good, R. A.: Subpopulations of human T lymphocytes. II. Effect of thymopoietin, corticosteroids and irradiation. *Cell. Immunol.* **34**:10–18, 1977.
13. Siegal, F. P. and Siegal, M.: Enhancement of human plasma cell production by irradiated T cells: dissection of helper and suppressor functions *in vitro*. *J. Immunol.* **118**:642–647, 1977.
14. Krakauer, R. S., Ilfeld, D. N., Gilhoed, G. and Waldmann, T. A.: Demonstration and partial characterization of human soluble immune response suppressor (SIRS). *Clin Res.* **25**:362A, 1977. (Abstract)
15. Talal, N. and Steinberg, A. E.: The pathogenesis of autoimmunity in New Zealand Black mice. *Curr. Top. Microbiol. Immunol.* **64**:79–103, 1974.
16. Gabrielsen, A. E., Lubert, A. S. and Olsen, C. T.: Suppression of murine lupus erythematosus by Dactinomycin. *Nature* **264**:439–440, 1976.
17. Fernandes, G., Yunis, E. J., Smith, J. and Good, R. A.: Dietary influence on breeding behavior, hemolytic anemia, and longevity in NZB mice. *Proc. Soc. Exp. Biol. Med.* **139**:1189–1196, 1972.
18. Fernandes, G., Yunis, E. J., Jose, D. G. and Good, R. A.: Dietary influence on antinuclear antibodies and cell-mediated immunity in NZB mice. *Int. Arch. Allergy* **44**:770–782, 1973.

19. Fernandes, G., Yunis, E. J. and Good, R. A.: Influence of protein restriction on immune functions in NZB mice. *J. Immunol.* **116**:782–790, 1976.
20. Fernandes, G., Yunis, E. J. and Good, R. A.: Influence of diet on survival of mice. *Proc. Natl. Acad. Sci.* **73**:1279–1283, 1976.
21. Fernandes, G., Friend, P. S., Good, R. A. and Yunis, E. J.: Prolongation of life-span of (NZB × NZW)F1 mice with calorie restriction. *Fed. Proc.* **34**:437, 1976. (Abstract)
22. Fernandes, G., Friend, P. and Yunis, E. J.: Influence of calorie restriction on autoimmune disease. *Fed. Proc.* **36**:1313, 1977. (Abstract)
23. Kincade, P. W. and Cooper, M. D.: Development and distribution of immuno-globulin-containing cells in the chicken. An immunofluorescent analysis using purified antibodies to mu, gamma and light chains. *J. Immunol.* **106**:371–382, 1971.
24. Cooper, M. D., Moretta, L., Webb, S. R., Pearl, E. R., Okos, A. J. and Lawton, A. R.: Diversity of defects in human B cell differentiation. *In*: Immunopathology: International Symposium, 7th, 1976 (P. A. Miescher, ed.). Basel/Stuttgart, Schwabe & Co., 1977. pp. 343–351.
25. Webb, S. R. and Cooper, M. D.: T-cells can bind antigen via cytophilic IgM antibody made by B-cells. *J. Immunol.* **111**:275–277, 1973.
26. Moretta, L., Ferrarini, M., Mingari, M. C., Moretta, A. and Webb, S. R.: Sub-populations of human T cells identified by receptors for immunoglobulins and mitogen responsiveness. *J. Immunol.* **117**:2171–2174, 1976.
27. Chiao, J. W., Pantic, V. S. and Good, R. A.: Human peripheral lymphocytes bearing both B-cell complement receptors and T-cell characteristics for sheep erythrocytes detected by a mixed rosette method. *Clin. Exp. Immunol.* **18**:483–490, 1974.
28. Chiao, J. W., Pantic, V. S. and Good, R. A.: Human lymphocytes bearing both receptors for complement components and SRBC. *Clin. Immunol. Immunopathol.* **4**:545–556, 1975.
29. Chiao, J. W. and Good, R. A.: Studies of the presence of membrane receptors for complement, IgG and the sheep erythrocyte rosetting capacity on the same human lymphocytes. *Eur. J. Immunol.* **6**:157–162, 1976.
30. Chiao, J. W. and Good, R. A.: Aggregated IgG receptors on lymphocytes detected with indicators coated with IgG and glutaraldehyde. *IRCS J. Med. Sci.* **4**:150, 1976.
31. Gupta, S. and Good, R. A.: Subpopulations of human T lymphocytes. I. Studies in immunodeficient patients. *Clin. Exp. Immunol.* (in press)
32. Gupta, S. and Good, R. A: Effect of thymopoietin, corticosteroids and irradiation on human T lymphocyte subpopulations. *Fed. Proc.* **36**:1240, 1977. (Abstract)
33. Gupta, S., Schwartz, S. A., Safai, B., Hansen, J. A. and Good, R. A.: Immunoregulatory T cell subpopulations in lymphoproliferative disorders. *Clin. Res.* **25**: 358A, 1977. (Abstract)
34. Janossy, G., Gomez de la Concha, E., Luquetti, A., Snajdr, M. J., Waxdal, M. J. and Platts-Mills, T. A. E.: T-cell regulation of immunoglobulin synthesis and proliferation in pokeweed (Pa-1) stimulated human lymphocyte cultures. *Scand. J. Immunol.* **6**:109–123, 1977.

35. Berry, C. L.: Histopathological findings in the combined immunodeficiency disease syndrome. *J. Clin. Pathol.* **23**:193–202, 1970.
36. Dardenne, M. and Bach, J. F.: The sheep cell rosette assay for the evaluation of thymic hormones. *In*: The Biological Activity of Thymic Hormones (D. W. van Bekkum, ed.). Rotterdam, Kooyker Scientific Publications, 1975. pp. 235–243.
37. Incefy, G. S., Dardenne, M., Pahwa, S., Grimes, E., Pahwa, R., Smithwick, E., O'Reilly, R. and Good, R. A.: Thymic activity in severe combined immunodeficiency diseases. *Proc. Natl. Acad. Sci.* **74**:1250–1253, 1977.
38. Twomey, J. J., Goldstein, G., Lewis, V. M., Bealmear, P. M. and Good, R. A.: Bioassay determinations of thymopoietin and thymic hormone levels in human plasma. *Proc. Natl. Acad. Sci.* **74**:2541–2545, 1977.
39. Lewis, V., Twomey, J., Goldstein, G., O'Reilly, R., Smithwick, E., Pahwa, R., Pahwa, S., Good, R. A., Schulte-Wisserman, H., Horowitz, S., Hong, R., Jones, J., Sieber, O., Kirkpatrick, C., Polmar, S. and Bealmear, P.: Circulating thymic hormone activity in congenital immunodeficiency. *Lancet* **2**: 471–475, 1977.
40. Meuwissen, H. J., Pickering, R. J. and Pollara, B.: Adenosine deaminase deficiency in combined immunologic deficiency disease. Birth Defects: Original Article Series, Vol. XI, No. 1, 1975. pp. 117–119.
41. Pollara, B., Moore, J. J., Jr., Pickering, R. J., Gabrielsen, A. E. and Meuwissen, H. J.: Combined immunodeficiency disease: an inborn error of purine metabolism. Birth Defects: Original Article Series, Vol. XI, No. 1, 1975. pp. 120–123.
42. Giblett, E. R., Anderson, J. E., Cohen, F., Pollara, B. and Meuwissen, H. J.: adesine-deaminase deficiency in two patients with severely impaired cellular immunity. *Lancet* **2**:1067–1069, 1972.
43. Giblett, E. R. Ammann, A. J., Wara, D. W., Sandman, R. and Diamond, L. K.: Nucleoside-phosphorylase deficiency in a child with severely defective T-cell immunity and normal B-cell immunity. *Lancet* **1**:1010–1013, 1975.
44. Stoop, J. W., Zegers, B. J. M., Hendricks, G. F. M., Siegenbeek van Heukelom, L. H., Staal, G. E. J., de Bree, P. K., Wadman, S. K. and Ballieux, R. A.: Purine nucleoside phosphorylase deficiency associated with selective cellular immunodeficiency. *N. Engl. J. Med.* **296**:651–655, 1977.
45. Biggar, D., Giblett, E. R., Ozere, R. L. and Grover, B. D.: A new form of nucleoside phosphorylase deficiency in two brothers with defective T cell function. *J. Pediatr.* (in press)
46. Holmes, B. and Good, R. A.: Metabolic and functional abnormalities of human neutrophils. *In*: Phagocytic Mechanisms in Health and Disease (R. C. Williams and H. H. Fudenberg, eds.). New York/London, Intercontinental Medical Book Corp., 1972. pp. 51–66.
47. Segal, A. W. and Peters, T. J.: Characterisation of the enzyme defect in chronic granulomatous disease. *Lancet* **1**:1363–1365, 1976.
48. Klebanoff, S. J.: Antimicrobial mechanisms in neutrophilic polymorphonuclear leukocytes. *Semin. Hematol.* **12**:117–142, 1975.
49. Marsh, W. L., Uretsky, S. C. and Douglas, S. D.: Antigens of the Kell blood group system on neutrophils and monocytes: their relation to chronic granulomatous disease (CGD). *J. Pediatr.* **87**:1117–1120, 1975.

50. Day, N. K., Moncada, B. and Good, R. A.: Inherited deficiencies of the complement system. *In*: Biological Amplification Systems in Immunology (N. K. Day and R. A. Good, eds.). New York , Plenum, 1977. pp. 229–245. (Comprehensive Immunology, vol. 2)
51. Prausnitz, C. and Küstner, H.: Studien über die Ueberempfindlichkeit. *Zentralbl. Bakteriol.* **86**:160, 1921.
52. Takatsu, K. and Ishizaka, K.: Reaginic antibody formation in the mouse. VII. Induction of suppressor T cells for IgE and IgG antibody responses. *J. Immunol.* **116**:1257–1264, 1976.
53. Kishimoto, T., Hirai, Y., Suemura, M. and Yamamura, Y.: Regulation of antibody response in different immunoglobulin classes. I. Selective suppression of anti-DNP IgE antibody response by preadministration of DNP-coupled mycobacterium. *J. Immunol.* **117**:396–404, 1976.
54. Eisinger, M., Kucarova, O., Sarkar, N. H. and Good, R. A.: Propagation of human wart virus in tissue culture. *Nature* **256**:432–434, 1975.
55. Horowitz, S. and Hong, R.: Selective IgA deficiency—some perspectives. Birth Defects: Original Article Series, Vol. XI, No. 1, 1975. pp. 129–133.
56. Wells, J. V., Michaeli, D. and Fudenberg, H. H.: Autoimmunity in selective IgA deficiency. Birth Defects: Original Article Series, Vol. VI, No. 1, 1975. pp. 144–150.
57. Fontana, A., Grob, P. J., Sauter, R. and Joller, H.: IgA deficiency, epilepsy, and hydantoin medication. *Lancet* **2**:228, 1976.
58. Rocklin, R. E.: Use of transfer factor in patients with depressed cellular immunity and chronic infection. Birth Defects: Original Article Series, Vol. XI, No. 1, 1975. pp. 431–435.
59. Schulkind, M. L. and Ayoub, E. M.: Transfer factor as an approach to the treatment of immune deficiency disease. Birth Defects: Original Article Series, Vol. XI, No. 1, 1975. pp. 463–440.
60. Kirkpatrick, C. H.: Restoration of cell-mediated immune responses with transfer factor. Birth Defects: Original Article Series, Vol. XI, No. 1, 1975. pp. 441–444.
61. Levin, A. S., Spitler, L. E. and Fudenberg, H. H.: Transfer factor I: methods of therapy. Birth Defects: Original Article Series, Vol. XI, No. 1, 1975. pp. 445–448.
62. Ballow, M., Dupont, B., Hansen, J. L. and Good, R. A.: Transfer factor therapy: evidence for nonspecificity. Birth Defects: Original Article Series, Vol. XI, No. 1, 1975. pp. 457–461.
63. Griscelli, C.: Transfer factor therapy in immunodeficiency. Birth Defects: Original Article Series, Vol. XI, No. 1, 1975. pp. 464.
64. Spitler, L. E., Levin, A. S. and Fudenberg, H. H.: Transfer factor II: results of therapy. Birth Defects: Original Article Series, Vol. XI, No. 1, 1975. pp. 449–456.
65. Ballow, M., Dupont, B. and Good, R. A.: Autoimmune hemolytic anemia in Wiskott-Aldrich syndrome during treatment with transfer factor. *J. Peditar.* **83**:772–780, 1973.
66. Bach, J. F., Dardenne, M. and Pleau, J. M.: Biochemical characterisation of a serum thymic factor. *Nature* **266**:55–56, 1977.

67. Goldstein, G.: The isolation of thymopoietin (thymin). *Ann. N.Y. Acad. Sci.* **249**: 177–183, 1975.
68. Schlesinger, D. H. and Goldstein, G.: The amino acid sequence of thymopoietin II. *Cell* **5**:361–366, 1975.
69. Schlesinger, D. H., Goldstein, G. and Niall, H. D.: The complete amino acid sequence of ubiquitin, an adenylate cyclase stimulating polypeptide probably universal in living cells. *Biochemistry* **14**:2214–2218, 1975.
70. Brand, A., Gilmour, D. and Goldstein, G.: Lymphocyte-differentiating hormone of the bursa of Fabricius. *Science* **193**:319–321, 1976.
71. Goldstein, A. L., Guha, A., Zatz, M. M., Hardy, M. A. and White, A.: Purification and biological activity of thymosin, a hormone of the thymus gland. *Proc. Natl. Acad. Sci.* **69**:1800–1803, 1972.
72. Goldstein, A. L., Low, T. L. K., McAdoo, M., McClure, J., Thurman, G. B., Rossio, J., Lai, C.-Y., Chang, D., Wang, S.-S., Harvey, C., Ramel, A. H. and Meienhofer, J.: Thymosin α1: isolation and sequence analysis of an immunologically active thymic polypeptide. *Proc. Natl. Acad. Sci.* **74**:725–729, 1977.
73. Good, R. A.: Cellular engineering. *MSKCC Clin. Bull.* **7**:33–39, 1977.

List of Contributors

Fernando Aiuti
    Department of Internal Medicine III, University of Rome, Italy
P. Ammirati*
    Department of Internal Medicine III, University of Rome, Italy
Tsugutoshi Aoki
    Department of Pediatrics, School of Medicine, Toho University, Tokyo, Japan
R. Michael Blaese
    The Metabolism Branch, National Cancer Institute, National Institutes of
    Health, Bethesda, Maryland, U.S.A.
S. Broder*
    The Metabolism Branch, National Cancer Institute, National Institutes of
    Health, Bethesda, Maryland, U.S.A.
L. Businco*
    Department of Pediatrics I, University of Rome, Italy
Max D. Cooper
    The Cellular Immunobiology Unit of the Tumor Institute, Departments of
    Pediatrics and Microbiology and The Comprehensive Cancer Center, University
    of Alabama in Birmingham, University Station, Birmingham, Alabama, U.S.A.
R. D'Amelio*
    Department of Internal Medicine III, University of Rome, Italy
M. Fiorilli*
    Department of Internal Medicine III, University of Rome, Italy
Yuji Fukumoto
    Teijin Institute for Biomedical Research, Tokyo, Japan
Richard A. Gatti
    Cedars-Sinai Medical Center, Department of Pediatric Hematology, Oncology
    and Immunology, Los Angeles, California, U.S.A.
Robert A. Good
    Memorial Sloan-Kettering Cancer Center, New York, New York, U.S.A.
Nagahide Goya
    Department of Pediatrics, Faculty of Medicine, Kyushu University, Fukuoka,
    Japan

391

Yoshihiro Hamashima
    Department of Pathology, Kyoto University School of Medicine, Kyoto, Japan
M. A. Hansen*
    Memorial Sloan-Kettering Cancer Center, New York, New York, U.S.A.
Junichi Hata
    Department of Pathology, Tokai University School of Medicine, Isehara,
    Kanagawa, Japan
Hiroshi Hayakawa
    Department of Pediatrics, University of Tokyo School of Medicine, Tokyo, Japan
Hideo Hayashi
    Department of Pathology, School of Medicine, Kumamoto University, Kuma-
    moto, Japan
Utako Hiei
    Departments of Pediatrics and Immunology, Toho University, Tokyo, Japan
Walter H. Hitzig
    Department of Pediatrics, University of Zürich, Switzerland
Makoto Hori
    Department of Pediatrics, The Jikei University School of Medicine, Tokyo, Japan
Nobuko Iizuka
    Department of Maternal and Child Health, University of Tokyo School of
    Medicine, Tokyo, Japan
Susumu Ikehara
    Department of Pathology, Kyoto University School of Medicine, Kyoto, Japan
Hiroshi Itoh
    Red Cross Hokkaido Blood Center, Sapporo, Japan
Benjamin M. Kagan
    Department of Pediatrics, Cedars-Sinai Medical Center, Los Angeles, California,
    U.S.A.
Yuji Kagosaki
    Department of Pediatrics, Hiroshima University School of Medicine, Hiroshima
    Japan
Tadashi Kanoh
    First Division, Department of Internal Medicine, Kyoto University School of
    Medicine, Kyoto, Japan
Tadashi Kawai
    Department of Clinical Pathology, Jichi Medical School, Tochigi, Japan
Kinya Kawano
    Department of Clinical Pathology, Nihon University School of Medicine, Tokyo,
    Japan
A. B. Kenny
    Department of Pediatrics, University of Zürich, Switzerland
Nobuyuki Kitani
    Department of Pediatrics, The Jikei University School of Medicine, Tokyo, Japan

Noboru Kobayashi
Department of Pediatrics, University of Tokyo School of Medicine, Tokyo, Japan
Yonosuke Kobayashi
Department of Pediatrics, Hiroshima University School of Medicine, Hiroshima, Japan
Yoshiyuki Kokubun
Department of Pediatrics, The Jikei University School of Medicine, Tokyo, Japan
Masakatsu Kubo
Department of Pediatrics, The Jikei University School of Medicine, Tokyo, Japan
Ataru Kuroiwa
Department of Immunology, Faculty of Medicine, Kyushu University, Fukuoka, Japan
Yoshigoro Kuroiwa
Department of Neurology, Neurological Institute, Faculty of Medicine, Kyushu University, Fukuoka, Japan
Benjamin H. Landing
Departments of Pathology and Pediatrics, Children's Hospital of Los Angeles, and University of Southern California School of Medicine, Los Angeles, California, U.S.A.
Alexander R. Lawton*
The Cellular Immunology Unit of the Tumor Institute, Departments of Pediatrics and Microbiology and The Comprehensive Cancer Center, University of Alabama in Birmingham, University Station, Birmingham, Alabama, U.S.A.
Wolfgang Leibold*
Institut für Pathologie der Tieraztlichen Hochschule, Hannover, West Germany
Tohru Masuda
Institute for Immunology, Kyoto University School of Medicine, Kyoto, Japan
Y. Masuho
Teijin Institute for Biomedical Research, Tokyo, Japan
Shuzo Matsumoto
Department of Pediatrics, Hokkaido University School of Medicine, Sapporo, Japan
Tadashi Matsumoto
Departments of Pediatrics and Immunology, Toho University, Tokyo, Japan
Kenichi Matsuo
Department of Microbiology, School of Medicine, Kyushu University, Fukuoka, Japan
Tyoku Matuhasi
Department of Allergology, Institute of Medical Science, University of Tokyo, Tokyo, Japan
Michael A. Medici*
Department of Pediatrics, Cedars-Sinai Medical Center, Los Angeles, California, U.S.A.

John H. Menkes*
    Department of Pediatrics, Cedars-Sinai Medical Center, Los Angeles, California,
    U.S.A.
Hideki Minami
    Department of Pediatrics, Hokkaido University School of Medicine, Sapporo,
    Japan
Mutsuhiko Minami
    Department of Allergology, Institute of Medical Science, University of Tokyo,
    Tokyo, Japan
Tsunenori Miyake
    Department of Microbiology, School of Medicine, Kyushu University, Fukuoka,
    Japan
Sumio Miyazaki
    Department of Pediatrics, Faculty of Medicine, Kyushu University, Fukuoka,
    Japan
L. Moretta*
    The Cellular Immunobiology Unit of the Tumor Institute, Departments of
    Pediatrics and Microbiology and The Comprehensive Cancer Center, University
    of Alabama in Birmingham, University Station, Birmingham, Alabama, U.S.A.
Ryoichi Mori
    Department of Microbiology, Faculty of Medicine, Kyushu University, Fuku-
    oka, Japan
Shizuo Muraoka
    Department of Microbiology, School of Medicine, Kyushu University, Fuku-
    oka, Japan
Michisato Murata
    Department of Immunology, Institute of Medical Science, University of Tokyo,
    Tokyo, Japan
Toshiro Nakagawa
    Department of Pediatrics, School of Medicine, Toho University, Tokyo, Japan
Kikuo Nomoto
    Department of Microbiology, School of Medicine, Kyushu University, Fukuoka,
    Japan
Susumu Ohmura
    Red Cross Hokkaido Blood Center, Sapporo, Japan
Shinya Ohtomo
    The Chemo-Sero-Therapeutic Institute, Kumamoto, Japan
A. Ohtsu
    Teijin Institute for Biomedical Research, Tokyo, Japan
Takeshi Okabe
    Department of Pediatrics, The Jikei University School of Medicine, Tokyo, Japan

A. J. Okos*
The Cellular Immunobiology Unit of the Tumor Institute, Departments of Pediatrics and Microbiology and The Comprehensive Cancer Center, University of Alabama in Birmingham, University Station, Birmingham, Alabama, U.S.A.

E. R. Pearl*
The Cellular Immunobiology Unit of the Tumor Institute, Departments of Pediatrics and Microbiology and The Comprehensive Cancer Center, University of Alabama in Birmingham, University Station, Birmingham, Alabama, U.S.A.

Jean-Louis Preud'Homme*
Laboratory of Immunochemistry and Immunopathology (INSERM U108), Research Institute on Blood Diseases, Hôpital Saint-Louis, Paris, France

Nancy Reinsmoen*
University of Minnesota Hospitals, Department of Laboratory Medicine Mineapolis, Minnesota, U.S.A.

Kimitaka Sagawa
Department of Internal Medicine, Kyoto University School of Medicine, Kyoto, Japan

Hideo Saito
Department of Oto-rhino-laryngology, Nihon University School of Medicine, Tokyo, Japan

Yukio Sakiyama
Department of Pediatrics, Hokkaido University School of Medicine, Sapporo, Japan

Maxime Seligmann
Laboratory of Immunochemistry and Immunopathology (INSERM U108), Research Institute on Blood Diseases, Hôpital Saint-Louis, Paris, France

Shoichi Shimotori
Department of Microbiology, School of Medicine, Kyushu University, Fukuoka, Japan

Toshikazu Shinbo
Department of Pediatrics and Immunology, Toho University, Tokyo, Japan

J. F. Soothill
Department of Immunology, Institute of Child Health, University of London, England

Erik A. J. Svedmyr*
Karolinska Institute, Department of Tumor Biology, Stockholm, Sweden

Machiko Sugawara
Departments of Pediatrics and Immunology, Toho University, Tokyo, Japan

Virginia L. Swanson*
Departments of Pathology and Pediatrics, Children's Hospital of Los Angeles, and University of Southern California School of Medicine, Los Angeles, California, U.S.A.

Tomio Tada
　　Laboratories for Immunology, School of Medicine, Chiba University, Chiba;
　　Department of Serology, University of Tokyo School of Medicine, Tokyo, Japan
Kiyoshi Takatsuki
　　Department of Internal Medicine, Kyoto University School of Medicine,
　　Kyoto, Japan
Toshitada Takemori
　　Laboratories for Immunology, School of Medicine, Chiba University, Chiba,
　　Japan
Kenji Takeya
　　Department of Microbiology, School of Medicine, Kyushu University, Fukuoka,
　　Japan
Norikazu Tamaoki
　　Department of Pathology, Tokai University School of Medicine, Kanagawa,
　　Japan
Masaru Taniguchi
　　Laboratories for Immunology, School of Medicine, Chiba University, Chiba,
　　Japan
Akira Tashiro
　　The Chemo-Sero-Therapeutic Institute, Kumamoto, Japan
Takehiko Togashi
　　Department of Pediatrics, Hokkaido University School of Medicine, Sapporo,
　　Japan
Katsuhiko Tomibe
　　Teijin Institute for Biomedical Research, Tokyo, Japan
Yusuke Tomita
　　Department of Pediatrics, The Jikei University School of Medicine, Tokyo, Japan
G. Torrigiani
　　Acting Chief of Immunology, World Health Organization, Geneva, Switzerland
T. Tursz*
　　Laboratory of Immunochemistry and Immunopathology (INSERM U108),
　　Research Institute on Blood Diseases, Hôpital Saint-Louis, Paris, France
Takashi Uchiyama
　　Department of Internal Medicine, Kyoto University School of Medicine, Kyoto,
　　Japan
Tomofusa Usui
　　Department of Pediatrics, Hiroshima University School of Medicine, Hiroshima,
　　Japan
L. B. Vogler*
　　The Cellular Immunobiology Unit of the Tumor Institute, Departments of
　　Pediatrics and Microbiology and The Comprehensive Cancer Center, University
　　of Alabama in Birmingham, University Station, Birmingham, Alabama, U.S.A.

Thomas A. Waldmann*
  The Metabolism Branch, National Cancer Institute, National Institutes of
  Health, Bethesda, Maryland, U.S.A.
T. Watanabe
  Teijin Institute for Biomedical Research, Tokyo, Japan
S. R. Webb*
  The Cellular Immunobiology Unit of the Tumor Institute, Departments of
  Pediatrics and Microbiology and The Comprehensive Cancer Center, University
  of Alabama in Birmingham, University Station, Birmingham, Alabama, U.S.A.
Kiyomi Yamada
  Department of Pediatrics, University of Tokyo School of Medicine, Tokyo,
  Japan
Eiji Yamagami
  Teijin Institute for Biomedical Research, Tokyo, Japan
Yuichi Yamamura
  Department of Internal Medicine, Faculty of Medicine, Osaka University,
  Osaka, Japan
Junichi Yata
  Department of Pediatrics, School of Medicine, Toho University, Tokyo, Japan
Kazuya Yoshino
  Department of Pediatrics, Teikyo University School of Medicine, Tokyo, Japan
Ida L. Yutuc*
  Departments of Pathology and Pediatrics, Children's Hospital of Los Angeles
  and University of Southern California School of Medicine, Los Angeles, Cali-
  fornia, U.S.A.
Koji Zaima
  Department of Pediatrics, University of Tokyo School of Medicine, Tokyo Japan

* Did not attend the symposium, but contributed papers.

In addition to the contributors listed above, approximately 30 pediatricians and
physicians, who were interested in immunodeficiency participated in the symposium.

Executive Members of Japan Medical Research Foundation